THE
SOCIAL
AND POLITICAL
CONTEXTS OF
FAMILY THERAPY

Contributors

The Social and Political Contexts of FAMILY THERAPY

Edited by

Marsha Pravder Mirkin, Ph.D.

Allyn and Bacon

Boston   London   Sydney   Toronto

Copyright © 1990 by Allyn and Bacon
A Division of Simon & Schuster, Inc.
160 Gould Street
Needham Heights, Massachusetts 02194

Library of Congress Cataloging-in-Publication Data

The Social and political contexts of family therapy / edited by Marsha
    Pravder Mirkin.
        p.   cm.
    Includes bibliographical references.
    ISBN 0-205-12455-0
    1. Family psychotherapy—Social aspects.   2. Family psychotherapy—
Political aspects.   3. Feminist therapy.   4. Refugees—Mental
health.   5. Poor—Mental health.   I. Mirkin, Marsha Pravder, 1953–

RC488.5.S63   1990
616.89′156—dc20   89-18235
                                                                                    CIP

Printed in the United States of America

10 9 8 7 6 5 4 3 2 1   93 92 91 90 89

To Mitch,
With love and gratitude

Contents

Foreword

The reader of *The Social and Political Contexts of Family Therapy*, intrigued as he or she may be by the diversity of topics encompassed, runs the risk of being overwhelmed by the picture it presents of the complex, turbulent, and angry world in which family therapy is practiced. Like psychoanalysis, family therapy created its own definition of the sphere within which it intended to operate. Psychoanalysis saw that terrain as the psyche of the individual, and family therapy saw it as the family in various forms, including the nuclear family and, sometimes, the extended family. But these definitions of worlds have proved to be tenuous, subject to a society that continues to change in ways and at a pace that the field did not anticipate.

When family therapy was first introduced, the psychoanalytic fellowship reacted defensively, fearing its discoveries were being attacked, and, possibly, that the professional community of scholarship, hierarchies, institutes, and economic reward that it had created would be eroded. In some ways, this did happen, but psychoanalysis survived, leaner and with new thinking and organization, including some cross-ties with family therapy. It is evident that family therapy is now facing the same trauma, not from another form of therapy, but from permutations in the world in which we live. By definition, systems therapies were on the border of the larger society, but who could have foreseen that the preoccupation in therapy with the double bind would give way to worry about the place of women and minorities and fears of nuclear holocaust?

To survive, family therapy must be relevant to today's world at the same time that it helps shape that world. And it will endure, even if some of the thinking growing out of these political and social concerns is challenging previously accepted notions such as the circularity of interaction, with no victimizer and no victim. It will not only survive but expand as a result of social changes, making room for people and institutions outside of the family to be brought into the territory of treatment and thereby broadening the definition from family to ecological.

Family therapy will also outlast the onslaught of arguments over epistemology, but will the family therapists themselves weather the storm? Some of these challenges have moved into the realm of basic interpretations of human relationships and of human experience. They bend, and even turn on its head, our understanding of the sexes, families, and reality. These ideas infringe not only upon the therapy we practice, but upon the way we live our lives—and indeed, that is what they are meant to do.

The thinking that is sampled in *The Social and Political Contexts of Family Therapy* must be considered a reflection of the social evolution our society is undergoing. As such, it merits the same thoughtfulness and skepticism that we give to the messages of today's prophet-scientists and social commentators. It is part science and part personal hunch, and very important.

Within our own field, our sense of ourselves and of our world is being called into question by theorists and practitioners with ideas, some new and some old. The flowering of family therapy will depend upon our being able to talk with one another with the openness evidenced in this book, but also with special attention to how this process is evolving, and a little humility and a lot of mutual respect as we wrestle with the difficult and important issues of our future.

—*Harry J. Aponte, A.C.S.W.*

Introduction:
Family Therapy
in Its Social
and Political Contexts

Editing a volume on the social and political contexts of family therapy has been both a personal and professional challenge. It has been a project of the soul: an attempt to integrate the issues that touch me and concern me profoundly in everyday life with how I conceptualize and practice my profession. I remember a college professor warning me of the potential pitfalls of becoming a clinical psychologist. He warned that I could be maintaining an inequitable and inhumane status quo if I chose to help wounded people conform to the system. But what were my alternatives, I wondered at age 20, and have wondered often since then. People were suffering; therapy can help alleviate pain. What were my choices?

When I began to learn about family therapy, the systemic conceptualization felt like the beginning of an answer to that dilemma. Finally, theorists and practitioners were working with people in a context; were looking at interrelationships; were seemingly not blaming an individual for problems but were instead redefining relationships and concretely helping to solve problems. The goals were appealing to me: families were being reunited on different terms rather than torn apart; children and adolescents with whom I worked were often symptom-free in relatively short periods of time; family pain appeared to be eased.

But there were troublesome questions that began to emerge once I felt secure enough in my skills as a family therapist to begin the never-ending questioning process once again. Although I worked hard at appreciating the uniqueness of each family, I continued to see the same pattern of what was labeled "overinvolved" mothers and "distant" fathers. Could it be just a coincidence that this pattern continued to reemerge? Did this pattern say more about the larger society than about each individual family? And what about work with the poor, and often minority, families that were labeled "multiproblem" families? When we work solely within the family context, are we simply changing the message from blaming the individual to blaming the family? What about the bureaucracy, frustration, and roadblocks experienced by the family as it tries to navigate through a system without having political and economic clout? I also found myself admiring the impressive ways in which families have managed to survive and start their lives anew after being traumatized by torture, war, death and relocation. How is it that these families are often viewed by their new community and therapists as disturbed rather than as strong? Then there is also the most frightening of issues: the omnipresent threat of nuclear war. When children or adults occasionally mention their fears of nuclear holocaust, whether in words or drawings, we have been trained to interpret these as concerns about their family falling apart, about their own destructive feelings toward particular family members. Our own perceived powerlessness in the midst of such an unspeakable threat makes it difficult for us to deal with our clients effectively.

It became clear to me that I needed to view families within a larger context: to look at how social, political, and economic factors affect families. The question was how. Where was the roadmap? It is intriguing and difficult enough dealing with my multiple-family group where five families meet to discuss family concerns. How would I begin to look at families embedded in so many complex systems?

The next step in this "search for meaning" in therapy was to begin to develop, and dare to ask, questions about the impact of the larger system on families and family therapy. From these questions, this volume was born. I spoke with colleagues throughout the country who were grappling with many of the same questions and ideas, and who agreed to contribute their thinking to this text. What resulted was a collection of the latest conceptualizations and treatment applications concerning the family in its larger context.

This book is divided into five sections. The first section provides an overview of therapy in its larger context. It sets the stage for understanding how issues concerning women, poverty, forced emigration, and the threat of nuclear holocaust fit together in a single volume. This section also helps the therapist make the leap to the larger system both by exploring the impact of systems on therapists and families, and by challenging our ways of thinking that may inhibit us from or facilitate our discovering more effective ways of viewing families.

The second section of this book focuses on women and family therapy. This section critiques current systems thinking and offers alternative models in which women can be treated respectfully and effectively within a family context. The gender-free nature of current family therapy, as well as its lack of recognition of the power differences between men and women, are two of the areas that are critiqued and reformulated. New understanding and treatment ideas concerning such unfortunately familiar issues as incest, eating disorders, wife abuse, and alcoholism emerge from a gender-sensitive framework.

The third section of the book discusses poverty and family therapy. These chapters provide a sensitive and compelling understanding of poverty, and its effect on families and service providers. Further, there is much discussion in mental health about the "underutilization" of services by this population. The contributors to this section instead grapple with how to change the services offered so that they are more useful for families struggling for economic survival in an often unresponsive society. The economic and political difficulties of the service-providing systems, as well as the innovative and creative development of these services, are described.

The fourth section is entitled "Forced Migration and Relocated Families." These families have been compelled to leave their country of origin and to resettle. This population has experienced the trauma of the loss of roots, and often of family members. Many have experienced or seen torture and other brutal forms of repression. They are also trying to come to terms with an un-familiar culture that is often unaccepting of cultural differences. For therapists to understand and assist these families, we need to understand cultural tran-sitions, trauma theory, and the climate of a society that makes it so difficult for the foreign-born to feel accepted and valued.

The final section of this volume concerns the threat of nuclear holocaust. The contributors to this section have managed to offer hope in the midst of this frightening, uncharted territory. What is the effect of the threat of nuclear war on therapists? On families? How can we help our clients with their fears when we are experiencing the same threat and are not objective observers/interpreters? Should this even be an issue that is discussed in the therapy situation? If we are indeed developing skills to intervene in larger systems, can we utilize these skills to help prevent nuclear war? Although the book cannot provide definitive answers, the hope comes from beginning to formulate and address these ques-tions, thus moving from a position of powerlessness to one of activism.

None of these sections are mutually exclusive, and the book is cordoned off into sections only for ease of organization. For example, the majority of poor in this country are women (NOW editorial, Fall 1987): the overlap between the poverty and women sections of this book is obvious. Similarly, much of the chapter on the legacy of slavery that appears in the forced-migration section involves poverty-level Black families, showing interactions among racism, cul-tural trauma, and poverty. If one goes further and looks at the interactions among sex, race, and poverty, the point is further driven home: Households headed by single Black women have a median income that is far below those headed by single White women (Institute for Puerto Rican Policy, 1986). It is not a major leap to state that political and cultural disenfranchisement go hand in hand with economic powerlessness.

In its entirety, then, this book is an attempt to challenge us to view families within a larger social, economic, and political framework. Further, it is a begin-ning attempt at developing more effective ways to intervene with families and individuals within families from this broader perspective. There are many ques-tions still to be asked, and many issues still to be struggled with. For every chapter that we included in the book, others need to be included. Because of space and time constraints, chapters on such topics as AIDS; the feminization of poverty; child care and the family; poverty and forced migration among Hispanic families; and single-parent families were not included. But then, my primary hope is to support thinking in these areas, and to read the many other books that will appear in the future as mental health professionals continue to grapple with issues of context.

Marsha Pravder Mirkin
Newton, Massachusetts

Acknowledgements

I am very grateful to the many people who throughout my life have influenced me, supported me, and made this book possible.

A warm thank you to my colleagues and dear friends Dr. Judith Libow and Dr. Pamela Raskin for their comments on the text and for all the discussion and debates that encouraged me to keep thinking. I'd also like to thank Dr. Benina Berger-Gould: although because of time constraints, Benina could not contribute her writing to this text, she certainly did contribute her support! I also appreciate Donna DeMuth and Faye Snider's unflagging enthusiasm and helpful suggestions throughout this process.

Besides the people who have supported me in the process of writing this book, there are many others whom I would like to thank for helping me develop the social and political consciousness that made this book possible. In particular, I would like to thank many of my friends, classmates, and professors from my undergraduate years at SUNY Stony Brook for for nourishing a fledgling awareness, and providing me with an intellectually stimulating and emotionally supportive environment in which I could grapple with these ideas. These individuals include Marsha Millstein Blodgett, Dana Bramel, Donald Bybee, Maureen Bybee, Claudette Charbonneau, Phil Chin, Robert F. Cohen, Paul Dolan, Stuart Eber, Ronald Hartman, Anne Singer Hartman, Dave McDermott, Blos Silberman, Ned Steele, Judy Horenstein Steele, Florence Steinberger, Karen Ginsberg Stutman, David Tilley, Irene Gilbert Torres, Al Walker, and Carla Weiss.

My sincere gratitude is extended to my parents, Ann Goldman Pravder and Sidney Pravder. My mother is my role model for community activism: Through her skilled and caring involvement, my mother demonstrates to me on a daily basis the meaning of social responsibility. My father helped ingrain in me an acceptance of people and high regard for human life and dignity. I am very grateful to both of them.

My deepest appreciation and heartfelt thanks go to my husband Mitch Mirkin, for his encouragement, unconditional support and unending patience, as well as for his suggestions and availability throughout this entire process. Finally, I want to express my gratitude to my daughters, Allison and Jessica. The birth of my children provided me with a sense of urgency that motivated me to edit a book on this theme. Watching them grow balances that urgency with hope and enables me to hold onto a feeling of optimism in spite of all the threatening issues addressed in this book.

—*Marsha Pravder Mirkin*

Part I
Therapy in Context: An Overview

1

MULTIPLE EMBEDDED SYSTEMS

Evan Imber-Black, Ph.D.

INTRODUCTION

A family was referred for family therapy by a public community health center. The family consisted of two parents, Mr. and Ms. Samson, and their three children, Ellen, 11, Dave, eight, and Shellie, five years old. The referral was made because Ms. Samson complained of having behavioral problems with Shellie. These problems, which had begun four months earlier, included temper tantrums. Shellie's teachers were also upset about her behavior.

A second family was referred by a private pediatrician for family therapy. This family also consisted of two parents, Mr. and Ms. Ellis, and three children, Cathy, 12, Bill, eight, and Sandy, five years old. This referral was made because Ms. Ellis had complained about having behavioral problems with Sandy, including temper tantrums, for about six months. Sandy's teachers were also upset about her behavior.

At first glance, these two cases appear remarkably similar. In fact, if one restricted one's inquiry to internal family interaction, one would see similar patterns involving a mother–father–child triad, with the mother more involved than the father with the temper tantrums. The first clue to any differences in the two families is found in the referral source, as the Samsons' referral came from a public clinic, whereas the Ellis's came from a private physician. Other differences emerged in the initial interviews.

Ms. Samson came to the first interview, at a public mental health clinic, with her three children. The family was Black and lived in public housing in the Bronx. Mr. Samson was working and could not get time off to attend the interview. He was frequently laid off, at which times the family received welfare assistance. When Mr. Samson worked, he earned just enough money that the family was ineligible for food stamps and Medicaid. His job did not include health insurance.

3

During a part of the interview devoted to a discussion of larger systems in the family's life, Ms. Samson said they had just finished a very intense involvement with the health-care system. Her son, Dave, had been diagnosed with a life-threatening illness a year and a half earlier, and had completed all of his treatments about five months previous to the interview. When he was diagnosed, the parents were told that Dave would not survive. They insisted on aggressive treatment, and Dave recovered. During Dave's illness, Ms. Samson was at the hospital constantly. The family could not afford child care, and Ellen at age 11 was put in charge of Shellie. Ms. Samson reflected that just as she thought she could relax a bit, Shellie began to have tantrums. She also said that she had become used to having many people from the health-care system to interact with, and felt a bit lonely, although she was becoming involved with teachers and others at school, because of the child's behavior in class. The school was planning to place Shellie in a special class. Ms. Samson did not know whether this was the right thing to do, and had no sense of what her rights might be. Her husband did not like the idea, but felt that school was his wife's province. She also remarked that during Mr. Samson's most recent layoff, her welfare worker had told her she should begin to look for work, as welfare reform would soon require her to do so. She had dropped out of high school at the age of 15 to have Ellen, and had no training. She stated that her own mother used to help her with child care when the children were smaller, but that her mother's attention was now focused on Ms. Samson's 17-year-old sister and her new baby. Finally, she said that she was surprised to be having problems with Shellie, as Shellie was her only child for whom she had had consistent prenatal care, (which she could not afford for the other pregnancies), that only Shellie was born at a normal birth weight, and that she had anticipated that these factors would make a difference in Shellie's behavior.

Mr. and Ms. Ellis, a white couple, came to the first interview without their children, whom they had left at home with their live-in nanny. The interview was held in a private-practice family therapy institute. Both Mr. and Ms. Ellis worked full-time at jobs they considered careers. They lived in their own suburban home outside New York City. They were approximately 15 years older than the Samsons, having postponed childbearing in order to launch their careers. Exploration of the family's involvement with larger systems yielded the information that the family had had only private-sector involvement at their own initiation. It included current individual psychotherapy for each of the parents of over five years' durations, and medical specialists (e.g., pediatrician and gynecologist) when needed, until the recent problems with Sandy, which were necessitating involvement with the school system. School officials insisted that Sandy be evaluated for hyperactivity, and were beginning to suggest placing Sandy in a special classroom. All involvements with the school were delegated to Ms. Ellis, by the school and also by Mr. Ellis, who stated that his own career path was more precarious and needed more attention. He also said that his wife was used to interruptions in her work, as she had stopped working with the birth of each child and then resumed here career. Ms. Ellis reluctantly agreed with him, but said she believed the school would pay more attention to his viewpoint. She also said that she believed that her work was not taken seriously by either her husband or the school officials, and that she felt angry with both.

While allowing that Sandy did have some problems, including what the parents referred to as "speech delay" and learning less rapidly than her siblings, Mr. and Ms. Ellis were adamant that Sandy remain in her present class, as special education might harm her later chances to go to an excellent university.

The differences in these two families with similar presenting problems were startling, and included finances, housing, educational opportunities, vocational possibilities, health care (especially prenatal and mental health care), child care, the children's futures, and options regarding interactions with larger systems. Although the initial referral information pointed to a meaningful system of family and school in each case, information gathered in the first interviews indicated very different meaningful systems in the two families. The Samson family's boundaries with outside systems were chronically diffuse, because of their required interactions with public housing and welfare, and more recently with the community health-care system. Interactions with the school system were familiarly stressful, and were regarded as one more system over which the family had no influence. At the same time, occasional kind and friendly interactions with helpers from larger systems provided Ms. Samson with people whom she considered good company and relief from a fairly isolated life. These boundaries were asymmetrical, as the larger systems could more easily enter the Samsons' family life, whereas the Samsons had much more limited access to the workings of the larger systems, and highly limited choices regarding with which larger systems they might interact.

The Ellis family's boundaries with outside systems were firm. They felt it was their right to choose when, where, and with whom to interact from larger systems, including health and educational systems, and believed that they could easily influence any interactions they might have with larger systems. They regarded representatives of larger systems as their peers or as public servants. Currently stressed by the school system, they saw private school as a viable option.

Both families also shared a similarity regarding interactions with larger systems, as both the large urban school system and the suburban school system seemed to be acting out of a belief that mothers are primarily responsible for their children's behavior at school, and that mothers should serve as the conduit between the school and the family.

These two case vignettes begin to draw the family therapist's attention to the need to examine multiple embedded systems when working with families. Recent literature has begun to conceptualize a macrosystemic level of assessment, interviewing, and inntervention for family therapists. This work has pointed to problems arising between families and specific larger systems, including hospitals and health-care systems (Bell & Zucker, 1968; Harbin, 1985; Imber-Black, 1988); public schools (Aponte, 1976; Coleman, 1983; Imber Coppersmith, 1982); probation (Schwartzman & Restivo, 19895); and child welfare (Schwartzman & Kniefel, 1985; Webb-Woodard & Woodard, 1983).

Specific presenting problems that lead to the emergence of particular larger systems, which, in turn, may inadvertently perpetuate the problem they were designed to alleviate, have been highlighted by several authors. These include families with handicapped members at various stages of development (Berger, 1984; Bloomfield, Neilson & Kaplan, 1984; Combrinck-Graham & Higley, 1984;

Imber-Black, 1987 b; MacKinnon & Martlett, 1984; Roberts, 1984); families with alcohol problems (Miller, 1983); families with eating disorders (Harkaway, 19893); and families with violence (Imber-Black, 1988a). Larger systems that simply locate the cause of the problem in the family or in the individual and eschew any focus on family–larger system interaction easily miss both their own contribution to the problem and expanded possibilities for intervention.

Patterns emerging between families and larger systems that function to perpetuate problems have been examined by several authors, who either implicitly or explicitly point to triads and boundaries as essential concepts within which to examine the macrosystem formed by family and helpers. Selvini-Palazolli, Boscolo, Cecchin, and Prata (1980) discussed what they called "the problem of the referring person," framing the issue as one caused by an "overinvolved" professional who had become "like a family member." Selig (1976) reframes the issue of multiproblem families to that of families with multiple agencies involved in their lives. Harrell (1980) expands on this multiagency phenomenon in research examining problematic triads formed by families and outside systems that interdicted therapeutic progress. Clinical approaches to the family–multiple helper system are elaborated by Imber-Coppersmith (1985).

Finally, the broader social, political, and economic levels of the macrosystem, within which families and larger systems are located, and which include issues of racism, sexism, poverty, nuclear war, oppression, and attitudes toward differences, have begun to be examined as a framework for effective family therapy (Bernal & Diamond, 1985; Gould, 1985; Imber-Black, 1986a, 1986b, 1987; Libow, 1985; MacKinnon & Marlett, 1984; Ritterman, 1985). The present chapter is offered as a continuation of the traditions of these works in which family issues begin to make a different kind of sense as they are examined in the context of the larger systems and the political, economic, and social levels in which they are embedded.

A FEW FACTS AND FIGURES

As professionals who work to enhance the daily well-being of families, family therapists are required to be aware of economic and social factors that affect families today. Such factors are not always visible in the immediacy of the consulting room, but are present and embue both families and the larger systems with whom they interact.

1. One-quarter of the nation's families are poor.
2. One-sixth have no health insurance.
3. Of small children, one in six lives in a family where neither parent has a job.
4. Fifteen percent of children born today are born into families where one parent works for wages below the poverty level.
5. Twenty-five percent of children born today will be on welfare at some point before reaching adulthood.

6. In 1955, the United States ranked sixth among 20 industrialized nations in infant mortality. In 1985, the United States tied for last place.

7. Between 1973 and 1979, one in five new jobs paid less than $7,000 a year (in 1984 dollars). Between 1979 and 1984, over half of the new jobs paid less than $7,000 a year.

8. In young women aged 16–19 with above-average basic skills and above-average incomes, fewer than one in 20 has given birth to a child. In young women with below-average skills and below-poverty incomes, more than one in five has given birth to a child.

9. From 1980 to 1992 (based on President Reagan's budget proposals), the budget for national defense will increase by 54.2 percent and the budget for low-income programs will decrease by 16.4 percent (Edelman, 1987).

What does all of this have to do with family therapy? The answer to this question lies in our responses to other questions. What does it mean to us as practitioners and to the families that we see that we live and work in a broader context in which the United States ranks first in arms exports, military expenditures, military bases worldwide, and nuclear warheads and bombs, but ranks fourth in literacy rate, tenth in public education expenditures per capita and in public health expenditures, per capita, and 22nd in population per physician (Sivard, 1987)? What do these facts and figures mean to health and human service workers in the larger systems designed to work with families? What does it mean to be embedded in a sociopolitical context in which "family" is a mythical concept increasingly owned by the right wing, and where the very definition of family championed by the right wing, in which there are two parents with mother remaining at home and father working outside the home, pertains to less than 10 percent of all families today? This broader context often eludes our grasp, and seems outside our responsibilities, as practitioners, but a family therapy theory and practice that ignore this broader context are, quite simply, a conservative family therapy.

ASSESSING FAMILIES, LARGER SYSTEMS AND THE WIDER SOCIAL, POLITICAL AND ECONOMIC CONTEXT

Large health, educational, and human service systems at once reflect and are shaped by sociopolitical systems and ideological beliefs of the wider culture. Such larger systems are also vulnerable to economic shifts, which, in turn, reflect political priorities. Standing between the family and the wider social context, many larger systems generally represent long-standing beliefs extant in the culture, including often unquestioned ideas and stereotypes regarding women, minorities, the handicapped, and the poor. The process of change in the culture at large tends to reach many larger systems slowly. At the same time, new larger systems may spring up in response to new ideas and needs, as, for instance, the larger systems designed to work with family violence, or the recent rise in larger systems whose *raison d'être* is to provide services to adult children of alcoholics. These newer larger systems are immediately cast into a competitive position with existing larger systems for economic support and clientele.

Much of our current human-service delivery system has roots in the post-World War II period, a time that glorified the nuclear family, focused on family togetherness, and defined variant family forms as aberrant. Other trends and developments have frequently been tacked on to the larger systems, often resulting in a "crazy quilt." For instance, whereas many larger systems may now offer services for single parents, such services are usually embedded in an unspoken and unexamined context that continues to suggest that single parents are a deficient family form, rather than a different family form with strengths that may either be supported or undermined, depending on the interventions offered.

Many larger systems do not have a perspective that affirms the historical, political, social, and economic context within which their work exists. Without an appreciation of this context, one is able to remain blind to the fact that the United States has no coherent family policy, thus enabling the creation of larger systems that often fragment families by the nature of the services offered. For instance, some states require that the father leave the home in order for the family to receive welfare support. Most larger systems tend to mirror the individualistic and competitive viewpoint that underpins the culture's mythology. A more collaborative perspective for both larger-system activities and human behavior is eschewed—including larger helping systems that affect family life, such as welfare, clinics, health care, schools and shelters; larger social control systems, such as probation, child welfare, and prisons; and work systems. Policies and practices of larger systems are seldom examined for their effect on family ecology. Funding to larger systems flows on an individual client model, and not on a family model. In short, many larger systems, wittingly or unwittingly, carry out an agenda that supports traditional sex roles; financial disparities between men and women and between middle-class and poor persons; a mythical, autonomous nuclear family that needs no help from anyone; and the value of productivity over relationship.

For family therapists working with families that are intensely involved with larger systems, which are embedded in the wider context, several key areas bear attention.

Assessment and Intervention

Here one is seeking to become aware that drawing a boundary around the family as client is a political act, which may both perpetuate distress and ally the therapist with broad social forces affecting families in general. The meaningful system often includes the family and the larger systems that mediate and translate the social agenda. This problem becomes particularly poignant in instances where a family or members of a family are working with two or more larger systems that may represent conflicting aspects of social policy, as, for instance, a family whose welfare worker is pushing the mother to assume work outside the home and whose child therapist from a mental health system is urging the mother to remain at home with young children.

The family therapist seeking to work from a macrosystemic perspective needs to find out both who the key actors in the family are and what larger systems interact with the family, and what beliefs in the wider context are being supported by any particular activity, such as referral, therapy, or reports.

Dyadic Arrangements in the Macrosystem

Clients and helpers from larger systems generally exist in a pre-defined complementary dyad of helper-helpee. Thus, there is a rigid definition of care provider and care recipient. If the client responds to this definition with a sense of helplessness, then the larger systems will usually respond with more and more help, in an escalating complementary pattern. This complementarity often replicates other aspects of the client's life, especially for poor or minority or women clients, in which the client lives in an enduring one-down position with the majority culture. At the same time, many helpers in the larger systems exist in this same one-down complementary position vis-à-vis decision and policy makers who affect the larger systems' operations. It is not unusual to behold clients who struggle with their workers, attempting to bid for a more collaborative relationship, marked by a sense of personal empowerment, and workers who insist on maintaining the complementary arrangement, as this often provides their only sense of empowerment, however tenuous.

Workers in many larger systems have been trained to examine clients for their deficits, rather than for their strengths. Ways of coping that do not match the norms and values of the larger systems are often ignored in favor of advice and direction preferred by the larger systems. If the clients continue to pursue their own methods, they will often be met by workers who push their point of view even harder, resulting in a macrosystem marked by conflict and symmetrical escalation over who knows best. Here relationships become marked by mutual blame and withdrawal.

Family therapists should avoid methods that further reify this rigid complementarity, as, for instance, assuming a one-up position with other helpers in the macrosystem, and seek methods that begin to introduce greater cooperative symmetry and collaboration into the macrosystem, as well as methods that offer new complementarities that highlight differing strengths of all of the participants.

Triads

Triads have been an organizing principle in many models of family therapy. When one moves to the family–larger system–wider context level, the concept of triads continues to prove useful, with modifications. Here, one may be examining the macrosystem for triads composed of family members and multiple helpers. Such triads may or may not replicate existing family triads. When triads do mirror internal family processes, helpers have likely not assessed the family ecology and their own effect on it, and behave in ways that perpetuate problematic patterns. Thus, in a family with a handicapped child in which the mother and child are especially close and the father is distant, the larger systems can easily exacerbate and replicate this pattern by interacting only with the mother. Never examining the social belief that the health and welfare of the child are the sole province of the mother, workers in the larger systems set appointments only for the mother, and impart their knowledge to her so that she becomes increasingly expert regarding the child and the father increasingly is left out. As the mother grows closer to professional helpers, the father may distance further, leading the helpers to interact even more with the mother.

Often, macrosystemic triads do not mirror existing triads in the family, but are a function of larger-system organization. Families may find themselves pressed to ally with two or more systems that are in conflict with one another, and may not, because of the survival value of each of the larger systems to the family, be able to leave. It is important to be aware that such triads are not composed of equal parts. Families that must interact with larger systems because of the exigencies of poverty or illness are not simply one leg of a triangle. Symptoms at the family level may be an expression of the experience of being caught between two larger systems with which the family is required to interact in order to receive food stamps, housing allowances, education, or health care. This viewpoint is not intended to conceptualize families as helpless victims, but to orient the family therapist to working methods that facilitate empowerment.

Triads at the macrosystemic level often contain hidden members, including supervisors, managers, directors and policy makers, to whom a given worker may be answerable. Family members can often be confused by what appear to be broken and betrayed alliances because workers in the larger systems have not informed them of particular mandate or policy shifts. As family therapists enter the larger-system terrain, it is important to discover who is answerable to whom in the macrosystem, in order to understand and anticipate triadic changes, and to be able to discuss these with families.

Boundaries

Boundaries between families and larger systems in the public sector are often marked by an unusual combination of diffusion and rigidity. Representatives of larger systems, especially social control systems, typically have much more access to the inner workings of families than families have to the inner workings of larger systems. Information about aspects of the family's life that are outside the appropriate interest of the larger system is often investigated, obtained, hypothesized about, or exchanged in gossip among workers. Information about the larger system, including crucial plans and policies, often is not known by clients. Many families have numerous representatives of larger systems, such as welfare workers or home health aides, literally going in and out of their homes, so that informal family processes are available for examination. At the same time, family access to the larger systems is organized by appointment times, formal procedures, specific meeting rooms, and the like. These asymmetrical boundaries can also be heard in the language exchanged by families and representatives of larger systems. Thus, both families and helpers may speak the informal language of the family, but only the larger systems speak the specialized languages of their disciplines. It is not unusual for such "foreign languages" to be employed at case conferences at which the family is present, thus drawing a rigid boundary between family and helpers.

The boundary issue is especially crucial in the immediacy of relationships between the members of poor and disempowered families and the individual workers from larger systems. Here, one frequently sees proximity between family and helpers, coupled with their mutual distance from actual decision makers with authority to implement real change in existing services and distribution of resources. Such proximity often contributes to a relationship marked by mystification, anger, tension, and mutual mistrust, as both families and helpers are unable to visualize their own similar positions in a wider social context that eschews justice and equality.

Finally, boundaries are crucial regarding the issue of access to needed services. Boundaries are shaped by economics, as when well-to-do families have access to private health and mental health services, allowing them to choose practitioners, whereas poor families may have access to public facilities, which allow no choice of practitioner, or may have no services available.

Myths in the Macrosystem

Family members and larger-system representatives often harbor myths about one another, and about their relationships that may preclude development and change. Just as myths in families limit observable information, so macrosystemic myths reify stereotypic relationships. For instance, if a family has had poor relationships with a health-care system in the past, it will tend to view subsequent interaction with this system (or other larger systems) with suspicion, ignoring more positive interactions, whereas the health-care system whose view of a particular family is negative will not be aware of transactions that do not fit this myth.

Family myths about larger systems come from the family's own intergenerational history of relating to outside systems, as well as from more current critical incidents involving larger systems that may occur at important nodal points in family development. Such critical incidents often relate to survival issues for families, at which points relationships with representatives of larger systems are remembered more vividly, and become the content of repeated stories, contributing to the family's mythology about larger systems. Any new helper entering the macrosystem thus enters a preexisting context that shapes new relationships.

Larger-system myths about families come from theories that become established as "truth," from prejudices regarding poor, minority, or alternative lifestyle families; from written reports about a family that are regarded as the "correct view" rather than as one opinion; by material shared at case conferences or network meetings; and by experiences with a specific family.

Myths in the macrosystem affect referral patterns, as for instance closing off certain referral options, when particular families are labeled as "unworkable" or "uncooperative," or when women are referred to mental health help but men are referred to the legal system for the same behavior.

Family myths and larger-system myths may also interact in ways that work against change. Thus, if the larger-systems myth is that single-parent families are deficit ridden and require a great deal of outside help coincides with a similar myth in the family, then a permanent family–multiple-helper coincides with a similar myth in the family, then a permanent family–multiple-helper system will be formed, establishing a rigid complementarity between single parent and outside helpers that ignores strengths, focuses only on problems, and bypasses elements of support in the family's natural extended system.

Binds

Since families and larger systems relate to each other while embedded in the wider culture, binds may easily result from the transmission of incompatible messages from multiple levels of the macrosystem. In the wider culture, families are told to be autonomous and that good families function without outside help. At the same time, many families are told by the larger systems that they need and should want to receive help from these systems. Thus, a family is simultaneously defined as "weak" or "broken" if it asks for outside help and "resistant" or "flawed" if it refuses to accept outside help. Families in poverty that require welfare assistance are told that they are entitled to such help, and are also told that they are bad for needing such help. Women are expected to organize their families to receive services from larger systems, and at the same time are criticized for overinvolvement.

Larger systems that operate by both social control and development or caregiving mandates easily generate binds with families, which are expected to trust the workers who may use information against them. Thus, a family may be expected to be open in a macrosystem where openness can lead the family into further difficulties. At the same time, the family's refusal to be open will also lead to problems in the relationship with the larger systems. In such systems, families are frequently ordered to treatment and expected to "show motivation."

As one examines binds in the macrosystem, the locus of explanation for behavior shifts from inside the family to the family–larger system–wider context level.

Labeling, Stigma, and Secrecy

Many larger systems utilize labeling. Such labels express current social norms and ideologies, but are frequently regarded as the truth. Particular labels provide access to particular larger systems. A child labeled "school phobic" will most often become involved with mental health services, whereas a child labeled "school refuser" will most often become involved with truancy or probation services. Labels provide access to payment for particular services from larger systems. Thus, a child labeled as "educationally handicapped" will be entitled to free special education services, but a child labeled as "lazy" will not.

Certain labels lead to a process of stigmatization at various levels of the macrosystems. When a family member is stigmatized by a particular label, it is not unusual for the whole family also to experience stigma; for instance, families with a member labeled "mentally retarded" are often treated as less than adequate by larger systems and the community. A family may respond to stigma by hiding its member, by turning inward and cutting off from potential sources of support in the larger systems or the community. Other families may respond to stigma by becoming angry and combative with larger systems, in defense both of the family member and of the family unit. The effects of labeling and stigma on the family's own sense of itself and on family–larger-system relationships are often ignored or unseen. Work that is done only within the boundaries of the family is often intervention at the wrong level of the macrosystem, as labeling and stigma generally require broad educational and social policy interventions.

Such labeling and stigma may combine in ways that generate secrets at multiple levels of the macrosystem. One may see replicating patterns of secret keeping, such as when a family tries to hide a labeled and stigmatized member from the community. The treatment services, in turn, develop secrets. An example may be seen in the pattern of care for the mentally retarded before deinstitutionalization. Families frequently hid their retarded members. Institutions for the retarded were hidden from the community and placed in distant locations. Finally, abuse of the mentally retarded in the institutions was kept secret from the public and from families. Intervention in this secret-keeping process began when the secret of abuse became known and publicized. A broad social movement then ensued to deinstitutionalize the retarded, to make their presence known and supported within communities near their own families, and to end the family's need to keep the member a secret. As mentally handicapped people became members of the community, families were also able to form self-help groups and handicapped rights movements. The process of labeling, stigma, and secrecy was replaced by a process of openness and advocacy at multiple levels.

WORKING WITH FAMILIES AND LARGER SYSTEMS

Following careful assessment of the macrosystemic issues involved in any given case, a family therapist's available working repertoire will broaden to include interviewing and interventions that reach beyond the boundaries of the family per se and include not only family problem solving, but family empowerment vis-à-vis the wider context.

Case Example—A New Report

A female-headed, single-parent family, consisting of a mother, Ms. Montero, and her two children, Ida, 11, and Joe, eight, came for family therapy on the advice of Joe's pediatrician. Joe, was born with congenital developmental disabilities, showed symptoms of angry outbursts. The angry outbursts had been going on since Joe was a small child but had worsened recently when the family moved into its own apartment, after several years of living with Ms. Montero's older sister. The father of Joe and Ida had left shortly after Joe's birth and had cut off all contact with the family. He did not call, visit, or provide support.

Ms. Montero was involved with several larger systems, including public welfare, a neighborhood health center, the public school, and now the mental health center where family therapy was taking place. In addition, she received advice from her family of origin—two older sisters and a mother. For many years, she had lived in an enduring complementary relationship both with helpers and with members of her extended family. Helpers and family members were the advice givers; Ms. Montero was the advice receiver. A similar myth was shared by both the extended family and helpers that Ms. Montero could not manage her family. A second myth, commonly held, was that Joe "lacked a male role model," and that his behavior would improve if such a role model could be found. In addition, Ms. Montero was criticized by family and helpers both for being overinvolved and for not doing enough for Joe as she had recently gone back to college and taken a part-time job. Her competencies as a single parent were not affirmed.

Initially, family therapy, which occurred within a large multiservice community mental health center, mirrored the other services given to the family. Ms. Montero was given advice regarding parenting. The complementary relationship between Ms. Montero and her family and Ms. Montero and helpers was replicated in the family therapy, culminating with the recommendation to have Joe tested psychologically. Believing that "experts know best," Ms. Montero agreed to the testing. The written psychological report was extremely pessimistic, predicting a future of patienthood for Joe and focusing heavily on his lack of a "male role model." The tester did not show the actual report to Ms. Montero, as he believed it would be "too upsetting." Other helpers in the macrosystem agreed, thus continuing to reify the definition of Ms. Montero as incompetent. Unaware of the position of the other helpers, Joe's pediatrician did go over the report with Ms. Montero.

The report provoked a crisis between the helpers and members of Ms. Montero's family, who insisted on a second opinion. Ms. Montero, wishing to be loyal to both her family and the helpers, was in a critical triangle, and did not know whom to support. She disagreed with much of the initial report, but she also did not see a need for more testing. She felt concerned about angering either her family or the helpers. At this juncture, the family therapist sought a consultation.

The consultation focused first on the macrosystemic relationships, clarifying Ms. Montero's ongoing one-down position with regard to the helpers and her family, the present triangle regarding the testing, and the myths about Ms. Montero, which reflected myths about single mothers in the culture at large. Sources of support that were never investigated came to light, as it emerged that Joe interacted regularly with two uncles. She declined a suggestion that she bring family members to a session, saying that she felt it was time to build her own family unit. During the discussion, Ms. Montero was clear and focused. She questioned the psychological report, pointing out that the findings did not fit with her views of her son. She spoke of many recent changes in their lives and wondered if these were not the source of the current stress, particularly the recent move from her family's home to her own apartment. During the interview, both children were well-behaved, and Joe spoke about recent improvements at school.

After the consulting interview, which framed Ms. Montero as a competent parent and normalized Joe's recent escalating anger as a response to shifts between the nuclear and extended family, an intervention was offered that was designed to empower Ms. Montero in the macrosystem, to shift the previous complementarity to a relationship marked by collaboration, and to interdict the triangle. Since a second opinion was being sought by the extended family, the first report was also termed an opinion by the consultant. Ms. Montero was then asked to create a new report, a third opinion, that would detail her point of view about the children, their relationship with each other and with her as mother and head of household, the family's relationship with the extended family, and the family's present and preferred future relationship with helpers. The consultant then suggested that this new report could form the basis for the direction of family therapy, in collaboration with the family therapist.

The consulting session and the intervention focused on strengths rather than deficits, introducing new information into the macrosystem. Instead of giving advice, a direction was set that would enable a therapeutic partnership. Larger systems were reframed as resources rather than as experts. The ritual of writing a new report, whose focus was relational rather than individual, served to empower Ms. Montero as a member of a macrosystem, organized now in her family's behalf, rather than as advice-givers to her (Imber-Black 1988a).

This consultation operated at multiple levels of the macrosystem, including intrafamily relationships, family-extended family relationships, family-extended family–multiple helpers relationships, and the wider social context whose messages and myths regarding single-parent, female-headed families served to shape and organize relationships at all of the other levels.

Although family therapists may not always have access to all of the participants in the macrosystem within which any given family exists, it is useful to assess each new case from a macrosystemic perspective, including a search for the meaningful system, and the generation of hypotheses regarding dyadic and triadic patterns, boundaries, binds, myths, labeling, stigma, and secrecy. Such an assessment can frequently be accomplished through a discussion with the family regarding past and present relationships with larger systems. A conversation of this type immediately orients the family therapist and the family to issues that reach beyond the family's own boundary for understanding current dilemmas and for shaping creative solutions. In addition, sessions may be held that include helpers from various systems and family members. Such sessions quickly move beyond assessment to intervention at the macrosystemic level. Often, several helpers involved with a family have never seen each other, or have done so at meetings that either excluded or mystified the family. Questions posed at such a meeting can orient family and multiple helpers to a sense of their interconnectedness and joint responsibility for problem solving within a macrosystem.

THERAPISTS' TRAINING FROM A
MACROSYSTEMIC PERSPECTIVE

Family therapy training can be conceptualized as a system, including established structures, patterns, and beliefs, and existing in relationship with family systems and larger service-delivery systems. Shifting from a focus on treating families in isolation from their broader contexts to a macrosystemic viewpoint requires a concomitant shift in the training of new family therapists, in both the recruitment and selection of trainees and in the content of training.

Family therapy has been an overwhelmingly White and upper-middle-class profession, dominated until recently almost exclusively by male leaders. Although these characteristics perhaps are not unlike those at most professions, family therapy began as an intervention, as a remarkable difference that made a difference, and has become a field in danger of promoting orthodoxies, professionalism, competition, and turf protection. Unchecked, this trend ultimately will find family therapy sucked in to the values and practices of the wider context.

Trainee recruitment and selection can function to reify the field through the selection of trainees who replicate current practitioners, especially with regard to race, ethnicity, and social class background, or can open the field through a deliberate affirmative-action process that brings together trainees of different backgrounds, including racial, cultural, ethnic, sexual orientation, and class differences. In so doing, a dynamic feedback loop may be established between training and practice, in which both move beyond established boundaries.

Current training frequently enables movement of trainees from the public sector to private practice, leaving poor and minority families with the lesser trained and the committed few. Curriculum content in family therapy requires shifts in order to facilitate a macrosystemic perspective capable of maintaining competent practitioners in the public sector. Thus, training in the complexities of the macrosystem, including effective ways to assess and intervene in the family–larger-system relationship, is required. Lacking such training, family therapists remain unempowered in the family–larger-system labyrinth, thus replicating the family's position. With such training, the capabilities increase for practitioners to navigate the public sector and raise the quality of services to poor families who are embroiled with larger systems.

New theories of human development that attend to gender differences and social theories that account for gender inequities and power imbalances in families and between families and larger systems must be a part of any family therapy training that seeks to educate a generation of family therapists who will be capable of effectively challenging conservative family organization and those larger systems that support such organization, wittingly or unwittingly.

Family therapy trainees require training in macrosystemic analysis that will enable an appreciation of their social and political roles as family therapists. Unexamined, family therapy can easily contribute to the homeostasis of larger systems, which are, in turn, messengers for the culture's rules regarding access to needed services, power, social startification, social control, mobility, and discrimination. Understanding the ways that models emerge out of a given social and historical context, and how work, no matter what its specific excellence, may be coopted by a broader and often hidden sociopolitical agenda can sensitize family therapists to question not only the family but themselves and their own context. Asking largely unasked questions regarding patterns of service delivery and the therapist's own place in the macrosystem can begin to facilitate intervention beyond the boundaries of the family, which is especially important when the locus of distress is embedded in the relationship with larger systems or at the sociopolitical level.

Finally, in a field in which pattern is the message, one must examine the structure of training and not simply the content. The very structure of a training system, when this replicates power, racial, ethnic, and gender inequalities in the larger systems and in the wider culture, via the exclusive promotion of hierarchy and competition, requires reorganization through training methods and structures that promote collaboration and empowerment for trainee and trainer alike.

SOME PERSONAL REFLECTIONS

As my own work with families has led me increasingly to focus on families' relationships with multiple helpers, and families' and larger systems' embeddedness in a wider social context that organizes and contributes both to a family's sense of itself and to the larger systems' mandates and relational possibilities with clients and other helpers, my own sense of human interconnectedness has grown. It seems to me that a macrosystemic perspective makes ignoring human suffering increasingly impossible, and thus the broadest view brings me full circle to a given individual and our involvement with each other.

REFERENCES

Aponte, H. (1976). The family-school interview: An eco-structural approach. *Family Process, 15,* 303–312.

Bell, N., & Zucker, R. (1968-69). Family-hospital relationships in a state hospital setting: A structural-functional analysis of the hospitalization process. *The International Journal of Social Psychiatry, XV,* 73–80.

Berger, M. (1984). Social network interventions for families that have a handicapped child. In E. Imber-Coppersmith (Ed.), *Families with handicapped members.* Rockville, Md.: Aspen Systems Corp.

Bernal, G., & Diamond, G. (1985). Notes on a socio-historical perspective of family therapy. *Journal of Strategic and Systemic Therapies, 4,* 42–47.

Bloomfield, S., Neilson, S., & Kaplan, L. (1984). Retarded adults, their families and larger systems: A new role for the family therapist. In E. Imber Coppersmith (Ed.), *Families with handicapped members.* Rockville, Md.: Aspen Systems Corp.

Coleman, S. (1983). A case of nontreatment of a nonproblem problem. *Journal of Strategic and Systemic Therapies, 2,* 62–66.

Combrinck-Graham, L., & Higley, L.W. (1984). Working with families of school-aged handicapped children. In E. Imber-Coppersmith (Ed.), *Families with handicapped members*. Rockville, Md.: Aspen Systems Corp.

Edelman, M.W. (1987). *A children's defense budget FY 1988: An analysis of our nation's investment in children*. Washington, D.C.: Children's Defense Fund.

Gould, B.B. (1985). Larger systems and peace. *Journal of Strategic and Systemic Therapies, 4,* 64–69.

Harbin, H.T. (1985). The family and the psychiatric hospital. In J. Schwartzman (Ed.), *Families and other Systems: d The macrosystemic context of family therapy.* New York: Guilford Press.

Harkaway, J. (1983). Obesity: Reducing the larger systems. *Journal of Strategic and Systemic Therapies, 2,* 2–14.

Harrell, F. (1980). Family dependency as a transgenerational process: An ecological analysis of families in crises. Unpublished dissertation, University of Massachusetts, Amherst.

Imber-Black, E. (1988a). *Families and larger systems: A therapist's guide through the labyrinth.* New York: Guilford Press.

Imber-Black, E. (1986a). Families, larger systems and the wider social context. *Journal of Strategic and Systemic Therapies, 5,* 29–35.

Imber-Black, E. l(1988b). The family system and the health care system: Making the invisible visible. *Journal of Family Psychotherapy.*

Imber-Black, E. (1987). The mentally handicapped in context. *Family Systems Medicine.*

Imber-Black, E. (1986b). Women, families, and larger systems. In M. Ault-Riche (Ed.), *Women and family therapy*. Rockville, Md.: Aspen Systems Corp.

Imber Coppersmith, E. (1985). Families and multiple helpers: A systemic perspective. In D. Campbell & R. Draper (Eds.), *Application of systemic family therapy.* New York: Grune & Stratton.

Imber Coppersmith, E. (1982). Family therapy in a public school system. In A. Gurman (Ed.), *Questions and answers in the practice of family therapy*, Volume 2. New York: Brunner/Mazel.

Libow, J. (1985). Gender and sex role issues as family secrets. *Journal of Strategic and Systemic Therapies, 4,* 32–41.

MacKinnon, L., & Marlett, N. (1984). A social action perspective: The disabled and their families in context. In E. Imber-Coppersmith (Ed.), *Families with handicapped members*. Rockville, Md.: Aspen Systems Corp.

Miller, D. (1983). Outlaws and invaders: The adaptive function of alcohol abuse in the family-helper supra system. *Journal of Strategic and Systemic Therapies, 2,* 15–27.

Roberts, J. (1984). Families with infants and young children who have special needs. In E. Imber-Coppersmith (Ed.), *Families with handicapped members*. Rockville, Md.: Aspen Systems Corp.

Schwartzman, H., & Kneifel, A.W. (1985). Familiar institutions: How the child care system replicates family patterns. In J. Schwartzman (Ed.), *Families and other systems: The macrosystemic context of family therapy*. New York: Guilford Press.

Schwartzman, J., & Restivo, R.J. (1985). Acting out and staying in: Juvenile probation and the family. In J. Schwartzman (Ed.), *Families and other systems: The macrosystemic context of family therapy.* New York: Guilford Press.

Selig, A. (1976). The myth of the multi-problem family. *American Journal of Orthopsychiatry, 46,* 526–531.

Selvini-Palazolli, M., Boscolo, L., Cecchin, G., & Prata, G. (1980). The problem of the referring person. *Journal of Marital and Family Therapyd,d 6,* 3–9.

Sivard, R.L. (1987). *World military and social expenditures* (11th edition). Washington, D.C.: World Priorities.

Webb-Woodard, L., & Woodward, B. (1983). The larger system in the treatment of incest. *Journal of Strategic and Systemic Therapies, 2,* 28–37.

2

TOWARD EPISTEMOLOGICAL TRANSFORMATION IN THE EDUCATION AND TRAINING OF FAMILY THERAPISTS

E. H. Auerswald, M.D.

It is evening in late autumn. The shadows outside the building I am in are growing and blending into darkness, and the lights are going on. I am sitting in a room with a small group of people of different ages and sexes. There are a couple of adults, one a man and the other a woman. There is a young girl in early adolescence, and two children, boys. There is also a toddler in the room who doesn't sit much in one place. When she does, she settles on the lap of the young girl. We are talking earnestly with one another. The conversation waxes and wanes. Voices become loud and strident, and then grow soft and tender. Then they become strident again. One person gets up and stomps out of the room. Another begins to cry. Then another. The person who left returns and, seeing the tears, throws up his hands. I talk with him, and he moves to embrace the first to cry. The crying ends. We talk some more, then they all get up, say goodbye to me, and leave. I sit for a short while, somber and thoughtful, and then go to the desk in the corner of the room. I take a folder out of a drawer, write in it for a couple of minutes, and put it back into the drawer. Then I turn off the video equipment and the room lights.

From the darkened room, I can see through the one-way mirror that dominates one wall. The lights have been switched on in the room on the other side, and I can see my new students, all eight of them, chattering away. They are excited. This is their first training seminar, and I have had them watch a family therapy session with the speakers in their room turned off. I have recorded the dialogue of the session, but they could not hear it. I want to expose them to the family's relatedness without letting them lock into the content of the conversation. This is the first step in my effort to open a window for them. I have also chosen to have them watch this family for a particular purpose. My reasons for beginning this way will become apparent as we move along.

I have already interviewed each of these students during the process of screening them for training, so I know their names, their professional training, and a little about their lives—very little. I don't really know them yet as people, so I watch them chatter for a moment, wondering what each of them will teach me. Then I walk out into the hall and through the door into the room where they are.

FIRST SEMINAR—THE EXPLICATE AND
IMPLICATE FAMILY

Fresh from the experience of the family they have watched, they want to ask me questions. They have, of course, figured out which persons are the mother and father in the family by their age, but they want to know how old the children are. Once they get the roles straight, they want to know what happened in the session, especially during the most visibly dramatic part. "What happened when the father got angry and left, and the mother, and then the oldest son began to cry?" one of them asks. I play dumb, and feign surprise. "You just told me what happened," I say. "The father got angry and disconnected from the family, but then he came back and reconnected. If you were watching his body language, you saw him disconnect and reconnect several other times without leaving his chair." Another student asks, "But what made the others cry?" By this time, they all look a little exasperated. They did not get it. The second student who had spoken up persists. "No," she says, "that's not what I mean. What were they *talking about?*" So I tell them, "They were talking about how the father is always going away to other pursuits and leaving the rest of them to get along without him, and then, when he is at home, all they get from him is lectures." Then I take them on another tack.

"Do you really believe there is any such thing as a family?" I ask. "If you do, raise your hand." They look puzzled and hesitate—trying, I am sure, to figure out what kind of a weird question *that* is. Then the hands all go up. Then I ask them if there is any such thing as a community. I get the same answer. I ask the same question regarding culture, and get the same answer. Then I tell them that I disagree with them, because a family is not a thing, nor is a community or a culture a thing. The students let out a muffled groan, and assert that my questions were trick questions and my assertion is a matter of semantics.

They are half right. The question *is* a trick question, but the answer is not a trivial matter of simple semantics. The issue it poses is not trivial at all. There are two answers to their question, Yes and No. Both can be correct, depending on what definition of family (or community or culture) is used to construct the answer. What makes the question and its answer profound is that these definitions, and thus the answer, come from differently structured realities. The other questions contain the same distinctions, and more. These students don't make these distinctions, and what I am up to is paving the way so that they will. I don't tell them this yet, because I want them to experience the distinctions before I put words to them.

The distinctions that I want them to learn to make are of different orders. The one that I was aiming at by having them watch the family without sound has to do with the nature of communication. It has been suggested by researchers of body language and human territoriality that from 80 to 90 percent of interpersonal communication takes place in the realm of the nonverbal (Scheflen, 1968). Nonverbal communication is often clearer and is devoid of most of the static that tends to obscure verbal communication. It is also more expansive in scope. Messages are "sent" that people have no verbal language to express. Messages about messages (metamessages) are also exchanged. And messages that originate in that which people consciously or unconsciously want to hide also sneak through. My students already communicate in this realm. They know some of these languages, those used by their family, culture, society, and community, but they use them without awareness, and they do not make conscious efforts to learn new ones. I want them to become acutely aware of nonverbal languages, so that they can read and respond in these languages at will. I will be showing them many videotapes, without sound, of various kinds of human situations.

I have also begun to prepare the way to teach them to make distinctions of other kinds, beginning with definitions.

After the students have accused me of playing a semantic trick on them, I say, "Well, stop and think for a minute about this. Do you *really* believe that a family is a thing?" I give them a full minute to think, and then I say, "OK. If you really think a family is a *thing*, raise your hand." No hands go up, so I rub it in a little. "C'mon now, You said my question was a semantic trick. If it was, some of you must believe a family is a thing." Still, no hands.

I once hoped that some students *would* raise their hands at this point to create a polarity in the class and facilitate discussion, but in all the years in which I have been teaching this way, it has never happened. At first, I thought it was so because they were intimidated by my one-up position as teacher, so I made this explicit. I would ask them if they were intimidated. None of them ever agreed to this notion, so I gave it up as a factor. What they did, they said, was to scan their experience, because they had no ready-made answer to the question, which is precisely what I wanted them to do.

No hands were raised because, like all of us, these students do not *experience* their own families as things. They experience their family ecologically. They experience their family of origin as a domain of relatedness, a patterned set of powerful and complex lifelong connections that were first established well before they had learned the word family or system or cybernetics, and well before they had connected these words with concepts. And, if, impelled by romantic love, they have formed a couple and, perhaps, produced children, they have added a new domain of relatedness, a new pattern of powerful connections to those that were there before. They have initiated the lifelong connections experienced by their children.

I have now reached a point in the sequence I am imposing on my students when I can begin to teach them what I consider to be a crucial distinction with regard to families. Then I can move on to additional similar distinctions concerning community and culture, and society, as well.

The next question I ask them is: "Okay, if a family is not a thing, then what is it?" Some of the students now are eager to answer. One says, "A family is a system." They know of the "systems approach," and they are sure this is what I want them to say. I ask, "Okay, can you define system for me?" This takes awhile, and many students participate. They give me an objective definition of a system. They describe it in terms of boundaries, subsystems, input, output, system characteristics, and so on. Once again, they describe a thing. (Often the students in these seminars have already delved into the family therapy literature. In recent years, some know a little about cybernetics, and they will throw in a statement about family processes being circular and not linear. Some of them have read Bateson (1972, 1979, 1987), and they mention "the pattern which connects." A few have heard of or read Maturana and Varela (1972, 1979, 1987) and they will add autopoesis [as a "property"] to their description. They add these concepts, however, as addenda. They do not use them as a core basis for their description.)

Given the system of thought they use to "make" sense, which they learned while growing up, had reinforced in their education all the way through graduate school, experience at work, and watch frequently on TV, it is unlikely that they would think any other way. They are trying to "make" sense as they answer my question.

While this is going on, I am also privately engaged in another activity. I am assessing the students in the class, looking for one who seems comfortable and articulate enough for me to call on next. I will be issuing a challenge to this student, and I want someone who can stand up well to the challenge. This time I choose a woman, whom I will call Sarah.

I ask Sarah to describe her own family. She "makes" sense by resorting to objective description. She describes the "parts" of her family—mother, father, brothers, sisters, grandparents, aunts, uncles. She identifies these family members by age, and sex, personality characteristics, and the like. Immanent in this description, again, is the definition of family as thing. She provides her description skillfully and with facility, matter of factly, displaying little emotion or affect. (The neophyte family therapy students I have asked to do this in various groups over the years have all behaved similarly. They are very skilled at "making" sense in this way.)

When Sarah winds down in her description, I issue my challenge. I ask, "Haven't you forgotten something?" She looks puzzled, and so does the rest of the class. She thinks for a moment, and then says, "Well, I haven't told you *everything* about my family. You want more detail?" "No," I say, "there's a whole aspect of your family about which you have told me nothing." The whole class looks more puzzled. "I'll give you a clue," I say.

I address the whole class: "You all agree that a family is not a thing, yet you persist in defining it as if it were a thing. You all told me it was a system, not a thing, but together you described a system as an objective thing. You didn't change its thingness. You just changed its name from family to system and threw in a few new words."

Then I again address Sarah: "Now, when I asked you to describe your own family, again you described it as if it were a thing. You broke it down into its parts and told me about them. If it's not a thing, an object, you could not reduce it to its parts. I think the reason that you agree that the family is not a thing is that you don't *experience* your family as a thing."

The class looks more puzzled than ever for a moment, but then, one by one, each of them lights up. When Sarah lights up, she says: "Oh, you mean the *relationships* in my family!" I answer, "You're close. You used a word that often denotes or connotes a thing. If you agree that your family is not a thing, then it's really not a thing made up of parts called relationships. You got what I wanted you to get, though. What you left out in the description you gave me is the domain of relations, the relational patterns that distinguish your family. Now, will you please describe that?''

The class is now alive, but Sarah is having a more difficult time. Her expression and general body language have changed. She looks distraught, though she tries to hide it. She also begins to use different language. She uses such words as love, and closeness and distance, and warm and cold, and those that describe congruence or incongruence of connecting attitudes and communication and patterns of events. As she attempts to describe her *experience* of her family, she does so thoughtfully and haltingly, often groping for words. No longer is she glib and organized in her description. She is struggling.

I let her struggle for awhile, and then I say, ''Forgive me. I am using you so I can make some distinctions for the class. I apologize because I know I have put you on the spot. What I asked you to do is difficult. You need to know that I chose you to have this conversation with me because I had already experienced you as one of the people here who could handle it. Thank you for hanging in while I did that. I still need you to help me make some more distinctions, but the rest is easier.''

Then I address the class. ''I think you all noticed that there was a change in Sarah's behavior and in the words she spoke after I asked her to describe her family in the relational domain. Before that, she seemed confident and articulate and at ease as she described her family as a thing, but now she seems much less confident and articulate and more ill at ease.''

I turn to Sarah and ask, ''Did you notice that yourself?'' She answers, ''Oh, yes.'' I ask, ''Can you tell us why? What created the change in you?'' Again, she thinks for awhile. Then she answers, ''Well, I couldn't be objective about it. I had to think very subjectively. Also, I'm not used to talking about such things in a group of people, some of whom I have just met and don't know.''

Were you afraid to expose information about your family that would reflect badly on you?'' I ask. ''Well, a little, I suppose,'' she responds.

''I noticed that you seemed to be groping for words,'' I say. ''Was that because of that fear?'' ''Not really,'' she says. ''I was having a hard time *finding* words. I was talking about things [things?] that contain a lot of feelings, and it's hard to find words that really express them. The usual words seem empty and not very precise.''

''Why did you care about being precise?'' I ask. Her answer is: ''Well, again, here I am in a class with a lot of people I don't know. I'm supposed to be smart here. Besides, you just told me I had been describing my family as a thing, and I was trying not to do that. I kept thinking of words that implied that.'' Her answer pleased me. I had been hoping she would say something like that. She had perceived the distinction I was trying to teach, and her answer was helping me. I had made a good choice.

''So you were having trouble making sense,'' I said. ''Oh, yes,'' she answered. ''I'm not sure I *can* make sense of my family even to myself, much less to the class.''

''Would you agree,'' I ask, ''that when you were describing your family as a thing you were in one realm of thought, and when you were trying to speak of your family in the relational domain you were in another?" She responds, "Oh, yes." I then ask, "What is the difference between the two realms?" She answers, "One is objective and the other is subjective." So I ask her, "What do you mean by objective?" She has to think about that one. Then she says, "Well, I guess what I mean is that I was thinking reasonably, in a way that I think makes sense to everybody." I say, "Well, you can't mean that you were thinking collectively and simultaneously *with* the class. Where was that thought going on?" "What do you mean?" she asks. "I mean, where is that thinking process located?" Well, inside me, in my brain," she says. I come back, "Isn't that subjective thinking?" She answers, "Well, yes." Then she hesitates, and adds, "But I knew that what I was thinking and saying would make sense to everybody."

"Would you agree then," I ask, "that what you call objective thinking is a form of subjective thinking in which you use some rules to organize and edit what you think and say that are used by everybody when they want to make sense to one another?" Sarah answers, "Well, yes, I guess so." "Were you thinking about those rules?" I ask. "No," she answers. "So," I retort, "they are immanent in your thinking. You use them automatically without thinking about them when you want to make sense in what you think and say." "I guess I do," she responds. "You agree?" I ask, to nail down the point. She thinks again for a moment, and then answers, "Yes, I agree."

I say, "Let me put this another way, and see if you still agree. When you want to make sense, without being aware of it, you have these rules you use. You have learned these rules. *You* did not construct them. But every time you use them to organize your thinking, you *construct* that which makes sense, and you call this being objective." Sarah once again hesitates while she thinks about what I have said, and then says, "I can go along with that."

"Okay," I say. "Now, would you agree that the rules you use subjectively to make objective sense are those that you use to make objective sense out of everything, out of it all, out of your world, even the universe?" Hesitation again. Then, "Yes, that's what I do." I move on. "So those are the rules you use to define reality?" She hesitates a long time. "Well, yes, when I need to make objective sense. There's a lot more I do, though." "Like what?" "Well," she responds, "most of what I think isn't sensible in that way."

To save time, I decide to distinguish that domain for her, so I say, "You mean when you are just sort of scanning what you experience or when you are creating and playing around with dreams and fantasies or when you are enjoying some experience without thinking much about it?" "Yes," she says. "I spend more time doing that than I do making sense out of things." "Right!" I say. Now I can make one of the distinctions I want the class to get.

"So your thought occurs in at least two very different realms," I say. "One is the realm of rational thought, of "making" sense, and the other is the irrational realm of experience and creativity and play. Right?" "Right," she answers. "Now," I ask, "in which realm do you invest your thinking with feeling the most?" She thinks again, "Well, not in the realm of making sense. In fact, if I really want to be rational, I can't let my feelings get in the way." "Right," I say.

I continue: "Now, you agreed with me that the realm in which you are making sense is the one you use to define reality. Does that mean that the other realm is unreal?" "She answers: "No, not really." Everyone laughs, picking up the pun. "So you live in two realities?" I ask. "I guess I do," she says, still smiling.

Turning to the class, I say, "How about the rest of you?" They think, and then nod agreement. "And they are very different?" I continue. They nod again.

Turning back to Sarah, I ask her, "In which of these realities do you experience the relational aspects of your family—the rational sensible reality in which your family is a thing, or the irrational, creative, feeling reality?" No hesitation. "The irrational reality," she says. "In which reality are your connections with your family?" I continue. "The irrational reality," she answers. "So, I say, "is it fair to say that if you *only* think about your family as a thing in the rational sensible reality, you are ignoring those connections?" "Yes, I guess I am," she responds.

I turn to the class. "Do the rest of you agree?" They all look pensive. They are pondering what I am saying. There is no ready response. They do not dissent, but they are thinking. What I am saying has a lot of implications for them. Like me, most of them have grown up with the concept that there is only one *real* reality. They have also been trained in disciplines that do not make the distinction I am making. A few of them are nodding. They sort of understand what I am saying, but they still want more, to convince them. I say to them, "Think back to the family you saw in action tonight. I turned off the speakers because I wanted you to focus on the shape of their relational connectedness, not on their words, which you could use to define them as a thing made up of parts identified by their characteristics, their so-called personalities. What you saw, among other events, was the father's disconnection. You saw him actively disconnecting, and you saw the response of the others when this happened, most dramatically in two of them, who cried."

"Sarah had a difficult time," I continue, "describing her family in this so-called 'irrational' reality because our language has been shaped by what we call common sense. It is well developed and very adequate to describe things, but it is not very useful to describe the irrational reality in which relational connections are located. We do have some words—such as love, and empathy, and altruism—but the tendency is to try to define these as things, too. As a result, they defy precise definition, and when we want to be "realistically" and "rationally" precise, we can't use them. Sarah wanted to be precise because she is in a class, and her experience is that one must try to be precise in class discussion. So she had difficulty.

"The realm of nonrational reality is the realm of creativity, and there are other languages there, some of them nonverbal. If we must use words there, the best medium is poetry. Lovers know this. They often try to say what they can't say in ordinary 'rational' prose by writing poems to each other. In a few minutes I will show you that we can make art to set the stage for using the words we have more creatively. But first let me give you a shorthand way of referring to the two reality domains we have been discussing. I have borrowed the words I want you to learn and define from the physicist David Bohm [1980].

"Bohm suggests that the physical phenomena available to our senses and their technological extensions that are amenable to empirical objectivity make up what he calls the *explicate* order of the universe. There is, he suggests, another order, not readily available to objective appraisal, from which the explicate order emerges. He calls this the *implicate* order. He suggests that empirical science must look to the implicate order of the universe as context for the explicate order.

"Bohm uses an experiment to illustrate this point. The experimental apparatus consists of a cylindrical container open at one end, balanced, with the open end up, on a motor-driven rotating axle so that the cylinder rotates at a steady rate without any lateral deviation. The cylinder is filled with glycerine. If one deposits a drop of India ink on the surface of the glycerine while the cylinder is rotating, the motion of the cylinder will pull the drop of ink into a circle of ink, which will then sink into the glycerine and disperse, so that it is no longer visible. Then, if the direction of rotation of the cylinder is reversed, the movement of the particles will reverse, the circle will again appear on the surface, and the ink will then coalesce to reform the drop. The visible ink, Bohm suggests, is analogous to the explicate order of the universe and the dispersed and hidden form of the ink is analogous to the implicate order. The explicate order in this experiment can be described 'objectively' using the language of 'common sense,' but the implicate order cannot be adequately described this way.

"I suggest that we use these terms in the following way: We will use the term *explicate family*, and also *explicate community, culture*, and *society*, to designate these entities defined as objects in 'sensible' objective reality, and the terms *implicate family* and *implicate society, culture, and community* to designate the experienced but difficult-to-describe nonobjectifiable definition of them as patterned connections in a domain of relations. I use explicate as an adjective or adverb to denote the state of objectifiability and the word implicate to denote a state of nonobjectifiability."

After I have introduced these terms, I tell the class that I now want to show them an artful way to communicate the implicate domain of a family using nonverbal language. I ask Sarah to sculpt her family while remaining silent. I tell her to use class members as representatives of the members of her family, and position them in a configuration in space in a way that feels right to her. I suggest that she might want to position some members higher or lower than others, and that she can stand them on a chair or have them stoop to accomplish this. I also suggest that she might want some to face toward others or away from others,, and that she will probably discover that to make the sculpture work, she will have to make it move, as families are not static entities. Their relatedness is constantly in motion. I may raise questions to assist her, but, except to tell the class members she enlists what person each represents and how to position themselves, I insist that she remain silent.

After Sarah has finished her sculpture, I ask those she chose to play the various family roles how they felt in the position in which they were stationed. They tell me, and I ask Sarah if it seems to her that the feelings described by the players are like those habitually expressed by the real family members they represented. From having done such exercises many times, I can predict that she will say that they are similar, or substantially the same.

Then I ask the class to make a sculpture together of the family they watched.

They put the mother and the oldest son, who cried, close together and facing each other, and the oldest girl and the toddler together, with the toddler sometimes moving about. They face the father away from the rest of the family and have him move alternately to a place distant from the rest of them, then closer, and then out again, all the while with his back toward them. They have the youngest son sit by himself, stationary, watching the others.

I ask the players how they feel in the position in which they are placed in the sculpture. The players representing the mother and the oldest son say they feel sad. The oldest daughter player says she feels annoyed because she is stuck with the task of taking care of the toddler. The toddler player says she feels helpless but relatively carefree, and the father and youngest son players say they feel very lonely. I ask them which family members they think are in the most trouble. At first, they are divided—some say the oldest son and the mother, and some say the father and the youngest son. After some discussion, they decide on the father and the youngest son.

I know this family, and they are right in their appraisal. I share with them the information that the family came looking for help for the youngest son, who is enuretic and failing in school. The father has a peptic ulcer. I end this first seminar on that note.

SECOND SEMINAR—REALITY SYSTEMS ON OUR PLANET

I begin the second seminar, a week later, by having the class recreate the sculpture of the family they had constructed at the end of the first seminar. Then I show them excerpts from the videotape of my session with the family, this time with the sound turned on. I ask them to use the information they already have and that they collect while watching the tape to construct a story about this family that includes and makes intelligible the distress they have expressed. There is not enough information on the tape, so I give them more. I tell them that the story consists of events that took place at different times and places, with different family members present, including some from different generations and extended family. Some events, which take place with *no* family members present, are societal and/or political events. I emphasize that all these events are affecting the family *now*. The story we are constructing is an "event-shape in timespace," not a history mapped on a linear time line.

There is one section of the tape that I do *not* show them, nor do I give them the information it contains. I explain that they are not yet ready to understand its significance, and promise that further on in their training we will come back to this family and complete the story.

I then deliver a lecture, which I preface by telling them that the ideas I will be describing have been expressed by many others, but that the way I put them together, the construct made of these ideas, is my own. I tell them that I want them to listen critically to what I have to say, and to see if they can agree. I also tell them that my constructs are incomplete, and that I am hoping that, if what

I have to say has merit in their view, they will add to them. My lecture (somewhat condensed) is as follows:

There are, of course, many definitions of family around and in use. Human societies on our planet operate with at least four discrete, though overlapping, sets of thought rules that are used by their proponents to edit what they consider to be real in the universe and what is not, and each has its own operational definition of the word "family." Three of these reality systems are in widespread use. These I will call Eastern/transcendental, aboriginal/animistic, and Western/mechanistic. One is relatively new and growing. This one I will call new science/ecological.

The Western/mechanistic reality system predominates in industrialized countries, and its use has been growing in so-called developing countries that want to reap the material benefits of industrialized society. The new science/ecological reality system also is growing and, as it was spawned in the industrialized countries, it is found in these places.

For our purposes, I will be concerned primarily with the definitions in these latter two. I want to make it clear that it is not my intention to give short shrift to the Eastern/transcendental and aboriginal/animistic reality systems. There is as much to be learned and discussed concerning these systems as there is concerning the others. I will not describe them now, however, because I can make the distinctions I want to make without attending to them.

The Western/mechanistic reality system evolved in the western segment of the northern latitudes. Its recorded origins can be found in the writings of the ancient Athenians, primarily in Aristotle. The major era of its development was during 17th, 18th, and 19th centuries, and it is solidly rooted in the science that flourished in those centuries.

In addition to being mechanistic, it is also objectivist, centripetally reductionistic, dualistic, and hierarchical. It uses concepts of linear time and linear casuality, and truth is considered absolute. It contains a formal logic, well developed in Western philosophical thought, which, in the service of brevity, I will call *mechologic*. By mechologic, I refer to the logic which Western/mechanistic thinkers generally refer to as "common sense." We adhere to it when we want to be "rational", to "make" sense. We saw this in Sarah's thinking in our last seminar.

In this edition of reality, family is defined as a complex object made of parts. The criteria used to identify its parts are gender, age, and roles. Parts and whole are considered bounded entities with identifiable location in space at a given point on a time line. Families are described as moving along the time line, changing as they go. Marriage contracts are made, children are born, grow up, and leave, and so on. These changes are defined as "family process." Plotted at a point on the time line already passed (past) is the family's future. The objective family is affected by its environment—by input, in the form of messages and supplies that cross its boundary—and it affects its environment by emitting output of the same genre. These effects come under the general definition of "forces." The tasks of the family as it moves along the time line are defined as maintenance of its own integrity and equilibrium and adaptation to its environment. This is, of course, the definition of what we have already defined as the explicate family.

In the evolution of ideas in the western portion of the northern hemisphere, the new science/ecological reality system also can be seen in rudimentary form in the writings of the ancient Greeks—first, I think, in writings of the pre-Socratic thinker Heraclitus, and later in some segments of the writing of both Plato and Aristotle. The system began to evolve in earnest in the latter half of the 19th century, and burst into full view in physics at the very beginning of the 20th century in the work of Max Planck (1900, 1936) and Albert Einstein (1905, 1938). It has grown rapidly in this century.

It has become the predominant reality system in use in the physical sciences, reinforced by some developments in 20th century philosophy. It is now taken seriously, though it is not predominant, in the biological and behavioral sciences, especially in family therapy. Ideas rooted in this reality system are expressed by all humans, but since the emergence of mechologic, such ideas have been relegated to the realm of the mystical or unreal, or to the realm of art. Until they appeared in physics, they were considered the content of play, romantic love, dreams, fantasy, or artistic creation, and they were not thought of as having serious adaptive utility. Although in mechological reality some latitude is given to artists, lovers, mystics, and, recently, "far out" scientists, those who regard such ideas as serious and adaptively useful are often considered deviant, even crazy.

The new science/ecological reality system is monistic, relativistic, centrifugally creative, patterned, emergent, connectionist, and evolutionary. That which is observed is thought of as relational differences that expose shifting, emerging, receding, patterned shapes of events in a timespace terrain, and truth is considered heuristic. This reality system has its own logic, which I will call *ecologic*. The formal (not formal in the sense that it creates fixed forms, but rather in the sense that there is widespread consensus) basis for ecologic is still emerging. I think it is important to recognize that the mechological thinker often cannot "make" sense out of ecological reality.

In this thought system, the family is defined as a patterned set of connected events in a relational domain. Changes and transformations in these connections occur in timespace. You will recognize this as the definition of the implicate family.

As you have already seen, because this system has emerged so recently, it has not yet developed a language sufficient to its description. The terms used are often confusing, because they are terms extracted from the language of mechologic. When these words are used in ecological discourse, their mechological denotations and connotations still hover in the background. Thus, their use is confusing because they often carry double meanings. For example, physicists have resorted to such terms as "charm" to describe a facet of the event shapes called quarks. What the physicists mean by charm and the usual meaning of the word in common sense differ.

The words that have come into descriptive use in ecologic are generally those borrowed to describe the evolution of patterned connections, words such as strong, weak, distorted, strengthening, weakening, emerging, receding, symmetrical, asymmetrical, synchronous, asynchronous, attrition, and disconnection. The same words used in mechologic to describe roles are used in ecologic to identify qualities of connectedness in observed patterns. To repeat, that which is experienced by humans in the relational domain is most richly expressed in art, at least until new language develops.

I have presented these definitions of family and their epistemological sources because both (mechological-explicate and ecological-implicate) are in use in the family therapy field, but the distinction as to which is in use when is seldom made. It is important in many ways, as you will see as we move along.

This distinction is epistemological, which means that it has to do with how we know what we think we know. It is the basis for the trickiness you recognized in my original question about whether you thought there was any such thing as a family. The answer to that question can be both "yes" and "no" depending on which definition you apply to the family. These definitions are rooted in differing thought systems that produce different editions of reality. The answer is Yes in mechological reality, and the answer is No in ecological reality.

The juxtaposition of mechologic and the logic of the other reality-defining thought systems requires a similar distinction. When family therapists adhere to mechological thinking in work with families who define reality in transcendental or animistic ways, their therapeutic work can be ineffective, and even damaging. This disparity is usually thought of as cultural—but it is more than that. It is also epistemological. However, that is another topic, which I will save for some other time.

End of lecture. End of second seminar.

THIRD SEMINAR—THE EXPLICATE AND IMPLICATE COMMUNITY, CULTURE, AND SOCIETY

Once my students have thoroughly learned the distinctions of implicate and explicate family and mechological and ecological thinking, my next goal is to expose them to an experience that will lead them to make these distinctions in their thinking as applied to community, culture, and society. Before I can do so, I have found that it is necessary to settle on some definitions of these words. In general usage their meaning is often very unclear, and if one consults a dictionary, one also finds considerable overlap in their definitions.

I begin by initiating a discussion. This exercise is somewhat less that democratic, as I rely on my position as teacher and moderator of the discussion to guide the process. I see to it that they come up with the definitions that I want them to use as we move on. I also make sure that they formulate the definitions in language that allows me to apply the distinctions I think important. Here are the definitions I get them to arrive at and short statements of the relevent points that usually come up in discussion.

I begin by pointing out the obvious, that all of these words denote groups of people who are connected in some way, and by suggesting that we look at the nature of those connections in order to arrive at our definitions. Then we tackle the word "community."

We arrive at the following definition. The word "community" denotes a group of people, who usually reside in a defined geographical area, who are relationally connected by a common intention to generate maximum conditions of well-being and relational harmony for the group's members.

In the course of discussion, the students decide that friendship networks are a specialized form of community, although they may not involve people who live in a defined geographical area.

The main objection that arises to this definition is that it is "idealistic" and that it is difficult these days to find a group that operates in this way. Communities, as thus defined, my students observe, seem to be disappearing. They agree, however, that the definition describes what a community could (and should) be, and they are willing to use it as a working definition.

The word "culture" denotes a group of people who are connected by a collectively held set of myths, beliefs, customs, taboos, modes of expression and communication, and practices that determine the manner in which members of the group comport their everyday lives in relation to one another.

In the discussion leading to this definition, there is usually mention of the more narrow definition of the word that denotes an appreciation of literature, music, and other arts, but this definition is rapidly discarded, and a mutual acceptance of the above definition is easily reached.

There is always a discussion of the word "ethnicity", and the conclusion is reached that it is a word that denotes common roots in one of various channels of biological evolution, and that although common ethnicity is often a characteristic of a given culture, it is not necessarily a basis for a definition of culture.

The word "society" denotes a group of people who are connected by a set of commonly learned institutions that are rooted in religious or secular ideology, that determines the political and economic organization of the group, and that are reflected in a system of laws that, in turn, prescribe the behavior of the group's members in formal ways.

As one might anticipate, the discussion that takes place regarding this definition is the longest and the most difficult for me to "guide." I have already written the definitions of community and culture on the blackboard, and, in order to arrive at this definition of society, as new elements for inclusion arise, I can refer to them. Many of the elements the students bring up are already included in the previous two definitions, so they are excluded. This process of exclusion leads us eventually to my definition.

Once these definitions are arrived at, I ask the class, now that they have made the distinction between the two thought/reality systems of mechologic and ecologic, to decide, in the context of their own life experience, which of these two thought systems would be most useful in contemplating community, and culture, and society.

They quickly decide that community and culture reside in the relational domain and are best contemplated in ecologic. They have trouble deciding, however, which logic is appropriate for thinking about society. They come to the conclusion that, though they would like to think about society in ecologic, the fixed nature of institutions makes this impossible. They decide that society can only be thought of in mechologic.

I then ask them to think of the distinction they have made between explicate and implicate family, and to try to distinguish explicate and implicate community, culture, and society. They have difficulty with this one. Finally, they decide to resolve their dilemma by adding another definition, that of "nation."

There is some objection at first, on the grounds that societies can span national boundries, but they get past that by recognizing that institutional configurations differ from nation to nation. They decide that a nation contains all of the entities we have defined—individuals, families, friendship networks, a culture or cultures, and what they now insist on referring to as institutionalized society. They further decide that the explicate nation is represented by institutionalized society, and that the implicate nation is represented by all the others. They also decide that what they are now calling institutionalized society is represented by bureaucratic structures—governmental, military, and corporate—and by a specific political system. These, they decide, are the ingredients of the explicate nation.

I pretend to agree with everything they say, and I end the exercise by asking them if they agree that the bureaucratic structures grew in the reality of mechological thinking, that they now support and sustain that reality system, and that citizens in a given nation, when in work roles in these structures, think and make decisions mechologically. They agree without dissent, and begin telling stories of their personal travails in contact with mechological bureaucrats.

In response, I tell them what I want them to understand now is that those same "bureaucrats" are participants in the implicate relational domain of family, community, culture, and friendship networks. Some of them make art in various media. They may even try to apply ecological thought in their work, but, in the end, in order to perform "sensibly" and "efficiently" and thus keep their jobs, they *must* think mechologically.

I remind them that mechologic is a system of thought that requires that people, communities, cultures, and societies be thought of objectively, as things, and that it also requires that, in order to understand these things, they be broken down analytically into parts. The result, I tell them, is that social planning, done by people who are required to think mechologically, is also broken down into parts. Knowledge, too, is segmented into specialities. Educational institutions are similarly organized, and they produce specialists, experts in fields of lesser and lesser breadth. The outcome is a fragmented institutionalized society divided into separate institutionalized systems and subsystems, and sub-subsystems, each constructed to deal with a part of the whole of human life, in a mechological reality that ignores the implicate relational domain.

In the domain of mechological thinking which is the domain of "common sense", these fragmented structures *are* reality, by definition. Creative thinking in the relational domain is accepted by that reality insofar as it can be assimilated and rationalized, and can be used to "make" sense. Otherwise, it is discarded in the making of policy as "non-sense" and labeled "unrealistic" or "idealistic" or just plain crazy. Furthermore, those ideas that originate in the creative relational domain that *are* accepted in mechological reality are converted from ideas with potential for expansion and growth to fixed concepts, which are then approached reductionistically and fragmented into parts.

The next charge I give to my students is to think about the entirety of both explicate and implicate domains ecologically, to imagine that the explicate society dominates the implicate, and then to imagine the impact of this on implicate relational connectedness.

In extended discussion, they decide that the rigidity, either/or dualism, reductionism, and hierarchicalization immanent in mechological thought/reality can only interfere with the ecological balance and flow of relational connectedness. Its use can only prevent the creative growth and affective investments of that domain. One student even goes to the blackboard and draws a time line and a hierarchical ladder, which she makes into a square. She superimposes it on a diagram of a network, pointing out how squares intersect the connections in the network. Summing up, they conclude that the edition of reality prescribed by mechologic in the explicate objective domain superimposed on the implicate relational domain results in fragmentation and disconnection.

I then ask them then if it is fair to say that mechological objective commonsense thinking and planning not only result in fragmentation of societal structures, but the social and political realities they create destroy relatedness and pull people apart. This is, of course, a rather shocking and radical assertion. They have always assumed that membership in a society only served to pull people together. They hesitate, and discuss it. In the end, however, they decide it is a fair statement.

I remind them that we are engaged in an educational experience designed to assist them to develop distinctions that they will be making in the context of an institutionalized health system and an institutionalized human services system. They will be expected and paid to perform as part of those systems and to play the roles prescribed therein. They will be defined that way by others who inhabit those systems, and the families they will work with will also define them in that way to start with.

I assert, that if they agree with and are serious about this appraisal of the destructive outcomes of mechological thinking and planning on relational connectedness, it will be necessary for them to learn to think ecologically, and to recognize that the domain in which they may have to intervene as family therapists extends well beyond the boundaries of the family. They will have to learn how to recognize when patterns that create distress in the family involve the social and political contexts that both they and the family share, and they will have to learn new ways of intervening there.

I point out that this can put them in conflict with the mechological society that provides the means of sustenance upon which they depend. They will have to learn how to make such interventions in the social and political surround in ways that will not evoke foreign-body reactions, if they are to avoid being ejected.

I end by telling them that in the next seminar they will be observing a meeting.

FOURTH SEMINAR—HEALTH CARE AND HUMAN SERVICES IN MECHOLOGICAL REALITY

The meeting the students observe is a networking meeting that is structured in a particular way for reasons that will become apparent. I call it a Chairman-of-the-Case Conference. It originated in the following way.

From 1965 to 1970, I designed, developed, and worked in a program that provided health care for impoverished families on the lower east side of New York City. There is a long history of helping agencies in this area, since so many immigrants began their life in the United States there. There were still many helping agencies in operation in 1965. Early in my work there, it became apparent that, with very rare exceptions, each of these various helping programs was operating autonomously, and they were largely disconnected one from another. Under these conditions, they not infrequently worked at cross-purposes.

To cope with this, we designed a meeting in which people or families (extended families when relatives were available) met in one place with representatives of all the helping agencies and, often, informal helpers with whom they had become involved in their immediate community.

We were able to hold these meetings because of funding from the Office of Economic Opportunity, which, during the war on poverty in Lyndon Johnson's "Great Society" program, was awarding grants for health programs for poor people with almost no predetermined program requirements. Our grant had been given with the simple instruction to "do something different which can make health care delivery for poor people more effective."

Before I arrived on the scene, the program had already been designed with a connecting idea in mind—to make families, instead of individuals, the primary unit to which health care would be delivered. This idea was what attracted me to the program in the first place.

I had come to this idea myself as a result of some previous work in which I could see how disconnected health-care practices had become from the total lives of people. I could see that specialized health-care professionals really knew very little about the people in their care. To a very large extend, health-care delivery is controlled by the needs of the health care system itself, and not by the needs of the people it serves. I had come to the conclusion that if this emphasis was ever to be reversed, a new basic definition of human distress was needed. It seemed to me that it would be interesting and useful to design a health-care system that defined all human distress, including that form of distress we call illness, as ecological phenomena. As the most immediate and continuous human ecological system for individuals is the family, the idea of designating the family as the primary target of health care was a step in that direction.

I was first hired as a planning consultant to design a program to respond to "psychosocial" distress. In order to foster connectedness, instead of designing departments of social work, psychology, and psychiatry, I designed what I called an "applied behavioral sciences" program. The idea was that people of these disciplines, public health nurses, and others, such as a group of "indigenous" people trained as "social health technicians," would work together as teams. Such teams would be joined with medical teams. Each combined team would serve one of the five census tracts that together made up the district for which the program was responsible.

I was asked to stay on and develop the program I had designed. As the teams were formed, I built my idea into their training as a guide to their work. I promoted the notion that, since poor people often had many problems other than those usually considered health problems, we might be able to do something different if we thought of human distress, including illness, as an ecological phenomenon. This, I hoped, would make us look at each family in a way that would take into account all of the difficulties with which they were struggling in the physical, biological, psychological, and social realms of their lives.

I then designed the meeting as a means of getting information simultaneously from the entire ecological field. The idea was to convene such a meeting whenever there was even a suspicion that the help provided by simple diagnosis and treatment of illness was inadequate.

We began these meetings by asking each of the helpers to express his or her view of the family's situation and to describe what the helper was trying to do about it. The first few times we did this, we were amazed at what happened. We had already discovered that many of the helpers went to extraordinary lengths to find reasons why they could not attend. When they did attend, we saw that many were reluctant to respond to our request. It turned out that they feared embarrassment. They felt that somehow their efforts with the family were less than successful, and they did not like to expose that. Then we saw that, when they spoke up because we insisted, each helper spoke from the vantage point of her or his agency. Each made the part of the family's problem that his or her agency was designed to address central to the definition of the family's difficulty. As a result, not only did each have a different definition of the problem, but collectively their view of the family was derived from negative problem-based assessments. Positive aspects of the family were seldom mentioned.

As each figuratively pulled out the reality view determined by his or her agency's rule book and the language contained therein, there were differences in the way the workers defined not only the problem they were addressing, but the family itself. Not infrequently, the differences were striking, to the extent that it sometimes was difficult to believe they all were describing the same family. We discovered that whenever we organized one of these meetings about a family involved with a lot of agencies, the same phenomenon occurred. We learned to expect it.

After we had heard from all the helpers, we interviewed the family members to get *their* view of themselves and their "needs." We then discovered that, with rare exceptions, agency representatives had not given much thought to the family as a whole. They almost never talked to all members of the family separately, let alone together. During the family interview, they learned much about the family they had not known before, just as during the first part of the meeting, they learned much about other helping agencies they had not known before.

After we interviewed the family, we enlisted the entire group, including the family, in the construction of a plan of assistance that included all facets of that which was needed to undo the distressful situation. Once the plan was agreed upon, we would determine the tasks that would have to be carried out to accomplish the goals of the plan, and each task would be assigned to a helper from an agency to which that the task was appropriate and which was able to carry it out. Finally, we held a kind of pseudo-election to decide collectively which helper would oversee the plan and ensure that all the tasks were carried out with dispatch. Hence, the title "Chairman-of-the-Case Conference."

Again and again, the same series of observations emerged in these meetings. One was that, despite the presence of representatives from a number of helping agencies, some tasks would arise in the planning phase of the meeting that could not be carried out appropriately by *any* single agency, and that, without the completion of that task, the efforts of at least some of the helpers would be ineffective. The opposite was also true. There was a lot of overlap of task capabilities in the body of agencies in this community. Sometimes two or more agencies carried out the same or similar tasks in different ways, to the confusion of the family. Workers in two or more agencies often worked at cross-purposes with a given family in other ways, as well.

To those families who needed aid from several programs, this fragmented scene very often emitted more than one set of mixed messages. The outcome was that, collectively, the very agencies that were trying to be of help were creating new problems for the families. Collectively, their work was sometimes very helpful, but, much too often, it was iatrogenic (a medical term that denotes a process in which that which is considered treatment creates disease, in this case, dis-ease).

The most astonishing observation was that when one took into account the vantage point helpers occupied and the agency rules they worked within, *all* of the descriptions presented by *all* the helping people, of *all* the families we saw in our Chairman-of-the-Case Conferences were objectively sensible. To those who presented them, and to anyone else who shared the same vantage point and information, they made common sense.

With this observation came the recognition that *everyone* whose thought and actions contributed to the development and maintenance of the structure and operations of the society in which these events occurred made their contribution by "making" common sense. Those who made social policy and those who carried it out "made" common sense. Those who designed and developed the helping agencies within that social policy "made" common sense. Those who administered and maintained them, and carried out their day-to-day operations, playing the various social roles defined therein, "made" common sense.

The outcome of all this common-sense thinking is a system that was (and is) not only totally incapable of responding with full effectiveness to the complex *relational* aspects of the situations encountered in these meetings, but was (and is) also frequently harmful to them. Until we brought all the appropriate elements of that system together in one place and stimulated the emergence of information concerning these relational connections, they were not even seen.

I bring students to meetings of this kind because I want them to observe what I have just described. I want them to recognize that, as family therapists, they must become sensitive to such observations. I also want them to learn a method for doing something about them. Over the course of their continued education/training, whenever I can arrange it, I have them observe such meetings, and we discuss them with the above issues in mind.

FIFTH SEMINAR—SOCIOPOLITICAL EVENTS IN FAMILY STORIES

My students and I spend the entire fifth seminar viewing excerpts of tapes of family therapy sessions that I have selected. I give them the task of spotting statements made by family members that detail events that originate in the social and political surroundings in which these families have resided over remembered generations. We make a list of these statements. Here are a few such statements taken from such a list:

"Well, when my wife's father *came home from the war,* he drank a lot, and when he couldn't reestablish himself at work, he turned into a drunk and treated my mother-in-law badly. I think my wife learned not to trust men."

"My grandfather, who left his family *in Germany because he was the youngest son and could not expect any inheritance,* settled here and built his own farming empire. He made good, and he was very proud of that, so when I said I didn't want to be a farmer, it made him angry. He said I was lacking in family pride."

"My father came *to New York* because *he was very poor and he hoped to find opportunities for a better life here,* but it didn't work out. We are still poor, and we live in the barrio, and he has turned bitter."

"My mother's family *left Russia to escape the pogroms,* so she was very upset when I wanted to marry a shicksa."

"It's very hard for me to like any *White.* After all, *my ancestors were slaves."*

The purpose of this exercise is fourfold. One purpose is to sensitize my students to recognize such statements, which can easily slip by in the welter of conversation with a family, and to give them practice in listening for them.

Another purpose is to demonstrate to them that the patterns of events that create family distress must include events that have occurred outside the boundary of the immediate family.

Another is to demonstrate to them that the events described in such statements continue to affect the lives of the family members they will encounter, regardless of their seemingly remote occurrence in time. In this way, they can learn to include such statements in the eventshapes and family stories I am teaching them to construct. They can practice locating these events in a timespace terrain instead of on a linear time line.

Finally, by keeping them focused on a field larger than the family, I am preparing them for the next seminar in which I will be enlarging the field even more.

SIXTH SEMINAR—APARTHEID IN MECHOLOGICAL REALITY

I begin the next seminar by referring to the family my students watched without sound at the very beginning of their training, reminding them that I had promised to give them the missing ingredient in the story of that family. We redo the family sculpture, and recall the story. Then I show them the segment of the tape that I had previously withheld from them. In this segment, I am working with the family on an issue that demonstrates the effect of mechological thinking on their relational connectedness.

The mother/wife is complaining that the father/husband never responds to her emotional needs, or to those of the children. He sometimes comes home from work late on a day when she has had a lot of silly little problems to cope with. She wants to share them with him, but when she does, he becomes annoyed and gives her a lecture about how to solve those little problems. His lecture makes her feel stupid, and it also makes her angry because she feels he does not really care about her as a person, about the way she feels. It also makes her sad that this happens so often. The children say they feel the same way.

The father, who spends his days as a construction engineer solving "one problem after another," angrily retorts that after a hard day's work solving problems, he does not need to be presented with more problems, especially petty ones. He is only trying to be helpful, and he is angered by their negative response to his effort.

At this point in the session, I step in and tell them that I think that the problem they are discussing arises because father brings his problem-solving way of thinking home with him, understandably, but that the rest of the family is operating in a different domain. They don't really want solutions for the problems they tell him about. They can solve them themselves. What I think they want, I say, is simply recognition that they have had a somewhat difficult day. They want a hug, not a lecture, but he is so caught up in his work logic that he misses that message. This, I suggest, is what creates their difficulty. The mother agrees, so I have them play-act the scene they have described. I have the mother tell the father about the petty little problems that have upset her while he was away, and I instruct the father to say, "That's too bad. I guess you haven't had a very good day," and to give her a hug. I ask the mother if that is what she wants to happen, and she says, "Yes, exactly."

I stop the tape here, and point out to the class that now that they have recognized the impact of mechological thinking on the ecological domain of relationships, they will recognize the distress of this family. The father has been bringing his mechological thinking home. When he uses it indiscriminately there, the outcome is severance of his relational connection with his family. Then I show them another very short segment of tape from a later session in which the mother and the oldest son say that the father has stopped lecturing and is now giving them lots of hugs, and they are getting along much better.

I use the rest of the seminar to deliver another, rather heavy, lecture. I begin by introducing and redifining the word "apartheid." This word usually refers to the separation of the races in South Africa according to government policy. In previous seminars, we have been confronting how mechological thinking creates apartness in the relational domain, and we need a shorthand word to denote that phenomenon. I think that apartheid in South Africa has the same epistemological roots as apartness everywhere, and so the word seems appropriate for this purpose. By making a distinction between explicit and de facto apartheid, I can tie together the widespread occurrence of the phenomenon throughout the mechologically defined world. I redefine the word to denote states of apartness in the relational domain of human life.

I also make another distinction, which I believe to be very important. I define two kinds of hunger. One kind of hunger could be called *somatic* hunger, the hunger we humans experience when we are deprived of adequate nourishing food. Social beings that we are, I think there is another kind of hunger that we also experience—*relational* hunger, the hunger for connectedness we experience as essential loneliness. I also think there is a distinction to be made between somatic and relational malnutrition, and between somatic and relational starvation.

It is known that among the symptoms of somatic starvation are intellectual constriction, emotional dulling, and dereistic thinking (private unshared thinking that is not subjected to consensual validation; in mechological psychiatry, usually associated with psychosis). I believe these same symptoms result from severe relational starvation.

Having introduced these notions, I move on by telling the following story.

I visited South Africa in 1984 to present at a conference on family therapy. While there, I visited Johannesburg, Pretoria, Durban, and Cape Town, and spent some time in rural areas talking to both "Blacks" and "Whites." (I also talked to "Colored," but, although this group is an important element in the South African story, I don't need to report these conversations to make the points I want to make.) I cannot claim much experience, but what I will say is not entirely lacking in first-hand observation.

South Africa is dominated by a numerical minority of Whites whose social organization has roots in Europe, and it is an industrialized country. The thought/reality system of this group is based on Western mechological "common sense." The Black majority is made up of people who edit reality animistically. (The animistic edition of reality assumes that "all that is" is endowed with universal and locally differentiated living spirit.) There is also language separation. Mechological thinking is embedded in the languages of Whites, and animistic thinking is embedded in the languages of Blacks.

Many of the Blacks I talked to seemed to understand the reality system of the White minority. Those who understood it were those who had learned the system by attending schools set up for them by the White minority. Some Whites also had a grasp of the predominant reality system of the Blacks, but their understanding seemed superficial. There is an underground system of illegal Black schools, but Whites do not attend them.

The Blacks, whose reality edit defines truth as relative, do not see the Whites' system as irrational and untrue. However, they resent the efforts of the Whites to force them to accept it and to live their lives within it. The Whites are mechological thinkers who think there is only one real reality, so they think the Blacks' system simply is wrong. Except for the family therapists I met, most of the Whites I talked to see Blacks, in general, as primitive irrational thinkers, although they recognize exceptions.

Social policies, including apartheid and all other policies that flow from it, are made, implemented, and enforced by the White government in power, based on their mechological system of thought.

In the context of that social policy, the White minority government has loudly proclaimed the intention to move the Black population to "homelands" where they can create their own governments and become enfranchised, leaving the Whites to pursue their own interests. Many Blacks *have* been moved to homelands, where most of them live in abject poverty. The duplicity in this proclamation is painfully obvious. First of all, there is no "homeland" for Blacks. What are called "homelands" are a number of separated areas consisting of the least fertile and least developed land in the region. Second, even if the homelands were consolidated and could support nationhood, the immense tasks of setting up an economy for a Black nation is far beyond the economic capacity of those who live there, and even of the South African government, so Blacks are simply dumped there with very little means of sustenance. Third, the economy of South Africa cannot be sustained without the exploitative use of cheap Black labor, so there is a another line of separation. Blacks are segregated into Black townships (unless, of course, such townships are too distant from their place of work when they are allowed to live outside the township).

The Blacks I talked to were outraged by four sets of conditions.

First was the widespread poverty, especially the lack of adequate housing and schools, and the lurking fear, if not the actuality, of somatic food starvation.

Second in order of ascending importance was the humiliation of their powerlessness in the arenas in which social policy is made, their position of nonenfranchisement, and the humiliation of the pass system (since abandoned), which gave the government total control of their movement.

The third was the degree to which the government's actions sytematically disconected the members of existing Black communities and cultures, and controlled what went on in the artificially created segregated communities they formed.

The fourth, which angered them the most, was that government policies systematically disconnect families by inventing pretexts to move people around, by recruiting men for work far away from their families under conditions they could not refuse, and by breaking up viable existing Black communities.

I came away from these contacts with the impression that the unmistakable primary concern of South African Blacks was the destructive havoc that governmental policies and activities were creating in the relational domain of their families and communities, and that the Blacks would not long allow that to continue. They were concerned about food starvation, but they were even more concerned about relational starvation.

The Whites to whom I talked, with the exception of most family therapists and of others who were against apartheid (a fairly large minority, I think), had a very different set of priorities when they talked about the problems of Blacks. Even those who clearly believed in the policy of apartheid admitted that the Blacks had a tough time, but the remedy, they maintained, is economic. Some way must be found, they said, to alleviate widespread Black poverty.

However, the pro-apartheid people I talked to never spontaneously brought up the issue most emphasized by Blacks—the breakup of families and communities. What happened when I mentioned these issues was frightening. They did not want to talk about them. I had to urge them to do so. I would describe what I was hearing from Blacks, and ask them, as diplomatically as I could, if they would not have similar concerns if they were in the Blacks' position. They would usually sigh or look angry, and it became clear that I had tapped an issue they would rather not think about. Although they said it in a variety of ways, their response boiled down to: "Well, the way things are, it's my family or theirs, and it's not going to be mine."

Like the Blacks, these people were primarily concerned with maintaining their relational family connections, but they saw the problem in mechological either/or terms. "It's them or us." Until I confronted them with that issue, they had kept it hidden. I am sure they considered me rude for even bringing it up. When I did, their friendliness often disappeared.

This experience taught me that Whites who espouse apartheid fear that dominance of a "Black consciousness," a nonmechological reality, will create relational disconnection for Whites. To prevent this, they construct and adopt policies and actions that create relational disconnection for Blacks, and, in this way, disempower them. Then they rationalize their thoughts and actions in standard mechological fashion.

My question challenged their rationalization. It created a paradox for them. And they did not like it. From a position of friendliness, they moved to one of polite animosity. They solved the paradox in the standard mechological way. They split it. "It's either them or us."

Tragically, what South African Whites who favor apartheid fail to understand is that relational connections exist in nonmechological realities, and that it is their own mechological system of thought that creates apartness and sustains it. They are trying to solve their dilemma with the very thought system that creates it.

Once the existence and intensity of *mutual* concern for maintenance of implicate connections are grasped, several phenomena now taking place in South Africa become understandable. The willingness of Blacks, as expressed by their leaders, to tolerate the economic famine that probably will accompany economic sanctions imposed on South Africa by other nations, such as divestment, becomes clear. Collectively, South African Blacks are willing to face somatic starvation in the service of forcing the changes that can alleviate and prevent relational starvation. Those who oppose such sanctions seem unaware of the power of the need for maintenance of relational connections. The relational famine created by attenuation or severance of those connections is more onerous than a famine of food and other material supplies. Also, the vicious behavior of some South African Blacks toward other Blacks who are perceived as pawns of the government can be seen as an extreme fueled by the specter of relational famine.

Before we leave South Africa, I must say that I did find Whites in South Africa, some of them Afrikaners, who understood the relational family and community issues. Most of them were among the group of family therapists I encountered who are in an unbelievably difficult position. In their work with families, they have opened a window through which they can see the importance of relational connections. This view separates them from the predominant view in their White society. Not only do they risk misinterpretation of their actions when they seek to establish and maintain a dialogue with Blacks, but they cannot communicate these issues to many in their own social and professional communities. When they do, the question I raised explicitly is implicit in their communication, and engenders an antagonistic response. Thus, when they raise these issues, they risk attenuation and severance of some of their own relational connections. When such attenuation and disconnections occur in their professional arena, they can lose the basis for their economic sustenance. They could join the Black poor, but in current conditions, they are fish out of water there, too. They are trapped in a kind of no-man's-land, and they may be among the most isolated victims of apartheid.

South Africa is hardly the only place where apartheid exists. De facto apartheid is a factor in most countries. It can be found wherever there are mechological thinkers in positions of power, and in the guise of development of so-called undeveloped nations, the mechological edit of reality seems to be gradually replacing all others.

Nonmechological peoples have a difficult time standing up to such an invasion. The technological capacity of mechologic to develop powerful machines, some in the form of sophisticated weapons, is too great. If nonmechological societies want actively to oppose such invasion, they are faced with an infuriating irony. They must learn to think mechologically, acquire or manufacture weapons themselves, and fight the mechological invaders on their reality terrain. When they do so, the outcome is war. Beginning as they do with a marked disadvantage, they are likely to lose such war. After many such losses, they have now, to a large extent, stopped trying.

They have discovered, however, that the certainties of mechological thinkers have certain vulnerabilities, and they are learning to exploit them. The methods they have learned we call guerilla warfare and terrorism.

Let us move our focus away from South Africa to the area of the world where mechologic originated. The cradle of mechological thought and reality, of course, was Europe, but as we live in the United States, I will, for the most part, be describing what I see here. Once the settlers from Europe moved to this continent and eliminated the animistic reality of the North American aborigines by nearly eliminating them, our national society was, by it very newness, free to develop its mechological reality without historical constraints. (Currently, we are seeing a similar situation in Japan, where mechological development has evolved without historical constraints.) The United States became the most powerful industrialized (developed) country in the world. Here, we can see the outcomes of mechological thinking all around us in the form of trends.

We have already contemplated the social fragmentation that has evolved in health and human services. In addition, de facto apartheid is to be seen everywhere—we have only to look at urban ghettos adjacent to affluent areas, at suburban enclaves protected by zoning laws, and at public housing for poor people who are required to stay poor to live there. Racial apartheid, despite efforts to erase it, is coupled with economic apartheid, and it persists. A bare majority of our lawmakers are willing to support busing of children in an effort to combat racial apartheid, but it is a fragmented effort. Few lawmakers are willing to support an attack on economic apartheid.

In urban centers, community connectedness in the relational domain has been largely destroyed, and in less populated areas, as these areas are developed, the same destruction of community is taking place. Shopping centers have replaced community connectedness, and in a state of relational malnutrition, citizens collect there to engage in a ritual frenzy of acquisition. Substitute connections are being made to pseudopeople who are images on television or in films. As a result of loss of connectedness, ethnic groups are also indulging in a kind of ethnic chauvinism, protecting their boundaries with prejudice. Families, deprived of community and, increasingly, cultural connections, have become vulnerable, and are disconnecting at an alarming rate. Fathers are becoming afraid to hug their daughters lest they be accused of sexual abuse.

Women are forced to fight for equality of rights in the competitive ladder climb. The numbers of homeless people and families without shelter are increasing. Both parents in many families spend long hours in the workplace in order to pay the mortgage and support their acquisitional frenzy, leaving a growing corps of latchkey children.

Aristotle defined politics as the art of community building. He would, I suspect, be dismayed by the mechological focus of many of today's politicians, who seem to define community operationally as turf, and community development as the development of turf. Many seem to spend most of their time acquiring, protecting, and developing various kind of turf. They focus on concrete physical development by seeking money for their districts (and, unfortunately, sometimes themselves), for development projects that will bring "in" money, jobs, and material comforts that will "upgrade" the standard of living of their constituents in material ways.

Many seek to develop and promote the abstract turf of political party, ideology, and so on. Their concerns and their actions seem entirely focused on the explicate. I no longer wonder where juvenile gangs got the idea of staking out turf and defending it. They have simply caught on to the game. People who work in government bureaucracies or corporate hierarchies or large educational institutions will recognize that the same political game goes on there, too.

There is even more evidence that what we are seeing in nations that espouse mechological reality is an insidious evolution toward more and more refined forms of de facto apartheid. Modern mechological societies are spitting out more and more disconnected people. The behavior of disconnected people is well known to clinicians.

In a person for whom disconnection and the onset of relational starvation begins very early in formative years, relational skills may not develop. Such a person cannot call on relational support in stressful situations, and so is likely to withdraw and resort to dereistic thinking and reification of an internal dialogue. Others, old enough to have developed relational skills but not old enough to have automatized them, will resort to the same form of withdrawal if subjected to sudden and intense relational starvation. When such people come into formal contact with mental health professionals, they often acquire diagnoses of "psychosis."

Some people who grow up in an atmosphere of attenuated implicate family relationality, and in sites lacking in implicate culture or community, do not develop a sense of ethical concern for the rights and integrity of others. As a result, they are likely to engage in behavior that is damaging to others in a variety of ways. These people, living in a society that bombards them with invitations to acquire consumer goods, will acquire such goods in ways that may violate the law. If they are affluent and educated, they may engage in so-called white-collar crime. If they begin in poverty, they may engage in street crime. They may sometimes engage in violence without much remorse. Some gravitate to criminal cultures and wind up satisfying some of their relational needs there. Regardless of other dangers, for some it is more relationally satisfying to be in prison than it is to be alone on the streets.

The use of "feel-good" or anesthetizing drugs is another way to escape temporarily from the distress of relational disconnection, used both by those who are trapped in the fast lane of acquisitional frenzy and by those who cannot escape the combination of material and relational starvation.

These people as groups are cemented into place in mechologically conceived social reality. They are reduced to "thingness" by the use of labels, both formal and informal. They are labeled psychotics or crazies, criminals or crooks, addicts or druggies. If we add "lazy" to this list, an epithet used by some of the economically secure to describe the poor, we can round out the list. The hierarchical social structure of mechological society is supported by these groups. If crazies, criminals, or druggies are also poor lazies, they represent the bottom rungs on the socioeconomic ladder. And without bottom rungs, there can be no ladder.

With regard to these groups, the policy of apartheid is more than de facto. The "common-sense" response to their disruptive impact on mechological society is to segregate them. When labeled and declared dangerous, they are relegated by law to mental hospitals and prisons. When the numbers incarcerated make the expense of maintaining these temporary "homelands" too great, they are allowed to inhabit "townships," or inner-city ghettos. In typical mechological fashion, we attribute the state of these people to things that exist inside their skins, to disease entities variously labeled.

When, trapped as they are, the behavior of these groupings of people persists over an extended period of time, we call them "chronically" ill. In a sense, we blame them, which is like blaming the messenger. Except for those with demonstrable anatomical damage or physiological deficit, I say that chronicity is not located inside people's skins. It is located in their social and political surroundings.

Such groups also support political activity. Political careers are made by decrying the plight of these bottom-rung dwellers, as well as by condemning them.

At the same time, many are probably aware of the total inadequacy of moral and monetary support for efforts to extricate members of these groups from their plight in the face of overkill support (beginning in 1987, more than a trillion dollars in three years) for the military. Equally telling is the observation that very little of the totally inadequate support that does exist is allocated to programs consciously intended to develop or support the implicate community or family, despite clear evidence that such programs are effective.

It is not that politicians who allocate resources this way are not concerned with the loving, cooperative, mutually supporting, emotionally connecting aspects of the implicate domain of our society. They support parks and community centers and libraries and art centers and multiracial and multicultural schools and other places where relational connections can be made and nourished. Most, however, simply do not see intense attention to these aspects of life as a feasible part of their jobs, as, to a large extent, it has been mechologically defined out of their jobs. They go home at night, often too late to be with their own kids, and it is often all they can do to keep their own implicate family intact. Sometimes they cannot even do that. Even if they did see the people-connecting aspects of community building as the focus of their job, they would have no time to attend to it. A few do make some attempt, but such efforts usually fizzle out rapidly for lack of public support. We cannot blame our politicians. They are, after all, us.

There is more, of course. There is the clearly known evidence that another outcome of mechological thinking/reality is the introduction of poisons into the environment that damage that which lives, including ourselves. We do not know the outcome of what has already happened, yet the polluting goes on. As far back as 1969, U Thant, who, as Secretary General of the United Nations, was in a particularly good vantage point from which to view this phenomenon, said that our species had ten years to reverse this trend, after which the trend would become irreversible. We do not know if he was right, but the ten years were up in 1979.

The most devastating poison of all is radiation, which, if enough is released, can spread across our planet in a matter of days. The northern hemisphere is currently encased in an envelope of nuclear weapons ready for activation. They are in submarines beneath the sea, in airplanes above us, and in silos and other sites on land. The two greatest nuclear powers, the United States and the Soviet Union, both have policies that, though euphemistically called policies of deterrence, contain a paradox that is easily exposed. The policy has been that in order to stop building nuclear weapons, we must build more. In the United States alone, five nuclear bombs come off the assembly line each and every day of the week (Cochran, 1987), and roughly 30,000 such bombs have been manufactured since the first one, enough to blow up our planet four times.

I have presented a veritable litany of evidence that the mechological thought/reality system we call common sense is bankrupt as a system for the creation of a viable and life-supporting planet. In the face of all this apartness, one question stands out: "What is holding our mechological societies together?"

Is it systems of morality, religious or secular? Only slightly. There is a plethora of value systems in mechological society, each of which its proponents rationalize to be right one. The rules of mechological thought are such that the system can rationalize *any* value system, even one that builds Auschwitz.

Is it patriotism? Some, within each nation. But nationalistic chauvinism also separates nations. On the international scene, it contributes to wars.

I think the most potent glue in explicate mechological society is provided by blame systems. Blame systems allow us to rationalize our anger at the above conditions and to live with them. If you look around, you will see that nearly everyone in mechological reality harbors pet blame systems. We use them to "make" sense out of what is happening.

Relational connections in the ecological domain? Yes! Like the Blacks, and, in their miscontextualized way, the Whites, in South Africa, we all fight to maintain those connections. It appears, as most people are willing to die for their loved ones, that the human response to the experience of relational starvation is even more powerful than the built-in biological response to that which threatens individual survival.

For this reason, even though linear projections made from the litany above would suggest that our species is doomed, I think we can be very optimistic. The universe does not work by linear projection, and the power of the implicate creative relational world society may yet prevail. The outlines of this evolutionary movement to reverse these trends can already be seen, I think. Participation in mechological reality has largely lost its potential for joy, and it is beginning to look like a caricature to an increasing number of human beings. A transformation, I believe, is under way.

On the other hand, we cannot be complacent about our evolutionary fate. The envelope of bombs still surrounds us. We continue to pollute our earth, and all of the above social and political conditions continue to multiply. Yet, we can observe that the majority of efforts to do something about these conditions, even those of disarmament negotiators, continue to be conceived in mechological terms. The very thought system that produced mechological reality is being used to solve the problems contained therein. Such efforts cannot work. In this regard, South Africa is not unique. Most of the world is trapped in the same dilemma. We remain an endangered species. We cannot sit around and wait for the needed transformation to happen. Our timing may be off. We may blow ourselves up before we make it happen.

I find it exciting that the solution to this dilemma has already surfaced—in what I have called the new science/ecological thought/reality system, which has been emerging in this century. In what happened in physics, we even have a model for the needed transformation.

Newtonian physics, which contributed heavily to the evolution of the mechological thought/reality system while developing within it, created a model of the universe that seemed, at the turn of the century, to be nearly complete. It was, however, never completed. It contained a couple of cracks, and Max Planck and Albert Einstein stepped through those cracks, laying the groundwork for quantum and relativity physics. As these domains evolved, a whole new thought/reality system emerged, and with it a whole new model of the universe.

The rules governing thought in this new edition of reality do not include either/or dualisms and the confrontations and paradoxes they create, nor do they require reductionistic fragmentation as a basis for understanding or the conversion of event shapes to objective things. They do not require hierarchical organization or adherence to linear time and causality.

Instead, they require that attention be paid to patterned shapes of events and how they are connected, and to the phenomenon of creative synthesis and synergy. These rules are ready-made for the task that faces us, which is the recreation and vitalization of the implicate domain of human existence, the domain of relational connectedness. Their use in planning for reorientation and reorganization of the planet can reverse the trends that are separating us, the trends that threaten relational starvation, conflict, war, and possible extinction.

It is important to note that the physicists did not throw out Newtonian physics. They simply stripped it of one of its assumptions, one of its rules. They threw out the rule that there could be only one reality that contained absolute truth. The concepts of Newtonian physics have continued to be highly useful. They are used, however, in the context of the new physics.

We must, I believe, follow their lead in this regard. We must not throw out mechological thought—to do so would create disaster. Mechological thinking is wonderful for the building of machines and as a system for planning sequences of action to get tasks done. Ecological thought is relatively ineffectual in this regard, though without its creativity, mechologic can take us nowhere. It is, I believe, necessary for us to continue to develop our technology and build our machines. There are now too many of us on the planet to thrive without them. It is possible to imagine the development of robotic technologies that could provide us time to attend to the relational and creative aspects of our lives.

However, we must follow the lead of the physicists, and use mechological thought in the controlling context of ecological thought.

That the transformation this represents is already in process is apparent. Philosophers, especially those who have been aligning themselves with and contributing to philosophical ideas of deconstructionism, constructionism, phenomenology, and hermeneutics, have been contributing much to the new thought/reality system.[1] Biologists have split into camps, one of which is producing research and ideas rooted in the ecological domain. Artists are registering protest against the apartheid that relegates their creations to museums, and to theaters entered only by an elite who can afford inflated admission fees. Many bring the art to the streets. In performance art and in community coalitions, artists have been attempting to integrate creative art into the fabric of our everyday lives.

For those who want to participate in this needed transformation, there is a movement to be organized, and some immediate tasks. We must apply ourselves, each of us, to the task of learning to think in two ways, in two reality systems. We are well trained to think in mechologic, but not enough of us have learned to think in ecologic in an organized way, and to distinguish one thought/reality system clearly from the other. (It is likely that ecologic will be drawing ideas from and merging congruent patterns of thought with transcendental and animistic thought systems.) Then we must teach others to do this, especially our children. Too, we will have to develop ways of thinking thus together. We might be able to develop a corps of transformational warriors, dedicated to forging the evolutionary transformation, to moving our species to a mode of existence beyond apartheid, and beyond the dualistic cycle of peace and war.

I have taken you far outside the primary focus for which we are gathered in this room, which is to give you the skills to be family therapists. I have taken you all the way to the physicist's view of the cosmos. Let us start coming back, so that we can get on with our primary task. To do so, let me talk in very general terms of how family therapy got started.

It began as a movement, founded by professionals in the behavioral sciences who wanted to open a window for the world on the implicate family and its

[1] The nature of philosophical discourse is such as to make facile reference to writings illustrating these trends without elaboration inappropriate. The following books are suggested as way of entering into the writings that make up the discourse. There are many additional books that could provide entry, and I have selected these largely because I have used them in this way, and not because they are necessarily better than others.

Howard, R. (1982). *Three faces of hermeneutics.* Berkeley and Los Angeles: University of California Press.

Krell, D. (Ed.) (1977). *Martin Heidegger—Basic writings.* New York: Harper & Row.

Skinner, G. (1985). *The return of grand theory in the human sciences.* Cambridge, New York, Melbourne: Cambridge University Press.

Watzlawick, P. (Ed.) (1984). *The invented reality.* New York: W. W. Norton.

Whitehead, A. N. (1925). *Science and the modern world.* Toronto: Collier-Macmillan Canada, Ltd.

importance in the genesis of various forms of human distress.[2] In order to do this, they broke the rules of mechological thinking. Many of them had become tired of having to think about psychopathological states, especially schizophrenia, as "things" that reside "inside" people and disrupt their adaptive machinery. They projected another reality, one in which symptoms and behaviors emerged from the distortions in and attrition of relational connections in families. Early in the game, they learned to induct families into their new reality using techniques of reframing, which, in turn, allowed families to redefine their reality, thus inducing behavior change and making symptoms irrelevant.

The epistemological shift immanent in this work was, in my view, the expression in the behavioral sciences of the transformation of thought/reality that has been taking place in this century. Hence, there was the quality of a movement.

The field of knowledge and practice of family therapy has grown rapidly since those early days, and the epistemological issues immanent in the early work have become explicit. They have stimulated a body of thought and literature, and the field has continued to grow at the forefront of epistemological, and, more recently, ontological exploration in the behavioral sciences. In these first seminars, I have tried to provide for you both experience and information that I hope will allow you to put this movement in the context of these epistemological developments, and to recognize their significance.

As in every transformative movement, those who are embedded in institutionalized orthodoxies will attempt to fit the information generated into their preexisting scheme of things. This happened in physics, and it is happening in the behavioral sciences and in the domain of family therapy. Currently, the field is split between those who would continue the epistemological explorations and transformation and those who would integrate the information generated in the field into their preexisting thought/reality structures. I don't have to elaborate on this statement. You will know now what I mean when I say that there is a mechological grouping in the family therapy field and also an ecological grouping.

What I want you to get is that now, as you begin your journey in this field, there is a fork in the road ahead. You have a choice. You can join the mechological grouping which considers family therapy to be simply a new modality of treatment to add to the many, perhaps replacing some. Or you can join the ecological grouping, which considers family therapy to be a way of thinking, indeed, a participant in a movement designed to ensure, reinforce, and hasten the evolutionary emergence of a new and generally accepted human view of reality—one that connects, not disconnects.

We will now move on to our exploration of the family therapy literature. Each of you will be sculpting your own family of origin in future seminars, and

---

[2] This body of work emerged in the 1950s and 1960s in several places in which ideas were expressed by a number of people in different ways using different languages in a manner that makes specific referencing difficult. It includes the work of such people as William Middlefort in Wisconsin; Nathan Ackerman, first, and then Sal Minuchin, Charles King, and myself in New York; the Mental Research Institute group in Palo Alto, Calif., which included Don Jackson, Gregory Bateson, Paul Watzlawick, John Weakland, Jay Haley, Virginia Satir, and others; Lyman Wynne, Margaret Singer, Murray Bowen, and Warren Brodey in Washington, D.C.; Theodore Lidz and Stephen Fleck in New Haven, Conn.; Carl Whittaker in Atlanta, Ga.; and Frederick Duhl in Boston, Ma. There were others.

we will all work with you to construct the story of your family most relevant to you as one family member. You will also begin to work with families, with our faculty, with one another, and by yourself. We will be watching you work and learn, and assisting you to develop your skills in this experience. Enough for today.

CONCLUSION

This the end of the first six seminars. I must here make a confession. Although I have carried out all of the exercises and given all the lectures contained in the education/training sequence, I have never done them in the order presented. This sequence is really my fantasy of how I think family therapy training *should* begin.[3] As the sequence is designed to provide context for the work the trainees have chosen to pursue, it contains discussion of the social and political contexts of family therapy. For this reason, I thought it appropriate for presentation here.

There is a big gap in this presentation. I have not presented the specific thought rules of mechologic and ecologic that govern the two thought/reality systems I have discussed. There is not room.

However, I would like you, the reader, to do a simple exercise as you exit from this chapter. I would like you to put on a watch with a second hand. Then, with your other hand, locate your pulse on the wrist with the watch and follow its beat.

Your watch, of course, is a product of the mechological domain, and it is the regulated passage of seconds, minutes, hours, weeks, and years of clock time that record the activities of the mechological world. Our pulses, on the other hand, beat out our lives, and the knowledge that they will eventually cease reminds us of our mortality. The pulse beats in the implicate ecological domain.

Are you in touch with both beats? Now I would like to ask you another question.

Which beat regulates your life, the tick of your watch or the beat of your pulse? Chances are it is the tick of your watch. That's the reality of modern life. Common sense tells us that. It makes sense to adapt to that reality.

Doesn't it?

---

[3] The work underlying the ideas in this chapter is presented in more detail in the following articles:
Auerswald, E. (1968). "Interdisciplinary" vs. "ecological" approach. *Family Process*, Z(2), 202–215.
Auerswald, E. (1972). Families, change, and the ecological perspective. *Family Process*, 10(3), 263–280.
Auerswald, E. (1974). Thinking about thinking in health and mental health. *American Journal of Psychiatry*, Vol. 2, Sylvano Arieti, Gen. Ed., Gerald Caplan, Vol. Ed. New York: Basic Books.
Auerswald, E. (1982). The Gouverneur Health Services Program: An experiment in ecosystemic community health care delivery. *Family Systems Medicine*, 1(3), 5–24.
Auerswald, E. (1985). Thinking about thinking in family therapy. *Family Process*, 24, 1–12.

REFERENCES

Bateson, G. (1972). *Steps to an ecology of mind*. New York: Ballantine Books.

Bateson, G. (1979). *Mind and nature—A necessary unity*. New York: E. P. Dutton.

Bateson, G., & Bateson, M. C. (1987). *Angels fear*. New York+ Macmillan.

Bohm, D. (1980). *Wholeness and the Implicate Order*. London: Routledge & Kegan Paul.

Cochran, T. (1987). *U.S. nuclear warhead production*. New York: Natural Resources Defense Council.

Einstein, A. (1905). On the electrodynamics of moving bodies. *Annalen Der Physik, 17*(b), 891.

Einstien, A., & Infeld, L. (1938). *The evolution of physics*. New York: Simon & Schuster.

Maturana, H., & Varela, F. (1972). *Autopoiesis and cognition*. Dordrecht, Holland—D. Reidel.

Maturana, H., & Varela, F. (1987). *The tree of knowledge*. Boston: Shambhala Publication.

Planck, M. (1900). Distribution of energy in the normal spectrum. *Deutschen Physiologischen Gesellschaft, Verlang Lungen, 2*(17), 245–257.

Planck, M. (1936). *The philosophy of physics* (W. H. Johnston, Trans.). New York: W. W. Norton.

Scheflen, A. (1968). Personal communication.

Varela, F. (1979). *Principles of biological autonomy*. New York: Elsevier North Holland.

Part II

Women and Family Therapy

3

A FEMINIST PERSPECTIVE IN FAMILY THERAPY

Marianne Walters, M.S.W.

There is no therapy, including family therapy, that can adequately reflect the range of human experience and conditions without including a feminist perspective. Yet a feminist perspective can never be monolithic or homogeneous as it will reflect the diversity of the complex social relations it addresses. A feminist perspective in family therapy is not limited to any particular methodology or technique, but rather is committed to exploring and elaborating the *context* and the *process* in the formation and transformation of any human experience.

Any feminist perspective in therapy has, I believe, four major components, each of which will be elaborated within a variety of theoretical and methodological frameworks. These components are (1) the conscious inclusion, in both theory and practice, of the experience of women growing up; developing; relating to each other, to men, and to social institutions; raising families; working; and growing old in a culture largely shaped and defined by male experience; (2) a critique of therapy practices, and the theoretical constructs on which they are based, that lend themselves to a devaluing of women, and of the particular social and familial roles of women—in other words, a critique of those practices and ideas commonly identified as sexist; (3) the integration of feminist theory, and the information derived from women's studies, into the knowledge base of psychological theory, as well as of methodological—and even pedagogical—frameworks; and (4) the use of female modes and models in the continuing expansion and development of theory and practice in the field.

WHAT *DO* WOMEN WANT?

This plaintive question has haunted such profound thinkers as Freud, to such mundane pundits as David Stockman. I would imagine Socrates himself pondering this dilemma as he framed yet another deductive question; or Nero dreaming of some answer to be found in the flickering flames of a burning Rome. Yet despite the best efforts of men to answer this question, it has remained largely a source of confusion, and perhaps concern, but certainly not resolution—partly, of course, because different women want different things, much as men do. But the answer is ultimately to be found in the construction of a society that equally represents the interests and aspirations and values of both sexes. To accomplish this task would mean rearranging power and privilege in our society—a difficult, if not for many, an unwelcome task. Yet, as a relatively enlightened microcosm of our society, it would seem that attempts at some rearrangement of that tiny piece of turf on which we therapists cavort would be welcome. Or so I thought when I first become interested in exploring with my family therapy colleagues the relevance of feminism to family therapy, and my own experiences as a woman therapist. What I learned (or perhaps already knew but chose to deny in order to get up the nerve to forge ahead) was that even in a field committed to change, and to representing the interest of the family and its members—both female and male—the subordination and devaluing of women were so strongly ingrained that even the wisest in the field had trouble broadening their vision.

Family therapists who have pioneered a feminist critique of the field have encountered all of the usual responses, everything from "We're all human, aren't we?" to "I've always loved women," to "But, I've always thought women were better than men!" Some therapists thought feminist family therapists should not be allowed to do family therapy because they would lecture and harangue their clients; others argued that a feminist theory was the antithesis of the "neutrality" and "objectivity" of systems theory. And there were those whose understanding of the issues could encompass nothing deeper than the tired notion of the "battle between the sexes." Some of our movers and shakers embraced the new ideas with benign neglect; others trivialized it by exploring the "complementary" plight of men. But perhaps more disappointing than the querulousness, or the opposition, was the tendency of the field to engage with the new ideas that feminist thinkers espoused, and then quickly assign them the significance of one, among many, issues in the field—which is exactly the problem. Although feminism raises issues for and about women, such as equal pay, child care, and maternity leave, its significance rests on its conceptual departure from a traditional, male-dominated perspective. Feminism, particularly in the field of family systems and family relations, suggests a fundamental rethinking of beliefs, principles, and practices. It suggests a search for new information, a conceptual dialogue, self-criticism. It is not about an issue, a symptom, or a segment of our society; it is about that society and the relationship of the two genders that compose it. As such, the feminist perspective challenges the field to restructure some of its practice and reconsider some of its assumptions. Such change is no easier for us than it is for our clients.

*   *   *

As a social worker, I learned a lot about human growth and development, about social systems and conditions, and some about the helping process. As my profession was mostly peopled by women (and never showed a profit), it was not highly valued by our society and was low in the hierarchical pecking order of the service delivery systems within which we worked, particularly those dominated by the medical profession, such as mental health. In this context, I often felt helpless and unclear about how to create change most effectively. And as the profession was often derivative—that is, flowing from and defined by professions higher in the hierarchy and with more power—social work did not evolve a distinct methodology of its own, separate from the roles and functions assigned by the prevailing power structures. Even within our profession, we tended to devalue much of what we knew and many of our tenets of practice—such as the ways in which process is used to inform and to convey a message; or that behavior is contextual and interactional; or that much of one's emotional development occurs within the family. Being devalued, lacking power, and thus devaluing ourselves, we internalized the negative social and professional attitudes that surrounded our work lives. We did not lay claim to a distinct methodology, and we shied away from explicit and direct techniques of intervention. Like many social workers, when I encountered family therapy, I embraced it eagerly and lovingly—and pretty uncritically. Here were methods, explicit and direct techniques for change, ways to work, ways to think. It had a conceptual framework—systems theory—a structure from which to view behavior and to tackle symptoms. And it did not take forever to see change occur. For the first time I felt truly instrumental in my professional functioning. Now I was not "merely" a social worker—I was a family therapist. It had a more authoritative ring to it.

When one feels instrumental and powerful, it is difficult to question some of the assumptions on which that instrumentality is based, or to understand that my own process of professional evolution mirrors the experience of women at every level in society and, of course, within families. Being in a woman's profession that was devalued and derivative, I was defined by others and began to devalue my own expertise. My roles and functions were prescribed within a male hierarchy. Unsureness, fed by a lack of power, undermined my effectiveness and self-esteem. Given the opportunity for instrumental functioning, I embraced that end without questioning the means by which it was achieved. I had forgotten that the ends seldom justify the means, that change without "due process" can indeed diminish the human endeavor.

What *do* women want? Perhaps the question can best be addressed through the process of asking them and listening to their answers.

WOMEN'S EXPERIENCE

At this stage in the development of the women's movement and of feminist consciousness, and considering the changes that have already improved the status of women, it seems almost redundant to discuss the continuing need to include the experience of women in our understanding of family dynamics and in the practices of family therapy. Yet perhaps in our field, more than many other of the social sciences and helping professions, it is necessary to emphasize this point. Systems theory and systemic modalities unfortunately have functioned to discount gender socialization and to blur gender differences. Systemic equations treat the *parts* as interchangeable, depending only on their configuration within the system for definition and explanation of their motivation and behavior. The fact that such configurations must have origins in larger contexts is acknowledged but goes largely unattended and unexplored. Systemic equations and formulations conjure up the illusion of an objectivity that obscures the value-laden reality that they are meant to represent. It goes without saying that representations of reality will reflect the prevailing order of things, the accepted hierarchy, the socially approved values—unless these are challenged and uncovered to reveal the subtext. And so our systemic formulations and interventions will represent—indeed will reproduce—patriarchal social, relational, and attitudinal structures unless the different, and often hidden, experience and reality of women in society, and in our families, are entered into the equation.

What is this experience? It is the everyday fallout—subliminal, explicit, and covert; direct and indirect; conscious and unconscious; accidental and purposeful; humorous and serious—of life for women in a male-dominated culture.

> She attends a wedding and hears jokes about entrapment and how *now* he will have to get rid of his sexy secretary. She leaves the wedding and goes to a bar where one of the drinks offered, along with the Singapore Sling and White Russian, is "the dreaded mother-in-law." She returns home and opens a magazine and learns that the best gift a woman can receive is a new Electrolux vacuum that will allow her to reach into the corners of the house she will clean. She reads an advertisement that tells her how easily she can be deceived if she gets something she wants in the end: "Promise her anything, but give her Arpege." She watches television and discovers that the only way a woman can get on the crew of a "love boat" is as cruise director, attending to the pleasures of the "family" of passengers—or failing that, as the daughter of the captain. She reads a popular novel and learns that success in the world of business is achieved by women who are bitchy. She turns to a history book where humans are referred to as mankind, work is described in terms of manpower, and the products of labor as man-made. Leaders are called chairmen and a skilled craftsman is called master (even when said expert is a woman). She calls a friend who describes a "cat fight" in the office, evoking images of people clawing at each other rather than landing a direct punch.
>
> She goes to a synagogue and sees that the most sacred, holiest of rituals there requires the services of 10 men. She enters a church and hears the words of the prophet Martin Luther: "if a woman dies in childbirth it matters not, because it was for this that she was created by God." She attends a dinner party with her husband where the women talk of children and schools and the men exchange information about their enterprises. As a girl, she is told the boys won't like her if she is too smart ("Men won't make passes at girls who wear glasses"). As a young woman, she is told she won't attract a man if she is too fat. As a wife, she is told she won't keep her man if she doesn't defer to his needs. She will be an old maid if she does not marry; but if she graduates from college, she will get a bachelor's degree as her reward. When her children marry, she becomes the stuff from which a whole genre of jokes are fashioned. Paintings will depict her goddesslike qualities when she is coupled with her infant child; journal articles will

describe her as smothering and hanging-on when coupled with her adolescent child. She speaks of "a rule of thumb," only to discover that this expression derives from an old English law that denied men the right to beat their wives with a stick larger than the circumference of their thumb!

Does the cumulative effect of such messages constitute a kind of psychological onslaught that shapes the way women experience themselves and each other? Do such messages effect the emotional and intellectual well-being of women? Of course they do; how could it be otherwise? These are the questions a feminist perspective will seek to address. Feminist family therapists have enlarged the theory of family functioning to include gender as a significant, if not fundamental, ingredient in the construction of family structures and interpersonal transactions. This challenges the idea that the family as a system is governed by its own internal regulatory mechanism within which all interpersonal transactions can be understood.

Women's experience is to be found not only in their encounter with the messages of a male culture and language, but within familial social institutions and structures. The institution of marriage, for instance, dramatically exemplifies the ways in which patriarchy, both implicitly and explicitly, organizes our lives. Marriage begins with the tradition of father handing his daughter over to another man whose name she will take, forsaking her own. (Of course, in a historical context, this quaint tradition would seem quite benign as it does not include purchasing a bride, a dowry, or some other form of economic barter, and the consent of the bride is almost always required!) The rituals of the marriage ceremony reflect the expected structure of the liaison to follow. The daughter is brought to her husband-to-be on the arm of her father while her mother quite literally stands to the side. The bride's face is often covered by a veil, suggesting humility. She wears white, symbolizing chastity. (And how does the groom demonstrate his humility and virginity?) In today's world, the bride may choose to keep her surname, but her formal social classification will change from Miss to Mrs. (his remains Mr.) and her person becomes, at least publically, identified with her mate. Her new career as a wife will be organizedl by roles and functions primarily identified with the *internal* life of the family.

Early life decisions for the newly married couple, such as where and under what circumstances they will live, will largely depend on the man's work or career. This begins to construct the context and rules for later decision making between them. A process is set in motion that will identify this wife, and later their family, by association with the work or career, the choices, the social and economic conditions of the husband, the man, the head of the household. (Women have head-of-household status only when there is no husband present.) This process, in which the life of one adult person is largely organized by, and identified with, the life and person of another, is at the very core of the institution of marriage and the structure of family life. In the life cycle of women, power is, for the most part, derivative: as daughter, father entitles; as wife, husband bestows.

How is it possible to conduct therapy with families, with couples in and out of marriage, with women, without understanding how this process constructs many of the problems, relationships, and conflicts that we encounter in our offices? How can we make *therapeutic* interventions—interventions that will create change without damaging self-esteem—and not be sensitive to the profoundly different meanings our words, tasks, and metaphors will have for men and for women as a result of their gender experiences? And how can we not but be aware that in a patriarchal culture life experience will be defined largely within a male frame of reference? These questions are not merely rhetorical. In fact, such questions, and the concerns that provoke them, surround the experience of women both as family members and as care givers within institutionalized frameworks.

WOMEN AND SERVICE DELIVERY SYSTEMS

Women are at both ends of service delivery systems, as consumers and as providers. As gatekeepers of the family, it is women who are largely responsible for seeking the services attendant to the general welfare of the family. Yet when seeking these services, women become both dependent on other women and in opposition to them. For instance, the working mother seeking day care for her child will feel both grateful to and displaced by the day care worker (over 90 percent of whom are women). In turn the day-care worker, while providing care for the child, will feel both commonality and conflict with the mother whose parenting needs often interfere with her own job performance. And both are caught up in a system that is underfunded and devalued, where their services are much in demand and in short supply, and where neither of their efforts, as the caretakers of the children, are signified by the larger society through the accepted signs of signification—money, power, access to resources, or public attention.

Or let us take the hypothetical case of a grade-school teacher (over 90 percent of whom are women) and a troubled young boy. His classroom behavior is disruptive and his grades are dropping. He seems to show no interest in school or in his peers. His parents are asked to come in for a consultation. His mother comes in alone because his father is working. She works, too, but only part-time, so she is able to manage the appointment. As the teacher describes the problem, the mother begins to feel failed, responsible, and overwhelmed. She has two more children at home, a younger child who has temper tantrums and a teenager who has been acting out of late. As the teacher inquires about family issues that might be affecting the boy's behavior in school, the mother begins to get the message that she may be causing the problem. She becomes defensive; perhaps indulges in some denial. She's afraid her son might get known as a misfit or trouble-maker. She defends him and feels protective. She feels alone in this.

The teacher has 30 other kids in her classroom and is a mother herself. She knows what this mother is going through, but she has her work to do and her job to protect. She begins to experience this child's mother as overprotective, defensive, even a bit resistant. The teacher recommends that the family seek help at a mental health agency.

The mother makes the call. The intake worker (the majority of whom are women) suggests she bring her husband with her on their first visit. He refuses; he does not think his son needs therapy. The mother, son, and little sister arrive for the initial session feeling irritable with each other. The intake worker sees an overloaded mother, who projects on others for the problem with her son: the school, her husband, her own mother. The worker finds the mother overprotective and overinvolved with her children; perhaps there is marital conflict. She suggests that the mother encourage her husband to come to the next session. Since the mother had already asked him to come to this one, she wonders if the worker thinks it is her fault that he didn't come. And thus a continuum is constructed along which women as caretakers, in a culture that devalues their services, begin to experience each other as adversaries.

Recently, at my training center in Washington, D.C., we worked with Lucy and her five children. They had been referred to us for family therapy by child protective services following the disclosure by the oldest daughter, Rose, age 17, that her stepfather had been sexually abusing her for six years. Lucy, a waitress, had alerted the authorities and had her husband removed from the home; Rose had been put in temporary foster care. The four other children were all under age 12. One had cerebral palsy, and another a learning disability. With the removal from the home of Joe, the father, and Rose, the eldest daughter, Lucy was left with no child-care support. She borrowed money from a brother in Detroit for the down payment for legal fees, and filed for divorce and for custody of the children.

Joe filed a countersuit, claiming that she was negligent of the children and sexually promiscuous. Joe, who was in a sexual offenders' group and was being seen by a court psychiatrist, continued to harass Lucy and to force entry into the house where she and the children lived. Whenever she called the police, they would get him to leave, but there was nothing they could do about keeping him from trying again, as he owned the house in which the family lived.

The foster care worker (a woman) received complaints from the foster mother that Lucy was inconsistent and demanding in making arrangements to visit her daughter Rose. When the foster care worker saw Lucy and Rose together, she felt there was a lot of unresolved conflict between them. She supported Rose in expressing her anger at her mother for not protecting her from her stepfather. The protective service worker (a woman) needed to determine if Lucy could protect her daughter in the future, care for her other children, and provide financially for the family. The worker was concerned that Lucy's work as a waitress resulted in irregular times at home with her children, and that her child care arrangements were haphazard. She thought that Lucy should arrange to stay home more to be with her younger children. But Lucy also needed to demonstrate that she could provide financially for her family.

The court-appointed worker (a woman) was concerned about Joe's allegations, and worried about whether Lucy could provide a proper home for *any* of the children. In agency case conferences, discussion centered on Lucy's problems with being a responsible, consistent parent; on her immature, narcissistic, disorganized behaviors; and on her financial credibility. In this context, Lucy was referred, with her children, to us for family therapy.

As a single parent, Lucy must provide for her children, but like many, if not most women in our society, is untrained and poorly paid. Like most families of divorcing parents, the father's child support is either nonexistent, unenforced, insufficient, or dependent on the vagaries of his financial situation. Lucy must work, but also provide adequate supervision for her children. The children must be cared for and nurtured. But public day care facilities have long waiting lists, and private ones are too expensive. Lucy needs to protect her daughter, but does not herself have access to legal protection. She is expected to begin to restructure her own life, but if she does so she is in danger of neglecting her children.

These are some of the familiar contexts within which women are defined and from which they will internalize ideas and attitudes that shape their sense of self. Women do not need to undergo these specific experiences to have them as part of what Jung would have called their collective unconscious, and I would call a universal consciousness. (Not that I would presume to compete with Jung, but we family therapists don't like to talk about the unconscious!) Attitudes and messages that devalue and subordinate women; social and institutional structures that diminish their instrumentality; double binds that hold mothers responsible for whatever happens with their children and overinvolved if they take that responsibility to heart; social realities that make women vulnerable to sexual abuse and rape while chiding them for being sexually repressed; economic conditions that place them in competitive, adversarial positions with each other in "spaces" where access to resources is limited—this is the terrain of women's experience that has been hidden from view and thus gone unnoticed in our theories of family functioning. Many of the methods and techniques of family therapy demonstrate a tunnel vision that sees only what is immediately apparent and never explores that which lies below the surface. "Meaning" is relegated to the margins or confined within the formulas of systems theory.

THERAPY, TECHNIQUES, AND WOMEN

It has been well established that theories of human development and scales of maturity and individuation have been based on male models. This also is true of theories of human systems. In many ways, these theories have pathologized women, particularly with respect to their roles in family life. In the practice of family therapy the very absence of a consciousness about gender, and the differences in the development of men and women in a patriarchal culture, serves to pathologize women. The following examples, taken at random from family therapy journals, publications, and workshops, illustrate interventions and techniques that, in their very lack of awareness of, and sensitivity to, the meaning they convey to women, reproduce sexist constructs that invalidate women's experience.

We can begin with the familiar pursuer wife and distancer husband, a typology frequently employed in conceptualizing conflict or lack of communication and intimacy between marital partners. While framing the pursuit and distance as a complementary pattern of interaction, maintaining the balance of power between husband and wife, a therapist moves to block the pursuer so the distancer can enter. He suggests that the wife is working too hard; that she should back off, take a rest. (To the degree that *she* works so hard, *he* does not need to work at their relationship. The more *she* pursues, the more *he* will distance. *She* fills their emotional space; if *she* backs off, it will create a vacuum that *he* will fill.)

Such a technique ignores the fact that women are socialized to be the purveyors of relationship, the articulators of feeling, the nurturers of intimacy. In a culture that does *not* put a premium on relationship and intimacy, that comes dangerously close to equating emotionality with irrationality, failure to validate the pursuit of these ends devalues the very behaviors that are socially expected of women. A double bind indeed! Asking a woman to "back off" from pursuit of intimacy and relationship will convey the message that *her* pursuit endangers the relational competence of her partner; that her pursuit causes his distance. And what a message for the man—that his capacity for intimacy is contingent on the degree of intensity his wife employs in trying to engage him; that he will withdraw in the face of too much pursuit.

A similar typology is that of the overinvolved mother, peripheral father, and acting-out or problem-bearing child. This time, a therapist uses the father to block the mother's concentration on the child, thus engaging the father in greater involvement with his child while freeing the mother to engage in more complex, adult activities. No matter that the relationships are conceptualized as complementary. The intervention carries the same message as the previous one: mother is overfunctioning, overinvolved, overprotective, and father's peripherality is connected to that. In her socially prescribed role as primary parent, she will be perceived as having failed. His primary socially prescribed role, as family provider, is not at issue; and as a parent, he need only *enter* to set things right. It may balance the system, but what is the effect on the self-esteem of its members? And what of the notion that child rearing is a less than complex or adult activity? This idea delegitimizes the very function that women are expected to perform. (Anyway, maternal functioning is less complex than what—selling used cars?)

Another therapist, faced with a disengaged, distant, often absent father, suggests to the mother that she pretend that she cannot handle the child anymore, that she act as if she has run out of alternatives and is giving up. Is this not isomorphic with generations of advice to women to "act dumb," or "fake it," so he will feel more competent and take charge? If we ask women to act incompetent on behalf of men, are we not conveying the message that their competence, at least with respect to their relationships with men, puts them at risk?

A therapist working with a couple in conflict because of the husband's infidelity uses a *meta* stance of tongue-in-cheek double-talk, suggesting that the wife might compete with her husband, perhaps "go into the business" and offer her husband good rates. What is the message? When a woman has an extramarital affair, it is likened to prostitution. I do not think the therapist thought this; I just think he did not think about the *meaning* his words would convey.

A therapist working with a sexually inhibited couple, in the same vein of playful prodding, asks the husband if he would mind if he—the therapist—had a little affair with his wife during the session, noting that she had been making eyes at him, and he would like to "retaliate". The message? Men ask each other for permission to "have fun" with "their" women; her consent is not even sought! (The word "retaliate" might have been a "Freudian slip"—it certainly conveys the message that the woman's flirtatiousness is experienced as aggression by a therapist whose experience of his own flirtation is benign.)

A therapist works with a couple who is fighting through their children, a boy and a girl, each of whom is allied with the same-sex parent. The therapist, using metaphor to dramatize the family system, suggests that the boy, who is older, has already removed himself from the parent's bed, only to be replaced by his younger sister. He wonders if the parents will ever let their daughter out, and asks them if she will have to stay home as an old maid forever to keep her parents apart. After all, the therapist remarks, their daughter is already 13 years old; it will be only three or four years until she has her first affair, or gets married, or has a sex-change operation. (So much for the possibilities for women in this world!) Here the therapist refers to a 13-year-old girl exclusively in terms of her sexuality, thus implicitly reaffirming a limited and stereotyped perspective of women and their psychosocial potential. His view of the daughter is expressed solely in terms of relations she might achieve with a man or, failing that, the prospect of becoming one!

A therapist works with a family in which the mother is depressed, the father is alcoholic, and the teenaged son is a high school dropout. The parents fight a great deal. The mother describes herself as the patient. The father says that he doesn't like to argue. The therapist, using circular questioning, asks the son what he thinks his mother does to get his father going. The message? Woman as provocateur—not so far removed from questions like, "How did she get him to hit her?" Later, the mother says her husband drinks and then he gets nasty. The therapist, taking a "neutral" position, suggests to these battling spouses that their fighting creates emotional intensity. He tells the wife that she was bored with her first husband, that the fighting is a game and she likes it. The message? Women in pursuit of intimacy, of emotionality, bring about their own destruction.

Then there is the therapist who is working with an intact family of four children. The identified patient is an eight-year-old girl who regularly wets her bed, having already ruined five mattresses. The therapist presses for inclusion of the mother's mother in the therapy. He wonders what the mother's life was like when she was her daughter's age. Assuming anger and defiance are connected to the bed wetting, the therapist seeks an answer to the child's anger. Using provocation to increase intensity, the therapist suggests that the child is like her mother; that she has her anger. The therapist comments that perhaps when the mother was pregnant, the daughter was swimming in her anger, in her belly. The message here is twofold. On the one hand, the daughter's bed-wetting symptom is defined and explained as somehow connected to her mother's anger, thus confirming traditional views of maternal destructiveness. This is compounded with ideas of inevitable intergenerational conflict and anger between the women in a family. In this respect, the therapist outdoes Freud by using a *prenatal* metaphor.

And then there is the therapist who uses trance with a father who was referred to him for beating his daughter when she returned 25 minutes late from a date. The trance is designed to help the father get in touch with the more expressive, trusting, and tender side of himself. The daughter is asked to quietly observe the process. The therapist then points out that the daughter brings her father a sense of trust by being there, quiet and accepting during the session, comparing this to the manner in which a puppy can evoke tenderness by being quiet and still. The message here is only too obvious: the way to a man's heart, the way to avoid being hurt, the way to take care of others, is to be there, quiet and still, much like a puppy. In orchestrating the daughter's quiet acceptance of her father as a remedy for his aggression, the therapist plays on an all-too-familiar refrain.

Of course, these examples are taken out of context— But what context can justify the use of interventions that replicate sexist thinking or that fail to take into account their effect on the sensibility of women in therapy?

The techniques, in and of themselves, are not the problem. It is only when they are put into words and behaviors that they reflect the sex stereotypes and gender biases, the values and belief systems, of the prevailing culture. Only an unused technique can be neutral. As soon as it is put into practice, it will convey meaning and impart significance that will be experienced in particular ways by the members of a family. And such meanings, no matter how much the intention of the therapist is to attach them to the systemic issues of the family, will be determined as well by the gender of the recipient.

INFORMED THERAPY

The literature and research that have been generated out of the past two decades of the women's movement has direct bearing on the practice of family therapy. A vast, and certainly rich, vein of writings by, for, and about women has gradually worked its way into the mainstream of research, study, and teaching, as well as into the popular media. Historians have delved into the past for evidence of the way in which women were hidden from view, and to rediscover the contributions of women in every area of human endeavor. Social scientists have studied social systems and institutions, uncovering the patriarchal structures that define the roles and functions of women. Ideologies that devalue women have been analyzed. The social, political, and economic processes that disadvantage women have been described. Mental health professionals have explored the psychological development of women and their emotional well-being—or lack of it—as this relates to the issues and conditions of their "second sex" status. Women have written about their lives, experiences, and relationships. Essays, letters, biographies, autobiographies, articles, novels, and anthologies of every description have enriched our literature. And people, for the most part, have become more aware of overt sexist language and behavior and make some effort to avoid it. Yet family therapy remained, until recently, largely indifferent to the significance this growing body of knowledge has for our own theory and practice.

As noted earlier, I think the reason for this lies within the limitations of systems theory itself. Systems theorists can become entrenched in the study of systems as if they have no political, social, or economic contexts. Systems practitioners can become so focused on the inner consistency of a given formulation that they lose sight of the larger realities that structure and shape it. And both theorists and practitioners can become so enamored of the internal logic of a system that they operate and think pragmatically, unaware of the values, subtleties, or meanings in what they do or in how they think. Within systems theory, some practices have evolved that are so focused on "what works," or on the "performance" itself of the therapist, that meaning and process are virtually ignored.

Every social, and every human, experience is at once personal and interpersonal; boundaried and continuous; specific and general; felt and understood. That which is internal to any system is also in process, moving within and between context, system, and person. If we continue to understand symptoms primarily in terms of their functions within the family system, then we do not need to understand the immigrant experience, the impact of poverty, the effect of overcrowded living conditions, the punitive classroom situation, the racial slur—or the gender stereotype—as determinants of dysfunctional interpersonal transactions and of familial structure. If we concentrate on hierarchal arrangements within the family, we do not need to worry about power arrangements and inequities outside of it. If we circle around reciprocal loops between marital partners, we need never concern ourselves with the sexist social conditions that organized and structured that partnership. If we look only at the complementarity in a parental relationship, we do not need to confront a society that assigns the woman the primary responsibility for the children and then blames her for their problems. If we focus on the medium, we do not need to struggle with the message.

Systems theory and systemic practices have, in the past generation, informed and transformed the field of psychotherapy in profound ways. Because of this, because systemic therapy continues to hold such promise for achieving the change human beings desire in their lives, their families, their work, and their relationships, it is important that our theory and our therapy continue to evolve with reference to the new information, meanings, and understandings that have been developed within the women's movement and feminist theory. Here is material that informs us in new ways about the very nature of the family system, and about the experience of women within it.

Most of us, in recent years, have become familiar with the statistics on women in the world of work, as single parents, in marriage and divorce. Most of us are aware that more women seek therapy for themselves and their children than do men; that married men report greater emotional and physical well-being than do married women; that, in fact, married women show poorer mental and emotional health than do either married men or unmarried women; and that for widowers the mortality rate is 61 percent higher than for married men the same age. We know that married men experience more dissatisfaction in the marriage if their wives work, and that women who work experience greater satisfaction in their marriage; that 92 percent of divorced women keep their children; and that single-parent families are really female- or mother-headed households, only one-third of which receive financial support from the father of the children. We are also aware that of violent crimes committed by a relative, 77 percent of the victims are women; that the divorce rate for women is higher among those with graduate education; that half of all women with children work, but earn 68 percent of what men earn; that 70 percent of full-time employed women work in occupations in which over three-quarters of the employees are female; that fewer women than men remarry after divorce—and on, and on.

Such information has a direct bearing on the way we frame a question, deliver an intervention, exercise power, develop a relationship, or offer a direction in the conduct of therapy with families. A brief example should suffice in making my point: In studies conducted in both primary and secondary schools between 1980 and 1986, American University education professors Myra and David Sadker found that boys get far more attention at all grade levels, be it praise or criticism from their teachers, than do girls. Interactions between the teacher and students in the classrooms studied were categorized, in relation to the teacher's response, as criticism, acceptance, remediation, and praise. In every category, the researchers found that boys received more attention from the teacher than girls, and that the domination of boys in the classroom grows as they get older. In films of teacher–student interaction, the observers noted that the boys were asked more challenging questions, were given more praise in response to correct answers, or were coaxed along toward the right answer. Girls were praised more for their neat handwriting and exemplary behavior than for their academic abilities. Boys, in the classroom, called out answers to questions without raising their hands eight times more often than girls. In addition, a review of books that have won the Caldecott Medal (the Pulitzer of the kiddie set) showed that for every girl depicted in the books there are 10 boys.

What then of interrupting women in therapy? And have we noticed the frequency with which we do this as compared with the frequency with which we interrupt men? Do we listen more to men? Do we block women from talking in order to give men a chance? Do we defer to a man who interrupts but object to a woman doing so? Do we validate a man's efforts in therapy more than a woman's?

Information such as that elicited in the Sadker study can filter into our work, helping us to evolve new techniques and refine old ones. For instance, recognizing that women are not accustomed to having their thoughts pursued, or to receive as much attention to their thinking as do men, we fashioned an intervention we call interior questioning, a way of referencing an emotional experience to the intellectual process that accompanies it. For example, a woman in therapy might talk about the way her husband's anger makes her feel helpless. She describes upset, distraught, sad, or conflictual feelings. To highlight how she *thinks* about how she *feels*, we might pursue a line of questioning that links these two processes: What do you mean by helpless? How did you arrive at that meaning? What other things make you feel helpless? Why do you think they do? What does being helpless look like? Can you tell when others feel helpless? Or: How do you define anger? How do you know when someone is angry? How do you think anger and helplessness are connected? And so on. Answers can be used to help the client elaborate her meanings and definitions by challenging her to expand, and to own, her thoughts, ideas, and beliefs. The idea—to integrate cognition and experience, understanding and feeling—is in fact, something of a compensatory intervention. In a world in which women have been trained to inquire of others whether they are cold rather than declare outright that "it is cold," it is important for therapy to provide them with the opportunity to make declarative statements and to identify their own belief systems. When people understand, they not only feel but *are*, more in charge. Self-definition is the key to empowerment.

WOMAN MODES AND MODELS

As male models of behavior and male modes of transaction are primary in our society, surely their use in therapy as translated into techniques of intervention needs to be reconsidered. If therapy is to give people a different experience, one that offers alternatives, it would seem important to look at our methodologies for the messages conveyed by the structure and ideology that underlie the methodology itself. For instance, many social analysts have noted that problem-solving modes are more associated with men. That men tend to go after problem resolution whereas women tend to go after the ways a problem is manifested. Men are more likely to be engaged in pursuing ends and women in pursuing means. Of course, these are dichotomized ways of thinking, and both men and women are found along the spectrum between these polarities. But the dichotomy does exist in the way in which modes of expression are perceived and models of behavior are experienced. Women are caretakers; men are doers. Such are the archetypes, the myths, built on many levels of social text and subtext that are internalized and reproduced by women and men, and by the systems within which they function.

Gender modes anad models provide a provocative context within which to consider the choices we make of interventions and techniques between the various methodological frameworks in family therapy. Is problem-solving therapy a male model? Does it affirm or give sufficient expression to female modes of processing experience? Will the therapy of prescription be experienced by women as affirming of relationship or as another expression of the privileged use of authority? Can even a well-worded directive fail to objectify women whose experience as objects has been so well documented? Can a functional hierarchy be achieved through behaviors that are at any level disrespectful? Can frames and formulations be used without reference to conditions of sex role stereotyping? Can we use techniques that exploit the greater access we have to women for creating change? Or, for that matter, can we use techniques that depend on the greater availability of women for compliance?

Again, such questions are not merely rhetorical. They force us to take a critical look at our theory and techniques; to examine the ideology underlying our choice of method. Beginning to make conscious use of female modes of transaction, and models of interaction, will offset the natural tendency to utilize modes and models that are more acceptable in our society because they are associated with authority and power. To help the women in family therapy not only to change, but to be empowered and feel understood, with their self-esteem not only intact but improved, we will need to pay attention to the meta-messages conveyed in the transactional modes we choose, as well as those conveyed in words. Such messages constitute a powerful means of transmitting values, meanings, and attitudes; more powerful perhaps than words because they are hidden, obscured by the structure and content of the technique itself, and so tend to be internalized without the filter of critical thought.

Perhaps the next stage in the evolution of family therapy will be the development of a methodology that is as congruent with the experience of women as of men. This will surely mean a focus on process, the use of relationship and engagement, a comfort with proximity and emotion, and a sensitivity to gendered meanings, differences, behaviors, and beliefs. It will mean not having to sacrifice instrumentality on the altar of power, or relationality on the altar of "reason."

CASE EXAMPLE

Although this discussion was not intended to be primarily clinical, a case example might be useful in illustrating a feminist rethinking in family therapy. I am reminded of a family I saw recently that was in treatment with a family therapist as part of an ongoing consultation group.

A couple, both in their late 30s, had brought their seven-year-old son for therapy because he had been found repeatedly going through his mother's clothes, touching her undergarments, and occasionally trying on some of her clothing. Although their son had not yet gone outside of the home in his mother's clothing, his parents were terrified that he would. Both parents worked outside of the home. They had been married for 12 years, and had been contemplating having another child before this problem developed. A family genogram revealed intact families of origin, with both sets of grandparents living nearby and visiting the couple frequently. Both grandmothers often provided child care. The father's younger sister lived and worked nearby; the mother was an only child.

The therapist, and the group observing the family, noted poor generational boundaries, an aggressive, sometimes seductive, mother, and a passive father who even described himself as a "milktoast." The patient's older brother, age 11, was, in size, behavior, and choice of heroes, reminiscent of a burgeoning Rambo. The therapist and the group agreed that sex roles were unclear in this family and the parental hierarchy was weak. There was concern about the number of women hovering around this boy, the youngest grandchild in the family. The mother wanted constant reassurance, and even brought in newspaper clippings about cross-dressers who were happily married! Both parents wanted to believe that nothing was wrong with their son, although the father seemed more prepared to intervene forcefully in the child's behavior if this was recommended. The mother, on the other hand, was protective, fearing that any intervention on their part would make her son feel more vulnerable or hurt his feelings. She did not want him to begin to think that something was wrong with him.

The therapist had four sessions with the family. He suggested that boundaries in the family were unclear, framing this in terms of too many open doors, so that their son was not sure where to enter and where not to enter. He suggested that the mother close the door to the master bedroom and that the father begin to monitor the boy's behavior, keeping him away from his mother's things. He worked with the father for more engagement with his son, and suggested the mother needed to stop working so hard for the whole family. During the session, the mother's intrusiveness was blocked with instructions that each member of the family was to speak for himself. The therapist suggested that the mother's protectiveness toward her son and the father's distance were interconnected. Both parents were encouraged to strengthen their own familial boundaries, together setting up some rules for interaction with their families of origin. The mother strongly objected to this idea. She saw the families as close, and their interchange as spontaneous. Moreover, their help with the children was indispensable. The father became more active around this question, suggesting ways to structure visits with their respective families.

In the fourth session, it became clear that the mother was not following through on the directive to close her bedroom door and she remained overly close and protective with her son despite her husband's objections. The therapist asked the son what he thought his mother was thinking, why he thought she didn't close her bedroom door, why she was not doing what had been asked of her. The mother became quite agitated and the session ended abruptly. The group felt there was a lot of resistance from the mother and that it would be necessary to secure the father's help in disengaging her from the overinvolvement with her son. At this point, I was invited to have a consultation session with the family.

Using a feminist perspective, I framed the family dynamics quite differently. I told the parents that their son loved them both very much indeed, but that his love was more complicated in relation to his Mom, than his Dad. I suggested that although their son wanted to be close to his mother because he loved her, he, like many little boys, was always getting conflicting messages. At school, at the movies, and on television, he heard that boys who were too close to their mothers were sissies or momma's boys—a fate worse than death! So he did not know what to do with all those good and warm and close feelings he had toward his mother. He sure did not want to be a sissy. And this made him begin to do some mixed-up things. The mother was right to be concerned and protective because her son really was feeling all mixed up. I suggested that both parents would need to reassure their son that it was good to love and be close to your mother, that it would not make him a sissy. But that mom would then need to help him find ways to be close other than wearing her clothes.

We spent much of the session talking about ways to be close that did not get people into trouble, reaching into the experience and repertoire of both parents for ideas and suggestions. Their thoughts about closeness were translated into behavioral and verbal interventions that they could use when their son got mixed up again and sought closeness by playing with or wearing his mother's clothes. The parents were asked to divide this work in an equitable fashion, that is, one that reflected the expertise and competence of each. I asked them to identify where they felt most competent with their son. Then I worked with them to negotiate where each would engage with their son during the week.

During the session, the mother's interruptions and overtalking diminished somewhat as the father was encouraged to express himself more fully. Feedback centered on their reactivity vis-à-vis each other and each was challenged to engage in the session from his or her own perspective rather than in response to the other. Within this framework, I could encourage the mother not to feel she had to fill in the silences left by her husband or the boys. And I suggested to the father that his wife probably often felt lonely, even within her family, and that was why she found it so hard to regulate contact with their parents. I suggested that future sessions might focus on how Dad could help Mom feel less lonely. During most of the session, the boys were excused after being asked if they had any questions or concerns they wanted to express. I thought that in future sessions their son might be seen sometimes with his parents and sometimes alone with the therapist, with the older boy being included on an as-needed basis.

At the end of the session, we talked together about privacy and boundaries versus closeness and spontaneity, and how to keep these from being opposites even though that is how they are so often experienced. I reassured both parents that their son's behavior was reversible but would continue to need their attention within the range of things we had discussed; some of which would not seem to be directly related to his problem. I congratulated them on being able to maintain close and often mutually satisfying relations with their own parents, even if these might need to become somewhat more structured.

I trust that this case illustrates some of the clinical approaches a feminist perspective will suggest. Each of us will do it differently, but always with a sensibility to the particular experience of women within a culture largely organized by men.

4

SCAPEGOATING MOTHERS: CONCEPTUAL ERRORS IN SYSTEMS FORMULATIONS

Michele Bograd, Ph.D.

Scapegoating mothers is a dubious but enduring tradition in psychotherapy. At first glance, family therapy seems immune to the pungent critiques that feminist theoreticians previously leveled against psychodynamic models. As a liberal theoretical framework, family therapists do not subscribe to essentialist notions of intrinsic, fixed, complementary male and female natures. As individual accountability is replaced by circular interactional patterns, there are few instances of blatant sexist characterizations of mothers. In fact, a small study (the only of its kind) suggests that a "new generation" of family counselors holds relatively liberal attitudes toward women and motherhood (Hare-Mustin & Lamb, 1984). Yet, as a theoretical and technical system, family therapy is developed and practiced at a specific historical time in a patriarchal social and political context characterized by the domination of men as a class over women. As participants in the dominant culture, family therapists cannot help but assimilate oppressive and sexist images and assumptions about women into their theory and clinical work (Goldner, 1985a, 1985b, 1985c; James, 1985; MacKinnon & Miller, 1987; Sherman, 1980; Taggart, 1985).

Feminist family therapists have begun to point out the most obvious and glaring examples of biases against women in family systems models and interventions (Ault-Riche, 1986; Bograd, 1984, 1986a, 1986b, 1986c, 1987, in press; Goldner, 1985a, 1985b, 1985c; Gurman & Klein, 1980, 1984; Hare-Mustin, 1978, 1980; Jacobson, 1983; James & McIntyre, 1983; Joslyn, 1982; Layton, 1984; Lerner, 1983; Libow, Raskin & Caust, 1982; Margolin, Fernandes, Talovic, & Onorato, 1983; Osborne, 1983; Taggart, 1985; Women's Project in Family Therapy, 1982, 1983). The goal of this chapter is to describe in greater detail more subtle but widespread conceptual errors in systemic formulations that promote scapegoating mothers in family therapy. This is not to suggest that family therapists adequately and nonjudgmentally understand the experiences of men. But as a feminist, my primary and explicit concern is elucidating the ways that women are defined, blamed, and oppressed by well-meaning care givers. I have chosen to focus on errors in family therapy formulations rather than on interventions because the goals and structure of interventions derive from how we conceptualize family process and dysfunction. Although clinicians express interest in learning "feminist" or "nonsexist" interventions, I believe that what distinguishes feminist family therapists from others is not the use of special techniques but how we think about and describe family life, which, in turn, influences the process and goals of clinical practice.

MOTHER BLAMING: SEVEN MAJOR CONCEPTUAL ERRORS

Seven major conceptual errors contribute to biases against women in systemic formulations. Although some of these errors are more likely to occur in a given family therapy model because of its theoretical assumptions, I will not focus on specific models (such as structural, strategic, or systemic) as my clinical experience suggests that family therapists commit these errors regardless of their particular theoretical persuasion. Although it is all too easy to cite examples from well-known family therapists and current literature, this approach too often leads to divisiveness and conflict, particularly when feminist issues are concerned. For this reason, illustrative examples throughout this chapter are composites of data gathered by review of the literature, case conferences, and local and national training workshops. For the sake of integration and continuity, the majority of examples focus on the concept of enmeshment (Minuchin, 1974; Minuchin & Fishman, 1981)—one of the most pervasive labels applied to women in families.

Seven conceptual errors lead family therapists to unfairly (if unintentionally) blame mothers: (1) confusion of individual and system levels of analysis; (2) sexist punctuation of transactional sequences; (3) confusion of fact with inference; (4) use of biased standards of adaptive family functioning; (5) privatization of the family; (6) neglect of social and material constraints; and (7) employment of oversimplified systems models. Although these errors co-occur and mutually reinforce one another, for heuristic purposes they will be distinguished conceptually.

Confusion of Individual and System Levels of Analysis

At face value, it would appear that family therapists would not scapegoat mothers as their theoretical frameworks direct them to describe interactional sequences that include the behavioral and emotional contributions of all family members. But in practice, family therapists often incorrectly apply systems terms to individuals. For example, although enmeshment is an organizational term describing a transaction pattern between two or more individuals, family therapists often refer to "the enmeshed mother." Through this common linguistic error, dimensions of the system are reified and placed inside the woman as static personal characteristics. Such statements inappropriately suggest that the mother alone has blurred boundaries and examine her in isolation from the interactional context of family life.

Sexist Punctuation of Transactional Sequences

Many family therapists are cautious in their use of systemic language and analysis. Yet the description of transactional sequence does not necessarily protect against scapegoating mothers as sequences can be punctuated in ways that subtly implicate the mother as a primary determinant of maladaptive family process. Take the following behavioral description of the beginning of a family therapy session:

> Mother glances at father, nonverbally suggesting that he begin the session. While he is talking, she silently monitors the behavior of her young daughter. She interrupts her husband to disagree with his assessment of the situation. As he begins to talk again, the mother touches her adolescent son (the identified patient), which leads him to pull away abruptly, disrupting the session.

This supposedly neutral description places the mother squarely in the center of family interaction, as if she is primarily accountable for the unfolding transactional sequence. Other family members are described almost as passive reactive players to the mother's moves, which are encoded in ways that suggest she is controlling, undermining of the husband, and oversensitive to nonverbal cues (Spiegel, 1982). The reciprocal influences of the husband's and children's behaviors on the mother are addressed in ways that minimize their effect on her. By highlighting negative characteristics of the mother, such formulations assume the mother lacks any competence, or take for granted her capable and valuable mothering skills (Bograd, 1987; Hare-Mustin, 1978; Hatfield, 1986; Imber-Black, 1986; Lerner, 1983; Women's Project in Family Therapy, 1982, 1983). This becomes more evident in a reformulation of the previous behavioral sequence:

> The father sits angrily and refuses to respond to the therapist's curiosity about why the family has entered treatment. In an effort to engage him, the mother nonverbally signals that he begin to talk. As the youngest daughter gets distracted from the conversation, mother watches her with concern. As the father begins to mock the adolescent son, mother interrupts him in an effort to redirect this destructive sequence. She touches the son reassuringly. Her son blocks this move by pulling away angrily.

This reframing suggests that family therapists make choices about how to highlight certain aspects of family process. Ignoring the temporal development of family patterns contributes to blaming mothers. By omission, systemic formulations often assume that how the mother is acting now, in the context of family distress, is the same as she acted before the distress became evident. Family therapists theoretically do not adhere to notions of unilinear cause, but their formulations focus disproportionately on the mother's current behaviors, implying that they are a primary cause of a child's distress, and minimizing the variety of ways a symptomatic child's behavior and the reactions of other family members may influence the mother.

Although family therapists adhere to a theoretical system that holds that each part of the system plays an important functional role in maintaining interactional patterns, formulations focus on the mother's involvement as if it takes place in an interpersonal and social vacuum. For example, the mother's intense connections with her children are often not linked to the father's intense involvement in his work. Although men's often peripheral engagement with children is sometimes tied to women's overinvolvement, formulations still give more weight to the mother's activity—although it can be argued that men's relative detachment from family life has major implications for the development of symptoms or dysfunctional patterns. Given the current structure of the nuclear family in society, it is undeniable that most women play central roles in family life—but this does not mean that they are, by fiat, more responsible for family dysfunction. Women's investment in family life, often labeled in pejorative terms, can also be viewed as women's positive and constructive commitment to their primary relationships. From this perspective, mothers' behaviors and feelings can serve as a model to others (including family members and family therapists) to value and cherish close and intense relationships, rather than to devalue or denigrate them.

Confusion of Fact with Inference: Assimilation of Cultural Ideologies About Women into Systemic Formulations

Even a casual review of the literature suggests that women are held accountable for the behavior of their husbands and children far more frequently than the converse (Spiegel, 1982). This systematic bias against women is based in part on the conceptual error of confusing fact with inference. The building blocks of family therapy are the descriptions of concrete, observable behavioral patterns that supposedly characterize key dimensions of the interactional field as objectively and neutrally as possible. Although family therapists often focus primarily on the mother simply because she is more involved with the children than is the father, are there clear, verifiable links between her behaviors and family symptomatology? There is little empirical evidence to suggest that this is so (Seiden, 1976), and thus it is more likely that family therapists often confuse fact with inference when they go beyond what is visually and empirically verifiable to draw conclusions, make interpretations, or convey pejorative judgments about women in families (Hatfield, 1986).

A woman makes repeated requests, for example, that her husband attend to her, and he responds with silence. This behavioral transaction is often coded in the formulation "wife nags and is overinvolved; husband withdraws." First, this formulation decontextualizes the interaction by highlighting the supposedly negative consequences of the wife's behaviors while ignoring the fact that her repeated requests evolved in a context of her husband's lack of responsiveness.

Second, this formulation reflects the man's view of the situation. That is, the husband experiences the requests as illegitimate or invasive, whereas the wife believes she has the right to expect responsivity and acknowledgment from her husband. Last, labeling the wife's requests as "nagging" moves beyond simple description of the sequence to assumptions about women, which, in turn, are based on cultural images of women as shrews or demanding, insatiable wives. Furthermore, identical behaviors by men or women may be labeled with different terms that convey different evaluative judgments: maternal enmeshment becomes paternal involvement or paternal disengagement becomes maternal neglect (Hare-Mustin, 1978).

The kinds of inferences family therapists make about women are relatively consistent and appear to reflect a systematic bias. How mothers are perceived and described by many family therapists may be due less to observable behavioral sequences, to a given family systems framework, or to idiosyncratic characteristics of the individual therapist than to facets of the current social and political context that strongly influence which behaviors, signs, or cues are deemed clinically important (MacKinnon & Miller, 1987; Taggart, 1985). Language is the most fundamental dimension of this context (Spender, 1980). Although family therapy has its own vocabulary, therapists also must draw from the linguistic repertoire of society. What is named, and so perceived and attended to, is primarily determined by the dominant class in any society. Throughout history, man have had the power to determine cultural meanings and symbols, which often distort, devalue, or render invisible the experiences of women. Our social knowledge is replete with derogatory images of women—such as the shrew, the nag, the hysteric, the seductress. The patriarchal context is sustained at the symbolic level through ideologies or sets of ideas and concepts deriving from unintended but systematically motivated distortions of reality that maintain the status quo (Bernal & Ysern, 1985; Ryan, 1971).

Of most relevance here is the ideological construction of motherhood that has developed in a patriarchal social context characterized by men's domination over women (Chodorow, 1978; Chodorow & Contratto, 1982; Dinnerstein, 1976; Goldner, 1985a, 1985b, 1985c; James, 1985; Oakley, 1976; Rich, 1976; Women's Project in Family Therapy, 1982, 1983). This ideology serves male interests by excluding men from the burdens of family life, by legitimatizing women's subordination, and by redefining social oppression as the expression of natural instincts (MacKinnon & Miller, 1987). Three major components comprise Mother as an ideological category: (1) mothers as larger-than-life perfect and naturally nurturant beings; (2) mothers as responsible for the well-being of intimate others; (3) mothers as all-powerful destructive beings who are the locus of blame.

In our society, mothers are defined as all-knowing, all-giving, all responsible, and all-sacrificing (Spiegel, 1982; Women's Project in Family Therapy, 1982). As women attempt to fulfill the dictates of culturally prescribed roles, the very capacities defined as necessary for mothering (such as constant availability, emotional responsiveness, sensitivity to the unspoken needs of others) are also those defined as problematic (Osborne, 1983). Yet it is still assumed that, under proper conditions, mothers can mother perfectly. Even therapists who do not subscribe to the notion that mothering is a natural innate capacity of women often believe that women could mother flawlessly if only certain internal, interactional, or social constraints were removed (Chodorow & Contratto, 1982). When mothers are assigned responsibility for the psychological or physical well-being of all family members, they are not given credit or recognition for the development of sensitive complex interpersonal skills, but are held accountable for any resulting breakdown in the functioning of individual family members or of the family as a whole. Within this belief system, everyone feels let down by mother, as the institution of motherhood finds all women more or less guilty of having failed their children (Spiegel, 1982).

By unwittingly incorporating cultural ideologies about mothers into clinical formulations, family therapists slip from fact to inference by assuming the mother's behaviors exert a powerful, primary, and negative influence on family functioning and so minimize the complexity of family interaction and development (Goldner, 1985c; James, 1985). As many women in families also employ these cultural ideals to judge their own performance, clinical assessment of mothers' presumed failures may intensify the women's self-blame. The link between mothers and psychopathology should not be assumed unless the clinical data clearly warrant it. Although mothers unquestionably influence their children and spouses, so do other systemic factors, including fathers, outside care givers, the economic level of the family, and the family's interactions with other social institutions such as schools and mental health systems.

Use of Biased Standards of Adaptive Family Functioning

Family systems terms and formulations appear objective, scientific, and neutral. But assessments of the health and pathology of family members and of the family as a whole are not free of gender stereotypes. Examination of the usually unarticulated values of family therapists reveals that many therapists adhere to biased prototypically male standards of adaptive or healthy family functioning (Bograd, 1987b; Broverman, Broverman, Clarkson, Rosenkrantz, & Vogel, 1970; Goldner, 1985c; Hare-Mustin, 1978; Layton, 1984; Luepnitz, 1984; Miller, 1976; Women's Project in Family Therapy, 1982, 1983). These standards can lead to (1) pathologizing women's typical relational styles, (2) pejoratively labeling "deviant" family forms, and (3) inaccurately describing family life.

Pathologizing Women's Typical Relational Styles

Embedded in the description that mother is enmeshed with her children is the ideal of some standard of appropriate involvement that the mother has breached. Although, formally, the term "enmeshment" is not supposed to connote dysfunction, in practice, labeling an interaction as enmeshed immediately suggests to many family therapists that this family structure needs to be modified. Until recently, this almost always entailed disengagement of the mother.

As there are no clear concrete operational definitions of clinical evaluative terms, the label "enmeshment" is based on the qualitative assessment of the family therapists. This assessment often rests on definitions of the "healthy" or "normal" self idealized in our culture as one who is relatively autonomous, achieves differentiation from relational systems, and utilizes reason and intellect rather than feeling and intuition (Broverman et al., 1970). The single standard rests on the assumption that men and women experience the self in similar ways. Given this standard, certain characteristics of mothering (such as responsiveness, sensitivity to others, and nurturance) are often assessed pejoratively.

But recent theoretical work by feminists proposes that women and men experience the self and interact in relationships in qualitatively different ways, which has major implications for how we assess adaptive functioning at both the individual and systems levels (Chodorow, 1978; Dinnerstein, 1986; Gilligan, 1982; Jordan, 1983; Miller, 1976; 1984; Rubin, 1983; Stiver, 1984; Surrey, 1983, 1984). These theorists do not assume that female development follows the same model as that of males. Instead, each sex tends to follow a different developmental path that has its own distinctive strengths and potential liabilities. This assumption rests on analyses of gender and family relationships. The self develops differently for boys and girls because of their different gendered relationships with their primary caretaker—who, in our society, is almost always a sole woman. Given gender differences between boys and mothers, sons' experiences of self are usually based on qualities of differentiation, separation, and autonomy.

In contrast, women's primary experience of self is relational, based on mothers' and daughters' both being female. The female self develops and is validated through reciprocal processes of understanding and empathy, in which mutual connectedness and empowering the other lead to further articulation of the self. Within this context, women develop complex interpersonal skills, such as highly developed cognitive and emtional capacities that facilitate their sensitivity to the emotional nuances and needs of others. This requires a strong sense of self that relies on emotion and reason and is characterized by flexible self/other boundaries, permitting intense closeness or caring distance, depending on the momentary and long-term needs of the other and/or on the situational context.

From this frame of reference, individual growth for women neither requires diluting intense relationships nor disconnecting from the system—as intense and pervasive interpersonal connectedness is not by definition dysfunctional. This is not to suggest that mothers' functioning should never be tampered with, but it demands that women's interactions with families first be understood in a nonpathological frame of reference (Bograd, 1987b; Layton, 1984). If men and women have qualitatively different experiences of selfhood, then assessing women by biased cultural standards leads to pathologizing women's preferred interactional styles—a phenomenon exacerbated by the fact that family therapy models lack a positive language of connection and intimacy (Bernal & Ysern, 1985; Bograd, 1987b; Luepnitz, 1984; Women's Project, 1982; Wynne & Wynne, 1986).

Although these beginning reformulations may help family therapists to conceptualize mothers' functioning in less derogatory and blaming ways, they are not an end in and of themselves. The glorification of women's capacities, in reaction to how women's prototypical styles of relating are typically semantically denigrated, poorly characterizes the dynamic quality of individuals and systems. Also, certain female capacities have developed, not only in the familial context of mothers and daughters, but in the social context of women's oppression. It is important to value women's capacities, but we must not lose sight of how they enable women to survive in contexts of relative powerlessness or covert coercion. As family therapists, assessments of the adaptiveness of women's preferred interactional styles (be they positive or negative) will be overly simplistic unless we examine women's relationships with family members in the larger social and political contexts of relationships in a patriarchal society. Furthermore, as women and men share many relational qualities, it is erroneous to highlight extreme prototypical exemplars of male/female differences on the basis of biological reality of gender. This can caricature the complexity of male and female experiences as they are structured and constrained by the current social context of inequality (Goldner, 1985a; Hare-Mustin, 1987; Hare-Mustin & Marecek, 1986; Hatfield, 1986; Miller, 1976).

Pejoratively Labeling "Deviant" Family Forms

The use of biased standards leading to scapegoating mothers also occurs when pathology is attributed to families that differ from or "deviate" from normative contemporary family structure. Although most family therapists state that a variety of family forms are healthy, adaptive, and functional, in practice many clinicians adhere to standards that reflect the structures and processes of the middle-class White family (Goldner, 1985a; Gurman & Klein, 1984). When families do not meet these standards, family therapists may critically highlight certain family dimensions in ways that are detrimental to women or may construct interventions that reflect and maintain traditional family roles that are oppressive to all family members, but particularly to women.

For example, in our society, a social norm and a cultural ideal are that wives do not surpass their husbands' educational or financial achievements. When faced with a family in which the woman is a professional and the husband a blue-collar worker, family therapists sometimes encode this social reality with the label "overfunctioning woman/underfunctioning man." This quickly redefines the woman's strengths and resources in negative ways and suggests that she "keeps" her husband in a maladaptive role. Even if a couple identifies status differences as problematic to their marriage, this may be more related to how outside people respond to the couple given social beliefs about "normal" marriages, than to any inherent difficulties between the couple simply because of status differences. Thus, it is an open question as to whether a woman's surpassing her husband on some dimension is empirically linked to family problems, whether it is an intrafamilial issue or related to the family/society interface, or whether it is taken as pathogenic simply because it breeches a social norm as well as taken-for-granted assumptions about appropriate roles of men and women in families.

Inaccurate Descriptions of Family Life

Clinical use of ideals of family functioning that are often based on interpersonal processes and structures valued by the dominant White middle class can also lead to biased or incorrect assessments of the adaptive and functional qualities of women and families that exist in different racial, ethnic, or class contexts.

Yet, even when family therapists employ more sensitivity in assessments of family functioning, cultural ideals may not accurately reflect the actual experiences of men and women in families (Eichenbaum & Orbach, 1983; James, 1985). For example, family therapists often tend to approach families with notions of appropriate interpersonal connection and distance, often presupposing that adult children should be relatively detached from parents, especially their mothers. In our society, it is often assumed that the adult children want and need this distance, and that it is the mother who resists it. Yet empirical evidence suggests that the reality is different from the cultural stereotype: exchange of resources, provision of assistance, and continuity of interpersonal connection exist across generations more commonly than is recognized, and mothers sometimes wish for more distance than their adult children desire (Cohler & Geyer, 1982). But if family therapists simply assume that mothers have difficulty separating from adult children since this is part of our taken-for-granted cultural knowledge about family life, it can lead to inaccurate assessments of what is actually going on in the family, to distorted descriptions of family life, or to interventions that do not correctly address the needs of family members—especially those of mothers.

Privatization of Family
Ignoring Mothers' Socially Structured Centrality

Most family therapists do not intend to blame mothers in a personal way or to isolate them as unilinear determinants of pathology. Instead, family therapists try to remain at the level of structure and interaction. For example, as an abstract theoretical term, enmeshment denotes a specific constellation of transactional sequences that deviate from normal family processes in ways that lead to symptomatic behavior. But if the structures and processes currently labeled enmeshment are standard features of the typical contemporary family, then it is erroneous to label them as dysfunctional. A major feature of family life that family therapists have not yet adequately accounted for, although they quickly label it pathogenic, is the consistent centrality of the mother's role. Given that the centrality of mothers is a socially structured fact of almost every family constellation, with or without dysfunction, then it must be questioned whether family therapists are adequately identifying the sources of family problems.

Because of the theoretical decision to focus primarily on intrafamilial life, family therapists approach each family as a novel interpersonal event. Such an analysis can beautifully illuminate the internal workings of the family, but it ignores that family structure does not evolve by chance (Goldner, 1985a, 1985c; James & McIntyre, 1983). It is no coincidence that, in most families, women are very involved in domestic life and intensely attuned to the emotional nuances of family relationships. These structures and patterns are not created de novo in each family, but result from the socially structured and predetermined interrelationships of men and women as a class (Gillespie, 1981). The contemporary family form is structured in ways that ensure the centrality and overinvolvement of women in families and the relatively more peripheral and instrumental orientation of men (James & McIntyre, 1983; Goldner, 1985a, 1985c).

Following the industrial revolution, the private and public domains became separate but not equal. With the sexual division of labor, women were relegated to the home to provide the devalued but socially necessary resources of nurturance and caretaking. The mother's identity became linked, in practice and in ideology, to the physical and psychological well-being of her family. The relatively new social structure of the nuclear family isolated the mother from peers and so intensified her connection to family members. Paradoxically, although women appear powerful in families, they often lack real control over family life, which is held by the husband with his access to social and economic resources. Even in families where the mother wields control over major decisions about domestic life, her intrafamilial power often exists in stark contrast to her relatively disempowered status in extrafamilial life. In fact, many women focus their energies solely on the family as it is one of the few socially sanctioned domains in which women can assert themselves.

The structural segregation and unequal power relationships of men and women are supported and rationalized through culturally constructed ideologies of the monolithic harmonious family with a woman at its core (Goldner, 1985a, 1985c; Imber-Black, 1982; Oakley, 1976; Shorter, 1982; Thorne & Yalom, 1982). Within this context of the socially constructed centrality of mothers, women are doomed to failure and subsequent blame. The contemporary family form requires mothers to perform "crazy" functions (Poster, 1978). In a position of almost total responsibility, she often wields little authority in contrast to her husband. When she is accorded power and uses it strongly, this role is often regarded ambivalently at best. At the same time that the mother is blamed for being too controlling of the lives of family members, she is also blamed for any difficulties. As mothers are by social definition at the vulnerable center of the family, any facet of their personalities or behaviors is exposed and available to criticism. Such scrutiny, coupled with cultural ideals of motherhood and the socially structured centrality of women in families, can lead to scapegoating mothers—especially if family therapists forget that the mother "is flawed simply because she is a unique individual with a characteristic style that inevitably has its limitations" (Goldner, 1985a, p. 40).

Neglect of Social and Material Constraints

In his brilliant exegesis of how people know, Bateson (1972) identified the conceptual error of creating an illusory explanation for a given state of affairs that confuses resulting consequences with contributing factors. For example, "Why do people sleep?" "Because of the dormitive principle." Similarly, pioneers of family therapy argued that psychoanalytic theories of the "masochistic woman" mistakenly attributed consequences of a complex interactional sequence to invisible psychic factors existing inside of the individual woman. Yet, paradoxically, family therapists themselves have tended virtually to ignore fundamental social and material realities that may strongly influence and constrain women's behaviors in families (Bograd, 1984, 1986a, 1986b, in press; Goldner, 1985a, 1985c; James & McIntyre, 1983; Lerner, 1983; Margolin et al, 1983; Taggart, 1985).

Family reductionism (Bernal & Ysern, 1986) leads to scapegoating mothers by placing the genesis of personal problems within the woman or family system when they are more properly attributable to situational or cultural factors (American Psychological Association, 1978; Brodsky & Holroyd, 1981; Weiner & Boss, 1985). If this is so, then systemic formulations focusing on transactional sequences may not be the most parsimonious or appropriate level of analysis and may contribute to scapegoating women (Sturdivant, 1980). This will be examined in the areas of material inequality between men and women, women and racism, and assessment of outcome.

Material Inequality Between Men and Women

Feminists strongly argue that a basic source of family problems is the material inequality between men and women in families that reflects and reinforces the gender-based distribution of power in the larger culture. Many of the behaviors of women in families—including so-called passivity, overinvolvement, intrusiveness, and dependency—result when women as a class are systematically blocked from equal access to education, employment, remuneration, and status (Ferree, 1984; Gillespie, 1971; Goldner, 1985c). Ample empirical evidence suggests that marriage as an institution is detrimental to the mental health of women and beneficial to that of men. Although employed women can have more power over some decisions than unemployed wives, this fact often does not reduce their active involvement in housework and child care. Upon divorce, sexual demographics reveal that the economic well-being for women drops precipitously whereas that of their ex-husbands increases (Goldner, 1985a). Although older divorced women often cannot pursue motherhood in subsequent relationships, men often remarry younger women who can provide them with children. Although men may be dependent on women (and not necessarily their wives), women are dependent on their husbands for economic support, status, and social legitimacy (Szinovacz, 1984). Even couples who reject traditional stereotypic roles may find that individual choice is not sufficient when faced with the demands of the marketplace.

For example, a couple enters treatment because of marital stress. The wife demands that the husband spend more quality time with her. The husband complains that the wife is too dependent on him, although she is assertive in her managerial role in a local business. Although both spouses adhere to values that each partner should be free fully to develop his or her personal and professional life, they were faced with a difficult decision. The husband was offered a promotion in his company in a branch that would require relocation to a different state. The wife is deeply saddened that she must leave family and friends, but she does not feel she can stand in the way of her husband's promotion, as her own job lacks opportunities for further professional and financial advancement. Although the husband understands his wife's wishes to maintain close relationships with family and friends, both partners accept the patriarchal culture's tendency to value individual development over loyalty to strong intimate connections. As the wife faces increased isolation within her nuclear family given the impending move, she becomes fearful of confronting her husband and of compromising her closeness with him. Her seeming passivity, from another frame of reference, is her effort to maintain a valued relationship. She tearfully recounts her fear that her husband will leave her and easily find a replacement, while she struggles to support herself and her children alone.

As the complex context of this couple's distress becomes evident, it is obvious that it is comprised of many interacting levels, including male/female individual differences, interpersonal dynamics, family values, cultural standards of success, economic necessity, and differential availability of professional, social, and financial resources for men and women. Many family therapists, with their primary focus on intrafamilial life, tend to ignore these dimensions. Without awareness of such dimensions, it is easy for family therapists to blame the wife for her neediness, her selfishness, her overdependence on her family of origin, and her overinvolvement with her nuclear family.

Women and Racism

The danger of the not-so-benign neglect of social and material constraints becomes even more obvious when we consider the interaction of sexism and racism (Pinderhughes, 1986). In analyzing racial issues, people often identify a problem, note existing differences between Blacks and Whites, and then label these differences as the original cause of the problem (Ryan, 1971). For example, before the civil rights movements, the documented unemployment of Blacks and their seeming lack of motivation to find work were attributed to an intrinsic laziness in the Black personality, rather than to the social conditions that spawned hopelessness and lethargy and that actively prevented Blacks from finding meaningful gainful employment. Even more liberal theorists, who analyzed Black/White interactions, tended to believe that it was possible for Blacks to modify their situation to take part in the dominant culture. It was not until the civil rights movement that the social structure itself was challenged.

Similarly, when Black women (who are usually the centers of an extended family) turn for help, they are often blamed for needing assistance at all. The clinical formulations of caregivers suggest that these women have castrated their partners, and so are blamed for failures of the social system. Minority women are asked to nurture and support family members while functioning in a social context that denies them valued social status and access to virtually all material resources. Social constraints make it difficult, if not impossible, for them to execute therapeutic tasks, as racism isolates the family from mainstream support systems. Therapists often view the Black mother as pathological, rather than highlighting her often fierce determination to provide for her family against all odds. Her adaptive strategies, which may become exaggerated under stress, are clinically redefined as factors contributing to family conflict and breakdown (Pinderhughes, 1986). Ignoring the social and material constraints on the Black woman and her family can lead family therapists erroneously to label the mother "resistant" which personally blames the individual mother.

Assessment of Outcome

Some family therapists suggest that it is not necessary to focus on extrafamilial factors because interventions that focus on intrafamilial functioning lead, in most cases, to effective and efficient change that benefit both men and women in families. Taffel (1986) challenges these assumptionss by suggesting that family gender arrangements and social structural variables limit the extent and nature of change possible through conventional family therapy approaches and techniques. If these arrangements and variables are not taken into account, then women in families can be blamed for factors beyond their personal control or family structures can be sustained that are ultimately detrimental to the wife and mother.

A structural family therapist, Taffel (1986) became intrigued by his clinical finding that many couples seemed to reach a plateau in their ability to change, in spite of their commitment to therapy and regardless of a wide range of effective structural techniques employed by the therapist. Because of his interest in feminist perspectives on family therapy, Taffel began to wonder whether the couple system's flexibility was constrained by extrafamilial social factors. To examine this, he correlated the relationship of outcome of 35 cases with several criteria emphasized by feminists as critical to understanding women's personal freedom in family life. He found that lack of therapeutic success correlated with the woman having a greater number of children of younger age at home, with lowered economic viability of the woman, and with lack of empathic support by her husband. Even compliant clients who were dedicated to treatment and had achieved some measure of improvement were unable to create "appropriate boundaries" or "a proper executive hierarchy" unless certain material resources were available to the wife. For example, a husband and a wife could not negotiate as equals about disciplining children when the husband retained unilateral financial control that gave him real power in the family as well as accorded him higher respect from other family members.

Through ignoring these social realities, family therapists and larger helping systems view family dysfunction from a too-narrow focus, which leads to blaming women (Imber-Black, 1986). When faced with an impasse in treatment, family therapists often refer to internal motivation of the woman (such as her inability to disengage from family members) or to resistance within the couple or family system. Attention to extrafamilial social and material factors suggests that the degree of personal freedom of men and women in families is not identical and that the family's potential for change at any given time may be related more to the family/society interface than to personal motivation or to intrafamilial factors. From this perspective, it is erroneous and dangerous to blame women who remain in unfulfilling relationships or who are willing to make major self-sacrifices for the well-being of other family members. These women may be following the dictates of rational choice given limited social and economic options, rather than blindly reacting to interactional patterns. Through ignoring material and social constraints on family life, family therapists reduce social powerlessness to intrafamilial transactional logic and confuse subordination of women as a class with personal enmeshment or overdependency.

Employment of Oversimplified Systems Models
Power, Gender, and Inequality

Although it is evident that family therapists unthinkingly assimilate misogynistic assumptions into clinical formulations and often minimize the impact of social and material forces on family life, these errors are not simply the result of careless thinking. Instead, systems concepts and terminology are based on oversimplified models of human social systems that preclude attending to certain information and so obscure aspects of power and inequality (Goldner, 1985c; James & McIntyre, 1983). The field of family therapy has been marked by the development of increasingly sophisticated and radical conceptual models, each of which suggests new ways of thinking about human interaction and family life. Although the significantly distinctive theoretical premises of the variety of systems models lead to important clinical differences—including how the therapists position themselves, how outcome is assessed, and the nature of intervention strategies—no model adequately addresses issues of gender and power. This, in and of itself, leads to blaming women.

Take, as an example, the fundamental systems construct of complementarity, which derives from early systems models based on the metaphor of families as organizations governed by homeostatic mechanisms. Complementarity means that each family member serves a functionally equivalent role in maintaining family structures and processes. Complementarity, by definition, assumes that parts are interchangeable, separate but equal. In this framework, the battered woman, the wife of an alcoholic, and the mother of a daughter who has been sexually abused by her father are all held as functionally accountable for the incidents as are the men themselves (Bepko, 1986; Bograd, 1984, 1986a, 1986c). These extreme examples are amplifications of how women are often blamed for more subtle, ordinary, less overtly coercive dysfunctional family patterns. Unless the power differential between husband and wife is acknowledged, the detrimental aspects of focusing primarily on the woman will not be correctly identified. As one seasoned feminist therapist cautioned a trainee who was scapegoating an emotional woman as her rational husband calmly sat by, "This couple is a steamroller and a doormat. Why are you jumping up and down on the doormat?" (Simon, 1984).

Although complementarity assumes that all family members have equal power to shape transactional patterns, there is no real parity between men and women in families (Women's Project in Family Therapy, 1982; Goldner, 1985a). This heuristic and clinically useful construct ignores the social origins of male/female relationships, the real material and symbolic power differential between men and women, and how the broader social context constrains their interactions. Based on formulations of complementary interactions, family therapists often guide each spouse to make equal changes that basically maintain the preexisting power balance between them—which, in the majority of families, is characterized by male dominance (Jacobson, 1983; Margolin et al, 1983). For example, a family therapist helps a couple to negotiate an agreement whereby the husband does the dishes every night and the wife is more physically affectionate with him on his arrival home from work. This seemingly innocent arrangement does not challenge the assumption that it is acceptable for a wife to trade off sexual favors for the husband's participation in domestic life. A more radical intervention, based on the assessment that the wife lacks marital power, would require the husband to make major compromises without his wife doing so as well.

Early family systems models that provided the basis for structural and strategic family therapies account for power and hierarchy between generations but rarely address the hierarchical relations between men and women in families. Because of this, structural family therapists often do not question the wisdom of repositioning family members into relatively traditional roles. Since conventional family roles are often detrimental to women, this can maintain the woman's personal stress and conflict, even while other family members become less symptomatic. In contrast, strategic family therapists often carefully analyze incongruous power hierarchies between husbands and wives. Yet, because of their theoretical focus on symptom relief, they can successfully accomplish short-term clinical goals without addressing long-standing family structures oppressive to women.

The new epistemology of systemic models seems to have the potential for addressing how the family as a social institution is constrained and shaped by the larger social system in ways detrimental to women. Yet, both because of its theoretical axioms and because of how they are interpreted and employed by its adherents, these newer systems models currently preclude adequate appraisal of women's position in families (MacKinnon & Miller, 1987; Taggart, 1985). For example, power itself is dismissed as a linear construct and as a theoretically unimportant, useless, or counterproductive way of punctuating reality. Since the newer evolutionary models do not rely on earlier notions of homeostasis and functional equivalence, systemic therapists do not explicitly hold women accountable for their participation in dysfunctional patterns. Instead, their self-consciously neutral stance implicates women by default (MacKinnon & Miller, 1987; Taggart, 1985).

This neutrality also applies to how the systemic therapist assesses outcome. Given their definitions about the nature of systems, systemic therapists do not believe they can know the best or ideal structure for any given family or that they are capable of unilaterally directing the people toward a healthier family form. Instead, systemic therapists hold to the theoretical axiom that families are autonomous systems that can utilize new information or perceptual categories to reorganize at higher levels of organization and adaptability. This more adaptive organization cannot be predicted by the therapist, who should remain neutral as to the end state achieved by the family. Yet, paradoxically, although systemic therapists give more credence to the social context of family life, they ignore how the patriarchal context strongly shapes and constrains the family structures that evolve from systemic interventions. In other words, families are not fully voluntary systems that can choose solutions that equally serve the interests of all family members. With the current powerful social forces that strongly constrain family life and the historical structures of families as social institutions, it is more likely that families will reorganize in ways that continue to be detrimental to mothers and wives (MacKinnon & Miller, 1987).

As feminists have critically examined the epistemological foundations of current family therapy models and found that they do not adequately address dimensions of power, gender, and inequality, other family therapists have charged that feminists are returning to outdated linear thinking. But 20 years ago, Buckley (1967) suggested that simple models from the natural sciences cannot adequately capture the complex, fluid, multifaceted nature of human systems (see also Bernal & Ysern, 1986; Goldner, 1985a, 1985c; James & McIntyre,

1983). Human systems may be poorly characterized through models that assume balanced, cooperative, mutually interactive functioning in order to achieve goals equally beneficial for all participants (Bogdan, 1986; Goldner, 1985c; Szinowicz, 1984). Regardless of the numerous significant differences among current family systems models, all of them still fail to account for how some systems variables have primacy or priority over others.

In contrast, a different *systems* model suggests that family life is composed of conflicting, although overlapping, needs of various subsystems attributable to patterned strain, disorder, or conflict that are an integral part of the system and that reflect varying degrees of connectedness to the system (Buckley, 1967; Goldner, 1985a, 1985c). The examination of the mechanisms that maintain systems in which one part governs or has primacy over another in adaptive and maladaptive ways leads to questions of power, ideology, and vested interest (Bernal & Ysern, 1986; Buckley, 1967). Feminists have added that a crucial sociocultural factor influencing the predictable and patterned nature of such systems is that of gender. From this perspective, models that rest either on assumptions of harmonious mutual interactionism or on polarities such as victim/victimizer or powerful/powerless are overly simplistic and inadequate (Buckley, 1967; Goldner, 1985a, 1985c).

CONCLUDING COMMENTS

Although therapists may deny that they make conceptual and technical errors that lead to widespread scapegoating of mothers, empirical evidence suggests that they do consistently focus on the mother as a major causal determinant of family dysfunction. In a review of 125 clinical articles from nine mental health and family therapy journals during 1970-1982 (Caplan, 1986; Caplan & Hall-McCorquodale, 1985a, 1985b), therapists held mothers responsible for 72 different kinds of psychological disorders; attributed children's pathology to mothers' behaviors 82 percent of the time and to fathers 43 percent (or at the level of chance); and applied judgmental terms to mothers in 74 percent of the articles and to fathers in 41 percent. Father absence or peripherality was noted but not connected to the pathology in 24 percent of the articles, but in only 2 percent of the articles was mothers' noninvolvement NOT labeled contributory to pathology. Over one-fourth of the articles evaluated deviation from traditional sex roles and family structure as pathogenic; nontraditional divisions of label were *never* regarded as normal or healthy.

Through elucidating the conceptual errors that promote mother-blaming in family therapy, it is hoped that clinicians will bring greater sensitivity to bear on their construction of systemic formulations. These formulations both reflect and shape our attitudes, beliefs, and values about men, women, and family life, and provide the ground for clinical interventions that have profound significance for the well-being of our clients. But sensitivity is not enough. Although many family therapy constructs and principles are not sexist in definition but misused in practice, others rest on questionable assumptions about the nature of intimate human systems. This requires the reconstruction of certain fundamental systems terms and the development of new models that can better illuminate the contradictions and consequences at the interfaces of gender, power, the family, and society. It cannot be forgotten that, as social beings, we can only draw upon culturally constructed assumptions about human nature, health, and pathology, and the meaning of intimate relationships. The gendered conceptual categories of the dominant cultural ideology are such a taken-for-granted context of our lives that men and women, feminists and nonfeminists, easily fall prey to their misogynistic predisposition.

REFERENCES

American Psychological Association. (1975). Report of the task force on sex bias and sex role stereotyping in psychotherapeutic practice. *American Psychologist, 30,* 1169–1175.

Ault-Riche, M., (Ed.). (1986). *Women and family therapy.* Rockville, Md.: Aspen Systems Corp.

Bateson, G. (1972). *Steps to an ecology of mind.* New York: Ballantine Books.

Bepko, C. (1986). Alcoholism as oppression: The dilemma of the woman in the alcoholic system. In M. Ault-Riche (Ed.), *Women and family therapy,* (pp. 64–77). Rockville, Md.: Aspen Systems Corp.

Bernal, G., & Ysern, E. (1986). Family therapy and ideology. *Journal of Marital and Family Therapy, 12,* 129–135.

Bogdan, J. (1986). Do families really need problems?: Why am I not a functionalist. *Family Therapy Networker, 10,* 30–35, 67–69.

Bograd, M. (1984). Family systems approaches to wife battering: A feminist critique. *American Journal of Orthopsychiatry, 54,* 558–568.

Bograd, M. (1986a). A feminist examination of family systems models of violence against women in the family. In M. Ault-Riche (Ed.), *Women and family therapy* (pp. 34–50). Rockville, Md.: Aspen Systems Corp.

Bograd, M. (1986b). A feminist examination of family therapy: What is women's place? In D. Howard (Ed.), *The dynamics of feminist therapy* (pp. 95–106). New York: Haworth Press.

Bograd, M. (1986c). Holding the line: Confronting the abusive partner. *Family Therapy Networker, 10,* 44–47.

Bograd, M. (1987). Enmeshment, fusion or relatedness?: A conceptual analysis. *Journal of Psychotherapy and the Family, 3,* 65–80.

Bograd, M. (in press). Feminist perspectives on family systems theory: Power, gender and the family. In M. Douglas, & L. Walker (Eds.), *Feminist psychotherapies: Integration of therapeutic and feminist systems.* Norwood, NJ: Ablex Publishing.

Brodsky, A., & Holroyd, J. (1981). Report of the task force on sex bias and sex-role stereotyping in psychotherapeutic practice. In E. Howell & M. Bayes, (Eds.), *Women and mental health.* New York: Basic Books.

Broverman, I., Broverman, D., Clarkson, F., Rosenkrantz, P., & Vogel, S. (1970). Sex-role stereotypes and clinical judgments of mental health. *Journal of Consulting and Clinical Psychology, 23,* 1–7.

Buckley, W. (1967). *Sociology and modern systems theory.* Englewood Cliffs, NJ: Prentice-Hall.

Caplan, P. (1986). Take the blame off mother. *Psychology Today, 20,* 70–71.

Caplan, P., & Hall-McCorquodale, I. (1985a). Mother blaming in major clinical journals. *American Journal of Orthopsychiatry, 55,* 345–353.

Caplan, P., & Hall-McCorquodale, I. (1985b). The scapegoating of mothers: A call for change. *American Journal of Orthopsychiatry, 55,* 610–613.

Chodorow, N. (1978). *The reproduction of mothering: Psychoanalysis and the sociology of gender*. Berkeley: University of California Press.

Chodorow, N., & Contratto, S. (1982). The fantasy of the perfect mother. In B. Thorne & M. Yalom (Eds.), *Rethinking the family: Some feminist questions*. New York: Longman.

Cohler, B., & Geyer, S. (1982). Psychological autonomy and interdependence within the family. In F. Walsh (Ed.), *Normal family processes*. New York: Guilford Press.

Dinnerstein, D. (1976). *The mermaid and the minotaur: Sexual arrangements and human malaise*. New York: Harper & Row.

Eichenbaum, L., & Orbach, S. (1983). *What do women want: Exploding the myth of dependency*. New York: Coward-McCann.

Ferree, M. (1984). The view from below: Women's employment and gender equality in working class families. In B. Hess & M. Sussman (Eds.), *Women and the family: Two decades of change*. New York: Haworth Press.

Gillespie, D. (1971). Who has the power: The marital struggle. *Journal of Marriage and the Family*, 33, 445–458.

Gilligan, C. (1982). *In a different voice: Psychological theory and women's development*. Cambridge, Mass.: Harvard University Press.

Goldner, V. (1985a). Feminism and family therapy. *Family Process*, 24, 31–47.

Goldner, V. (1985b). The feminist critique: Its influence on the future of family therapy. Keynote presented at Harvard Medical School Continuing Education Department conference, "What Works in Family Therapy?," Cambridge, Mass.

Goldner, V. (1985c). Warning: Family therapy may be hazardous to your health. *Family Therapy Networker*, 9, 18–23.

Gurman, A., & Klein, M. (1980). Marital and family conflicts. In A. Brodsky & R. Hare-Mustin (Eds.)., *Women and psychotherapy*. New York: Guilford Press.

Gurman, A., & Klein, M. (1984). Marriage and the family: An unconscious male bias in behavioral treatment. In E. Blechman (Ed.), *Behavior modification with women*. New York: Guilford Press.

Hare-Mustin, R. (1978). A feminist approach to family therapy. *Family Process*, 17, 181–194.

Hare-Mustin, R. (1980). Family therapy may be dangerous for your health. *Professional Psychology*, 11, 935–938.

Hare-Mustin, R. (1987). The problem of gender in family therapy theory. *Family Process*, 26, 15–27.

Hare-Mustin, R., & Lamb, S. (1984). Family counselors' attitudes toward women and motherhood: A new cohort. *Journal of Marriage and the Family*, 10, 419–421.

Hare-Mustin, R., & Maracek, J. (1986). Autonomy and gender: Some questions for therapists. *Psychotherapy*, 23, 205–212.

Hatfield, A. (1986). Semantic barriers to family and professional collaboration. *Schizophrenia Bulletin*, 12, 325–336.

Imber-Black, E. (1986). Women, families and larger systems. In M. Ault-Riche (Ed.), *Women and family therapy* (pp. 25–33). Rockville, Md.: Aspen Systems Corp.

Jacobson, N. (1983). Beyond empiricism: The politics of marital therapy. *American Journal of Family Therapy*, 11, 11–24.

James, K. (1985). Breaking the chains of gender: Family therapy's position? *Australian Journal of Family Therapy*, 5, 241–248.

James, K., & McIntyre, D. (1983). The reproduction of families: The social role of family therapy? *Journal of Marital and Family Therapy*, 9, 119–129.

Jordan, J. (1983). Empathy and the mother-daughter relationship. *Work in Progress, No. 82–02*. Wellesley, Mass.: Stone Center Working Papers Series.

Joslyn, B. (1982). Shifting sex roles: The silence of the family therapy literature. *Clinical Social Work Journal*, 10, 39–51.

Layton, M. (1984). Tipping the therapeutic scales—Masculine, feminine, or neuter? *Family Therapy Networker*, 8, 20–27.

Lerner, H. (1983). Female dependency in context: Some theoretical and technical considerations. *American Journal of Orthopsychiatry*, 53, 697–705.

Libow, J., Raskin, P., & Caust, B. (1982). Feminist and family systems therapy: Are they irreconcilable? *American Journal of Family Therapy*, 3, 3–12.

Luepnitz, D. (1984). Cybernetic baroque: The hi-tech talk of family therapy. *Family Therapy Networker*, 8, 37–41.

MacKinnon, L., & Miller, D. (1987). The new epistemology and the Milan approach: Feminist and sociopolitical considerations. *Journal of Marital and Family Therapy*, 13, 139–155.

Margolin, G., Fernandes, V., Talovic, S., & Onorato, R. (1983). Sex role considerations and behavioral marital therapy: Equal does not mean identical. *Journal of Marital and Family Therapy*, 9, 131–145.

Miller, J. (1976). *Toward a new psychology of women*. Boston: Beacon Press.

Miller, J. (1984). The development of women's sense of self. *Work in Progress*. Wellesley, Mass.: Stone Center Working Papers Series.

Minuchin, S. (1974). *Families and family therapy*. Cambridge, Mass.: Harvard University Press.

Minuchin, S., & Fishman, C. (1981). *Family therapy techniques*. Cambridge, Mass.: Harvard University Press.

Oakley, A. (1976). *Woman's work: The housewife, past and present*. New York: Vintage Books.

Osborne, K. (1983). Women in families: Feminist therapy and family systems. *Journal of Family Therapy*, 5, 1–10.

Pinderhughes, E. (1986). Minority women: A nodal position in the functioning of the social system. In M. Ault-Riche (Ed.), *Women and family therapy* (pp. 51–63). Rockville, Md.: Aspen Systems Corp.

Poster, M. (1978). *Critical theory of the family*. New York: Seabury Press.

Rich, A. (1976). *Of women born: Motherhood as experience and institution*. New York: Norton.

Rubin, L. (1983). *Intimate strangers: Men and women together*. New York: Harper & Row.

Ryan, W. (1971). *Blaming the victim*. New York: Pantheon Books.

Seiden, A. (1976). Overview: Research on the psychology of women. (No. 2: Women in families, work and psychotherapy.) *American Journal of Psychiatry*, 113, 1111–1123.

Sherman, J. (1980). Therapist attitudes and sex-role stereotyping. In A. Brodsky & R. Hare-Mustin (Eds.), *Women and psychotherapy: An assessment of research and practice*. New York: Guilford Press.

Shorter, E. (1975). *The making of the modern family*. New York: Basic Books.

Simon, R. (1984). From ideology to practice: The women's project in family therapy. *Family Therapy Networker*, 8, 28–40.

Spender, D. (1980). *Man made language*. Boston: Routledge & Kegan Paul.

Spiegel, D. (1982). Mothering, fathering and mental illness. In B. Thorne & M. Yalom (Eds.), *Rethinking the family: Some feminist questions* (pp. 95–110). New York: Longman.

Stiver, I. (1984). The meanings of "dependency" in female-male relationships. *Work in Progress, No. 83–07*. Wellesley, Mass: Stone Center Working Papers Series.

Sturdivant, S. (1980). *Therapy with women: A feminist philosophy of treatment*. New York: Springer.

Surrey, J. (1983). The relational self in women: Clinical implications. *Work in Progress, No. 82–02*. Wellesley, Mass.: Stone Center Working Papers Series.

Surrey, J. (1984). The self-in-relation: A theory of women's development. *Work in Progress, No. 84–02*. Wellesley, Mass.: Stone Center Working Papers Series.

Szinovacz, M. (1984). Changing family roles and interactions. In B. Hess & M. Sussman (Eds.), *Women and the family: Two decades of change*. New York: Haworth Press.

Taffel, R. (1986). Revolution/evolution: Feminism forces us to reconsider our expectations about dramatic cures. *Family Therapy Networker*, 10, 52–58.

Taggart, M. (1985). The feminist critique in epistemological perspective: Questions of context in family therapy. *Journal of Marital and Family Therapy*, 11, 113–126.

Weiner, J., & Boss, P. (1985). Exploring gender bias against women: Ethics for marriage and family therapy. *Counseling and Values*, 30, 9–23.

Women's Project in Family Therapy. (1982). Mothers and daughters. *Monograph Series, 1*.

Women's Project in Family Therapy. (1983). Mothers and sons, fathers and daughters. *Monograph Series, 2*.

Wynne, L., & Wynne, A. (1986). The quest for intimacy. *Journal of Marital and Family Therapy*, 12, 383–394.

5

EATING DISORDERS: A FEMINIST FAMILY THERAPY PERSPECTIVE[1]

Marsha Pravder Mirkin, Ph.D.

> The body holds meaning. A woman obsessed with the size of her body, wishing to make her breasts and thighs and hips and belly smaller and less apparent, may be expressing the fact that she feels uncomfortable being female in this culture.—Chernin, 1981, p. 2.

In a sudden, rising wave that has swept through high schools, colleges, and households across the country, eating disorders have reached epidemic proportions in Western society over the past 20 years. The vast majority of victims are female: 90-95 percent of anorexics and at least 87 percent of bulimics are women (Halmi et al., 1981). Given the magnitude of the problem, and the finding that eating disorders differentially affect women, three apparent questions emerge: (1) Why women? (2) Why now? (3) How can we, as mental health professionals, conceptualize this problem and intervene effectively?

This chapter addresses these questions by integrating feminist and structural family therapy concepts within the context of eating disorders. It is beyond the scope of this paper to discuss all the schools of thought concerning family therapy, eating disorders, and feminism. Therefore, the focus will be on structural family therapy, since the family therapy pioneering efforts in treating eating disorders, and some of the most successful outcomes, come from this conceptual framework. Although the primary focus of this chapter is on anorexia nervosa, and in particular as it affects female adolescents, the reader is invited to draw from these ideas to formulate how gender issues and context can further our understanding and treatment of other eating disorders (for a detailed discussion on these issues, see Chernin, 1981, 1985). A more comprehensive review of many of the theories and interventions with both anorexic and bulemic patients may be found in Garner and Garfinkel's (1985) and Emmett's (1985) edited works.

This chapter will address the questions outlined above by defining the major

[1]I'd like to thank Judith Libow, Ph.D., Pamela Raskin, Ph.D., and Catherine Steiner-Adair, Ed.D. for their thoughtful comments and suggested revisions for this chapter.

eating disorders and their prevalence in our society, and examining the structural family therapy conceptualization of anorexia, as well as the larger societal context and female developmental theory. A discussion of how structural family therapy can be integrated with a feminist perspective toward anorexic patients and a case example follow.

The position taken in this chapter is that eating disorders are a response to unrealistic and often conflictual expectations placed on women in this society (Chernin, 1981; Steiner-Adair, 1986; Surrey, 1984). Eating disorders symbolize the difficulties in being female in our society, including the belief that adulthood is marked by unbearable isolation. The loss of weight in anorexia is a metaphor for the loss of connection the anorexic believes is a necessary part of adulthood. It also represents an extreme reaction to society's demands for female thinness and suppression of female needs. The taking in of food, and then discarding it, is a metaphor for the bulimic's belief that relationships cannot be maintained. It is her symbolic effort to juggle the conflictual and impossible expectations set for women in this society. Structural family therapy, therefore, needs to be utilized in a manner that highlights the interface between eating disorders and the larger societal context. The therapeutic goal becomes one of demonstrating that there are gains possible in adulthood: that new types of interpersonal connections can develop and relationships do not have to be lost.

DEFINITION AND PREVALENCE

Anorexia Nervosa

According to the third edition of the *Diagnostic and Statistical Manual of Mental Disorders* (DSM-III) (1980), anorexia nervosa is characterized by self-starvation, with a weight loss of 25 percent of body weight (or, in the case of adolescents, a loss of 25 percent once the projected weight gain is taken into account). This is accompanied by an intense fear of becoming fat and a distorted body image in which the woman sees herself as fat even when she is emaciated. The anorexic refuses to maintain normal body weight, often excessively exercises, and typically invokes rituals around food. Vomiting, laxatives, and diuretics may be used to facilitate the weight loss. Peak ages of onset are 14 and 18, although anorexia can affect a person at any age. According to Anorexia Bulimia Care, a self-help organization in Massachusetts, 10 percent of cases are fatal.

The physical and medical disorders associated with anorexia are severe. The body tries to maintain functioning of the heart and brain by slowing down or stopping other vital processes. As a result, heart rate, body temperature, blood pressure, and respiratory rates are lowered; thyroid functioning is diminished; constipation occurs; and lanugo (newborn baby) hair appears to preserve body heat. The woman feels weak, tired, and faint. Her skin dries out, heart abnormalities may be seen, and electrolytes may become imbalanced. She becomes amenorrheic, and her body apears prepubescent. (Spack's chapter in Emmett's, 1985, volume provides further details.)

Behaviorally and socially, many of these women report becoming isolated, no longer choosing to be with friends, breaking up with boyfriends, withdrawing from husbands and other family members, losing interest in sex, feeling restless, and experiencing labile moods.

Studies indicate that as many as one in 100 16- to 18-year-old girls in British private schools are anorexic (Crisp, Palmer, & Kalucey, 1976). When all British girls of that age, rather than private school students only, are taken into account, the incidence was reported to be one in 250. Nylander (1971) reported similar results with a population of female Scandinavian adolescents: one in 150 were reported to be anorexic.

Bulimia

Bulimia is defined by DSM-III (1980) as episodic binge eating, fear of not being able to stop eating voluntarily, food consumption of high-calorie foods, and ending the binge by vomiting, abdominal pain, sleep, or social interruption. The bulimic often has depressed and self-deprecating feelings following the binge, which are relieved by purging.

As with anorexia, the medical effects of bulimia can be very serious. They include, but are not limited to, swollen salivary glands, facial swelling, scars on hands and fingers, hoarse voice, tooth decay, tooth enamel deterioration, seizures, electrolyte disorders, and injury to the esophagus (Spack, 1985).

Behaviorally and socially, it is often harder to distinguish bulimia than anorexia. Although the former may be more isolated because of her demand for privacy during binges and purges, the rest of the time she can be with friends, have a boyfriend, and, unless medically unstable, concentrate without being restless. She also generally maintains her body weight. There is a subgroup of bulimics who show symptoms of depression and such behaviors as stealing, drug and alcohol abuse, promiscuity, and gambling (Hudson, Hope, Jonas, & Yurgelun-Todd, 1983).

A sample of the studies on incidence of bulimia indicate that 13 percent of college students (Halmi, Falk, & Schwartz, 1981) and 11 percent of women under 21 (Cash et al, 1986) are bulimic.

Although DSM-III (1980) differentiates anorexia and bulimia, the two eating disorders are not always that clearly separable. In fact, it is reported that up to 50 percent of anorexics have bulimic episodes (Guttman, 1986). Incidence reports indicate that "bulimarexia," the name given to a pattern that combines anorexia and bulimia, affects from 3.8 percent (Stangler & Printz, 1980) to 13 percent (Halmi et al., 1981) of college students. Since the 1960s, the incidence of all eating disorders has been increasing (Theander, 1970).

STRUCTURAL FAMILY THERAPY

Given the frighteningly skeletal appearance of anorexics, as compared with the more robust presentation of most bulimics, it is not surprising that anorexia was the first eating disorder to be identified and studied in detail within the mental health field. The initial outcome results were disappointing. For example, Hilda Bruch, the mother of contemporary theory and treatment of anorexia, reported that only 40 percent of her sample of 10- to 17-year-olds who were ill for less than one and a half years recovered. Two of the adolescents died. When follow-up studies were initiated with the recovered group, it was reported that two children were in state hospitals, one was anorexic, and the others were "restricted" in their functioning (Bruch, 1973, in Minuchin, Rossman & Baker, 1978). Although some of the outcome studies yielded greater success, many clinicians began to view anorexia as a chronic illness (see Minuchin et al., 1978, for a summary of early outcome studies).

At this point, when the outcome was pessimistic and the incidence was rising, Minuchin, Rosman, and Baker published their ground-breaking work, *Psychosomatic Families* (1978). This critical volume is the basis of most family systems treatment of anorexia nervosa and bulimia today. Minuchin and his colleagues view anorexia in a systems framework. The locus of the problem is not seen as residing in the individual but as behavior symptomatic of a dysfunctional family structure. Minuchin labeled families with a member displaying psychosomatic symptoms as "psychosomatic families," and found similarities among anorexic, diabetic, and asthmatic families, as well as differences between these families and families presenting with nonpsychosomatic disorders.

Characteristics of Psychosomatic Families

Minuchin and his colleagues observed four characteristics shared by anorexic families: enmeshment, overprotectiveness, rigidity, and lack of conflict resolution.

Minuchin defines enmeshment as "an extreme form of proximity and intensity in family interactions" (1978, p. 30). A corollary of enmeshment is weak subsystem boundaries. In an enmeshed family, individuals get lost in the system. The excessive togetherness leads to a lack of privacy. For example, an anorexic family with which I worked did not close doors in the house, a commonly cited issue in families described as enmeshed. The parents' bedroom door was always open so that "we can hear if the girls need us for anything" (the girls were 13 and 16 years old). Neither the children nor the adults were permitted privacy. There were no clear boundaries around the couple subsystem. In another family, an 18-year-old daughter went out with her parents each Saturday night, and reportedly enjoyed spending the time with her parents and their friends. Nobody questioned this behavior, reflecting the weak boundaries around the couple subsystem. Both families had difficulty with differentiating between the spouse subsystem and the parent-child subsystem, and establishing boundaries accordingly.

A second characteristic of anorexic families is overprotection. There is tremendous concern within the family for each member's welfare, and extreme sensitivity to any signs of distress. According to Minuchin et al., overprotectiveness slows down the child's development of autonomy and hinders establishment of interests outside of the family. It should be noted that the overprotectiveness goes in both directions: parents to child as well as child to parents. These youngsters often feel a tremendous responsibility to care for and protect their parents. For example, a family with which I worked had a 14-year-old anorexic daughter, as well as 16- and 18-year-old sons. None of the teenagers were allowed to be out after dark, because of the "dangers that lurked in the night." This rule may have been appropriate several years earlier, but it made it difficult for adolescents to pursue interests outside of the family. Reciprocally, the 14-year-old would clean the entire house, so that her mother would not "tire herself out."

A third characteristic is labeled by Minuchin et al. as rigidity, or an effort to resist change and maintain the status quo. These families have difficulty traversing the waters of change that are an inherent part of the life cycle. If a certain issue—for example, negotiating a curfew that would result in coming home after dark—threatens to lead to change (i.e., movement from the child to adolescent phase of the life cycle), the status quo is preserved by not allowing the issue to surface. Thus, a mother of a 16-year-old continued to choose her anorexic daughter's clothing, a fact of life accepted and encouraged by her daughter, who would not go shopping without her mother.

The final characteristic, closely related to the third, is conflict avoidance. These families often present as not having any difficulties other than the one child's medical problems. Frequently, the family insists that "we don't get angry" or "we never fight." When family members begin to express conflict, a third member often attempts to intervene, thus diffusing or altering the conflict. The illness can serve to detour conflict for a couple: rather than focusing on their own conflict, the couple is united in its efforts to help the anorexic daughter. According to Minuchin et al. (1978), "The key factor supporting the particular symptom was the child's involvement in parental conflict" (p. 32). In a case illustrating this point (Mirkin, 1983), Mr. and Mrs. R. didn't socialize with each other or go out without their children. Their daughter Cathy's anorexia provided a way for them to unite in their mutual caring for their sick child, thus avoiding their own conflict and leaving it unresolved. It was only when the marital dyad was united with clear boundaries, a hierarchy was established so that the parents were in charge of the teenagers, and the family was able to negotiate change, that Cathy recovered from anorexia.

Minuchin observed that the anorexic family is typically child oriented, with parents vigilantly watching over and protecting the at-risk youngster, who learns to be hypervigilant toward herself and her parents: "The child develops as a keen observer of intrafamilial operations, dependent on parental assessment, and highly loyal to family values" (p. 59).

Anorexia becomes the "perfect symptom," given the characteristics described above. Even if the adolescent cannot begin to take control of her own life through age-appropriate independent activities, she can control her body and make it the arena for the battle for her independence. In this way, she is not betraying her parents: they can still protect her since, because of her illness, she still requires caretaking; conflict does not surface since the symptom is perceived as an illness rather than as rebellion; and the developmental status quo is maintained since the adolescent is able to maintain or revert to a prepubescent body.

Within the framework of the structural model, the focus of therapy is on changing the structure of the family system so that boundaries within the family are less diffuse and boundaries between the family and outside world are less rigid; that enmeshment and overprotectiveness are modified; and that conflict is recognized and addressed.

Minuchin's work, as well as many of the articles written after his book (cf., Mirkin, 1983; Todd, 1985), focus on adolescent anorexics. Clearly, this is a problem that also affects many adult women. These women often describe characteristics in their families of origin that parallel certain of the characteristics described by Minuchin, and at times are replayed with their husband and children.

Dynamics in Bulimic Families

In recent years, more attention has been paid to the problem of bulimia and to the characteristics of bulimic families. Root, Fallon, and Friedrich (1986) offer a typology of bulimic families. They posit three types—the perfect family, the overprotective family, and the chaotic family—and suggest that the symptom is developed in order to maintain the family homeostasis. They suggest that, regardless of type, all bulimic families have individual and subsystem boundary problems, believe that weight and appearance are critical factors, and have unequal power distribution within the family. Unlike anorexic women, many bulimics report substance abuse and sexual abuse within the family, which Root and her colleagues routinely include in their assessment of the bulimia. Further, these authors discuss bulimia within the sociocultural as well as family and developmental contexts.

Guttman (1985) reports that bulimic families tend to share the psychosomatic characteristics of anorexic families, especially the enmeshment and lack of differentiation. She states that these families can be intrusive and verbally abusive, and that generally one parent is aggressive while the other parent covertly supports the spouse. Schwartz, Barrett, and Saba (1985) agree that the interactional patterns found in anorexic families are evident in bulimic families. However, they found that the issues over which enmeshment, overprotectiveness, and so on, have been played out are related to the degree to which families consider themselves "Americanized" as compared with having a strong ethnic identity.

My own experience has been that although the characteristics of bulimic families can be very similar to those of anorexic families, there are also some substantial differences. There are some bulimic families who fit the anorexic mold of the "perfect family," where each family member appears to have succeeded in all that he or she has undertaken, and where each member relates that until the anorexic became ill, there were no conflicts or arguments within the family. The families tend to be enmeshed, overprotective, and rigid, and to avoid conflict.

More frequently, I have seen a very different pattern emerge. Many bulimic patients, and anorexics who have bulimic cycles, have reported that their prior life was not conflict-free. Just the opposite—many of these women were traumatized by events that left them feeling violated and not in control of their bodies or the rest of their personal world. The binge/purge cycle comes to represent the out-of-control nature of every aspect of the bulimic patient's life.

Many of these women report having been sexually abused before the onset of bulimia. The perpetrator varied: it could be a father, close relative, unknown male, or male friend. The type of abuse also varied, from fondling to rape. In each of these cases, the woman felt violated and experienced a situation in which she had no control over her body, where her protests were unheard, her assertive "no's" were unheeded.

Many of these women also reported feeling out of control because of substance abuse in the family. A pattern emerges where one parent (often the father) is an alcoholic, the other parent has difficulty acknowledging the alcoholism and/or dealing with it openly with the daughter, and the daughter finds her world to be out of control and unpredictable. She learns early on that her needs are unacceptable and unacknowledged, as the family revolves around the needs of the alcoholic father. Like other children of alcoholics, these daughters often feel responsible for the alcoholism in the family, and, therefore, for taking care of their alcoholic parent in the vain hope that this will win the parent's approval, if not abstinence. Other adolescents identify with the alcoholic parent by becoming substance abusers themselves. Both types of adolescents share an experience of the out-of-control family life, symbolized by the out-of control binge/purge cycles.

The third type of out-of-control pattern that is symbolized by bulimia is the chaotic family. No rules govern the behavior of the children. No rules govern how conflict is managed or how differences are negotiated. Upon first seeing these families, I feel that I am in a free-for-all, and my first step is often to get them to be silent and take turns speaking long enough for me to organize my own thoughts.

While anorexic patients often feel that they have no control over their lives because expectations are so high and deviation from these expectations is seen by the family as disloyal, bulimics often feel out of control because of too much disorder and unpredictability, because of contradictory or absent expectations. This is clearly a generalization, given the diversity among eating-disordered families as well as the overlap between anorexia and bulimia, but can be helpful in guiding treatment. For example, although it appears that chaotic bulimic families are not avoiding conflict—they are arguing all the time—the arguments can be a diversion from the conflict that is being avoided. The areas of conflict avoidance often are substance abuse, sexual abuse, marital discord, maternal loneliness, and the adolescent's transition into adulthood.

FEMINISM AND THE STRUCTURAL MODEL

The treatment model that follows from the structural family therapy conceptualization of eating disorders has been a major breakthrough in the field. By clarifying boundaries, modifying overprotectiveness, increasing flexibility, and identifying and negotiating conflict, these families have been able to change dysfunctional structural patterns and to eliminate the anorexic symptom. However, there are problems, as well as strengths, with the structural approach to eating disorders.

In many ways, this framework is compatible with a feminist conceptualization of eating disorders. The social context, in this case the family, is seen as a primary determinant of behavior (Libow, Raskin, & Caust, 1982). No longer is the locus of the problem rooted within the person; rather, it is seen as an aspect of relationships. The focus that family therapy places on relationships is also very respectful of the relational model of female development (cf. Miller, 1976). As will be detailed later, female development is based on development in relationship. Working with the entire family respects and validates the importance of women in relationship.

Feminists and structural family therapists share their mistrust of diagnostic labels (Bograd, in press). Minuchin calls anorexia "a Greek word," and prefers to be descriptive rather than use diagnostic labels. Both models assume competence and health, and focus on eliminating the symptom (Bograd, in press). Both models look for observable, verifiable change. Both utilize modeling as a therapeutic tool, and both see power as an important dimension in therapy, although the definition and use of modeling and power are very different between the two frameworks (Libow, et al., 1982).

Structural Family Therapy's Unanswered Questions

In spite of the compatibilities outlined above, several questions central to feminists working with eating-disordered women have been neither asked nor answered by family therapists. Why has an epidemic of eating disorders escalated over the past 20 years? Why does this epidemic primarily affect women (Chernin, 1981; Steiner-Adair, 1986)? In an effort to address these questions, the following concerns about structural family therapy, as traditionally applied, are outlined and subsequently detailed.

First, family therapists have taken a major leap from a linear to a systems model by moving the locus of the problem from the individual to the family. However, a systems approach needs to go beyond the family and take into account the larger context of society and culture, within which the family is the primary socializing agent. Therefore, a more complete systems perspective would see the family as one important system embedded in a larger culture that forms a feedback loop with the family (Bograd, in press; Imber-Black, 1986; Raskin, 1984). The societally sanctioned rules governing women's position and behavior dictate that women have little power, be giving and nurturant, not express anger, and conform to society's standards for physical appearance. The expectations become more impossible and contradictory as women are expected to take on careers but not increase their power base, work but not take time away from the family, and make decisions that will support and appease everyone. Eating disorders are one way of dealing with these many levels of impossible expectations.

Second, by working with families, family therapists have developed a format that potentially can accommodate the relational model of female development (Miller, 1976; Gilligan, 1982). However, the way that family therapy is applied to eating disorders instead emerges from a male model of development. The goal of most accepted theories is separation and individuation, in spite of the female developmental focus on connection. Therefore, separation may be an inappropriate goal for eating-disordered women, and the development of mutually enhancing relationships and growth within the context of those relationships may be a more useful goal.

Jordan (1986) suggests that this mutually enhancing relationship is defined by:

> An interest in and cognitive-emotional awareness of and responsiveness to the subjectivity of the other person through empathy; 2) a willingness and ability to reveal one's own inner states to the other person, to make one's needs known, to share one's thoughts and feelings. 3) the capacity to acknowledge one's needs without . . . manipulating the other . . . 4) valuing the process of knowing, respecting, and enhancing the growth of the other; 5) establishing an interacting pattern in which both people are open to change in the interaction. (p. 2)

The third difference between feminist and structural family therapy that will be addressed here is that of observation and interpretation. Minuchin and those who followed him have made some keen observations of patterns and successful interventions with anorexic families. There are, however, other ways of interpreting these observations and interventions that are more compatible with an integration of feminist and systemic frameworks.

These three issues—the broader context, female development, and reinterpretation of observations—will be elaborated upon in order to develop a more integrative feminist family systems approach to eating disorders.

THE LARGER CONTEXT

By focusing solely on the family, structural family therapists often ignore the larger societal context. The family is probably the most powerful structure for maintaining society's standards, as these standards are enacted and passed on from one generation to another. In turn, cultural standards influence how thoughts, feelings, and values develop within family members.

A Historical Perspective

The links among cultural expectations, the fashion industry, and women's bodies are strong. Boskind-White (1985) points out, for example, that the "wilted flower" and "weak and delicate" Victorian women, in trying to achieve the admired hourglass figure, wore such painful attire that they often fainted or broke their ribs, thus making fashion a statement of a crude reality.

Boskind-White also delineates the link between thinness and class issues. In an interesting proposal about prejudice in our society, Boskind-White suggested that the pursuit of thinness came about as a way of differentiating people who already were living in America from the immigrants. The immigrants, who remembered their privation, perceived body weight as a symbol of plenty in their new land. In addition, fattening foods were cheaper and more available than fresh fruits and vegetables, and so more accessible to the poorer immigrants. Robust women thus became associated with the lower classes and were deemed inferior by their middle- and upper-class counterparts. As a way of dissociating themselves from the immigrants, the wealthier Americans embraced slimness. The fashion industry, which was geared toward that population, also began to value this new standard. Young women trying to escape poverty by working in the mills hoped that if they looked like rich women, they would have a better chance of attracting a wealthy husband. Often, their hard-earned money was spent on fashionable clothing, and they were thus placed in the position of emulating the body type for which the fashions were made. The striving for thinness took root in the culture, and only during short periods of crisis—such as world wars—were women again more voluptuous.

Boskind-White's last observation in itself raises an interesting question: Why, during times of strife, were women again allowed to gain weight? Perhaps during these hard times, women were needed in the work force, and thus had more personal power, which was symbolized by their more substantial weight. The absence of men during wartime may have also freed women from concerns about attracting men and placing the needs of men above their own. When men returned home, and demanded back their jobs and power, the loss of status and power was again reflected in women's loss of weight.

The Pursuit of Thinness

Anorexics are known to pursue thinness with unequaled perseverance and discipline. However, during the past 30 years, Western society as a whole also has pursued thinness with growing fervor. A 1978 Neilson survey found that 45 percent of American households had someone dieting in the course of a year, and that 50 percent of all females between the ages of 25 and 54 diet. Dieting is obviously a result of displeasure with one's body, and a 1984 Glamour magazine poll of 33,000 women reported that 41 percent of respondents were moderately or very unhappy with their bodies, and 80 percent felt that they had to be thin in order to attract men. Many of these women went to unhealthy extremes to become thinner: 50 percent used diet pills, 18 percent used laxatives, 18 percent used diuretics, and 15 percent induced vomiting in order to lose weight.

Rosenbaum (1979) asked 30 "normal" adolescents for their three magical wishes. The majority chose losing weight and keeping it off as their number one wish. Surrey (1984) reported that many non-eating disordered college students showed extreme concern about their relationship with food and scored as high as anorexics on an eating-attitude test.

The fact that women are extremely concerned about their bodies is evident in many Western countries. A study of 2,370 Swedish adolescents, for example, indicates that most of the females felt fat at some point between 17 and 19 years old, and 40 percent of the 18-year-olds were dieting (Nylander, 1971).

The weight issue for women is correlated with other social and personal concerns. Self-esteem, self-confidence, and anxiety levels fluctuate more in women than in men on the basis of body image (Fisher, 1974), and the female adolescent's body build is correlated with prestige and popularity (Clausen, 1975).

Thus, although eating-disordered women may display more extreme methods of coping with this obsession, Western society as a whole is obsessed with thinness. Given this perspective, anorexia can be viewed as taking society's message "the thinner, the better" literally, and as a way of excelling in an area in which the majority of women feel like failures. Many anorexics reports the admiration they receive from other women as they lose weight. They feel that they have accomplished a difficult task, and have shown discipline and perseverance where others gave up. Bulimia in this context is a desperate effort to conform to a standard of thinness: women succumb to the lure of food, but cannot allow themselves to keep that food as it would mean deviating from the pursuit of thinness.

Distortion of Body Image

In addition to the relentless pursuit of thinness, anorexics are known to experience distortions of body image. However, many studies indicate that even women who are not experiencing an eating disorder view their bodies inaccurately. In one study (Cash, Winstead, & Janda, 1986), 47 percent of average-weight women reported themselves as overweight, and 40 percent of underweight women reported themselves as within average weight limits (based on new Metropolitan Life Insurance Company charts). The men in the study by Cash and colleagues were more accurate than the women in classifying their weight.

Another recent study (Thompson, 1986) supports the Cash data. Thompson asked women to guess the size of their waists, hips, thighs, and buttocks. Over 90 percent of those studied overestimated their body size. On the average, women reported themselves as 25 percent larger than they really were. In addition, the more inaccurate a woman was about her body size (the heavier she thought she was), the worse she did on a self-esteem questionnaire.

Finally, in a study conducted by Surrey (1984) at Wellesley College, 72 percent of the women reported a moderate to extensive concern about reaching their ideal weight, and 36 percent were very concerned about their eating patterns. Yet, the average student studied was within five to ten pounds of her ideal weight, and her eating patterns were generally normal.

Once again, in an extreme way, eating-disordered women reflect the concerns and distortions of a majority of women in this society.

Acceleration of the Trend

Not only are women required to look thin, but they are now expected to be thinner than their counterparts of 30 years ago. Glass (1980) reports that fashion mannequins with plastic bodies are shaved down yearly so that the new fashions are shown on thinner bodies. A review of *Playboy* centerfolds and Miss America contestants from 1959 through 1978 indicates that the average weight of the women declined throughout this period (Garner, Garfinkel, Schwartz, Thompson, & Johnson, 1980). More extreme was the finding that, after 1970, winners of the Miss America crown have weighed less than the average of the other contestants, who already weigh less than the population mean. The same authors reported actuarial data indicating that the average weight of women increased by a few pounds during the same time frame in which the glamorized ideal woman became thinner.

The United States spends $10 billion per year on the diet and glamour industry (Millman, 1980). Garner and his colleagues (1980) reported that the number of diet articles published has increased significantly over the past ten years. Mail surveys of how people spend their leisure time at times include dieting in a list of hobbies. In a contradictory message, magazine covers often show pictures of rich cakes side by side with headlines about the latest diet.

Once again, a parallel can be drawn: the incidence of eating disorders is increasing, along with the expectation that women should weigh less each year!

Beyond the Fashion Industry

To blame women's relationship with food, and eating disorders specifically, on the fashion industry would be misleading. The fashion industry is also a reflection of society. The question is, what is it reflecting? In part, the pursuit of thinness can be seen as a reflection of the unrealistic expectations and multiple roles cast upon women in our society. Whether it is a small dress size or multiple roles, women are struggling to fit into something that just does not fit. Most women cannot resemble the fashion models, even if their weight loss is maintained. An alternative would be to reject this expectation, and to make decisions based on more realistic goals. However, rejecting a societally imposed expectation contradicts the way in which women are socialized and rewarded, and thus is extremely difficult for them.

The expectation of thinness can also be seen as a reflection of women's relative powerlessness, and society's mechanism of maintaining women in that position. The message is that women should take up less space, thus symbolizing less power and less of a threat. It is not surprising that as women became more educated and take steps into the business world, the corresponding push is for them to become more diminutive, to negate these steps.

Finally, obsession with thinness may be a reflection of society's devaluation of women's priorities. As will be discussed later, women place a great deal of importance on relationships, which they try to maintain, often at great personal cost. Given the importance of maintaining relationships, women often try to please others. The unrealistic demand for women to be thin leads them to "dance around in circles," endlessly trying to please others by yielding to this demand, but finding that they cannot succeed in doing so, or "succeeding" at tremendous personal cost—that of self-denial and ultimately, their physical well-being.*

*Dr. Judith Libow, in a personal communication, asked whether anorexia nervosa is as prevalent among all cultural groups and as common in the lesbian community as in the heterosexual community. Although I could not find any confirming studies in the literature, Dr. Catherine Steiner-Adair (personal communication) and this author both noted that we rarely saw minority women or lesbian women in treatment for anorexia. We speculated that the women who were free from cultural mainstream expectations for women, who were not "buying into" the patriarchal message to please men or conform to standards imposed by men, and whose culture supported "strong" women, were less likely to suffer from anorexia.

FEMALE DEVELOPMENT AND EATING DISORDERS

Structural family therapy is potentially compatible with a greater emphasis on the relational aspects of female development. By focusing on the family, rather than on the woman in isolation, family therapists recognize and validate this dimension of relational development for all family members. Minuchin and colleagues (1978) state that the goal of structural family therapy with eating-disordered patients is to "facilitate the growth of a system that encourages the freedom to individuate while preserving the connectedness of belonging" (p. 91). However, the work of therapy itself often focuses on issues and goals of separation and individuation to the exclusion of connection and relationship. Minuchin et al., described the goals of the therapists in their study who worked with anorexic adolescents as "to develop autonomy, individuation, and independence" (p. 132). Further, with older adolescents and young adults, therapists worked with families initially, but quickly moved to individual sessions with the patient (as well as couples sessions with parents) to "foster disengagement" (p. 132). For this group, the therapy focused on issues involving separation from the family.

Therefore, although Minuchin mentions connection as one of the goals of therapy, the goals stated by the practitioners in his study (16 family therapists), as well as subsequent structural family therapists, focus on separation and individuation, on autonomy and leaving home.

The researchers and authors in the forefront of female developmental theory (cf. Chodorow, 1978; Gilligan, 1982; Miller, 1976; Surrey, 1984) view women as developing through attachment to others, as relational beings. The core structure in women is seen as the "relational self": "The 'self' is discovered, experienced, and expressed, in the context of human bonds and relationships" (Surrey, 1984, p. 6). The goal of development, according to Surrey, becomes relationship differentiation, and other aspects of development, such as initiative and industry, occur within the context of relationships.

For example, Gilligan (1982) demonstrated that separation, individuation, and autonomy without the context of maintaining relationships is not central to female development in the same way as it is to male development. Instead, when confronted with moral development tasks, girls attempt to negotiate solutions that include everyone, and work to everyone's benefit.

Given that girls are socialized to value relationships, Steiner-Adair (1986), in a study of anorexic girls, asks a compelling question: "Are girls also socialized to value the values they are given for relationships?" (p. 99). Her answer is a loud and poignant No. This devaluation of female values is reflected by many mental health professionals. Broverman and her colleague's classic research (1970) indicated that mental health professionals equated being a valuable human being with having stereotypically male characteristics. The "female" traits (those involving relationships), as well as women themselves, were devalued. Kohlberg's (1976) work on moral development views males as more highly developed morally for using nonrelational, individual concepts of justice to solve moral dilemmas (Gilligan, 1982).

In a society that values independence and devalues the relational self, it is not surprising that there is such a high incidence of eating disorders. These young women are often extremely loyal to their families, and often view their mothers as isolated and unhappy. How can the adolescent leave a depressed mother in pursuit of her own development when she has been socialized to take responsibility for other people, and to nurture others? Further, why should she want to enter the world of adult women given the unhappiness, isolation, and lack of fulfillment she has seen in that world? Why venture out of the nest when you feel your wings have already been clipped?

The unhappiness and isolation experienced by many mothers of eating-disordered teenagers can also be understood in the context of female development. Often, there is an unacknowledged rift between spouses. Because the wife in these families places such importance on the relationship with her husband and on her job as a mother, she often finds that she has lost or never made friends. Since the relationship may be important, but not central, in the life of her husband, he can focus on career and hobbies. In the absence of close friends or a meaningful career, a close relationship with her husband takes on added importance for the wife, and she tries harder to attain it. The more she pursues, the more he withdraws, and the more he withdraws, the more she pursues. If she loses hope that even her pursuing will effect change, she may feel depressed but have no friends to turn to. At the same time, her daughter is growing up, and the mother may feel that she is being forced into retirement from the one job that made her feel worthwhile. With the real and impending loss of relationships, these mothers feel alone and isolated.

The extreme weight loss of anorexia can be seen as a metaphor symbolizing the loss the adolescent believes she will experience as she moves into adulthood. To her, adulthood means isolation, the loss of close relationships. Who would want to enter that bleak world? Simultaneously, anorexia represents the desire to return to the more familiar and comfortable childhood where dependence was accepted, and even encouraged. Finally, by staying a needy child through the eating disorder, these girls are able to keep their mothers "employed", and, in some way, limit the maternal isolation.

The Wise Woman and the Superwoman

The fear of loss and isolation is an extremely important piece in the puzzle of eating disorders, but there are even more complex parts to this puzzle. The contradictory expectations that society places on women, along with the lack of validation of women's relational priorities, are also critical in understanding and treating eating-disordered women.

In a telling study, Steiner-Adair (1986) proposed that eating disorders have erupted because of an overemphasis on autonomy in women, which makes it difficult for girls to integrate and value relationships. She interviewed and gave questionnaires to 32 teenage girls at a private girls' school, and found two patterns of responses with regard to societal and cultural values concerning women. The "wise woman," as one pattern of answers was entitled, recognized that there are new cultural expectations for women that involve autonomy and independent achievement in careers and appearance. The wise women rejected that image, and differentiated their own ideal of women from the societal one. Connectedness and relationships were central to their vision of adulthood. The "superwoman" pattern was significantly different: these girls did not identify the new cultural values of autonomy and success for women, but instead felt that the expectation was that women should be caring and sensitive. They identified the superwoman, who could also be independent and autonomously successful. Their own ideal for women was congruent with society's ideal superwoman. The superwoman was described as tall, thin, carrying a briefcase, and having a high level of independent achievement. Relationships were seen as appendages, and not central or well integrated into the lives of superwomen.

Interestingly, all the wise women scored in the non-eating-disordered range of the questionnaire, whereas 11 of the 12 superwomen scored in the eating-disordered range. Therefore, the central finding was that:

> Girls who are able to identify contemporary cultural values and ideal images of women that are unsupportive of core female adolescent developmental needs and who are able to reject these values in choosing their own female ideal image are not prone to eating disorders. Girls who are unable to identify the societal values that are detrimental to their developmental needs, and who identify with the ideal image that is projected by these values are at risk for developing eating disorders (p. 107)

This study poignantly expresses the risk of eating disorders in a society that denies and devalues what is central to women—the relational self—and which imposes multiple contradictory expectations on women.

Conclusion: Why Women? Why Now?

Although structural family therapy can offer effective strategies for intervening with eating disorders, it has not been able to answer the questions "Why women?" and "Why now?" These questions are better understood in a larger systems context. In a society that does not value the interconnectedness and nurturance of women, and yet expects independent (isolated) achievement from women, women are in a profoundly difficult situation (Steiner-Adair, 1986). They can either conform, as their training, and lead isolated lives foreign to their core selves, or they can rebel, which is an important instrumental act but is foreign to their socialization. There are further paradoxes as women are expected to climb the corporate ladder, but to remain subordinate to men; as they are placed in more professional positions, but the actual fabric of the society remains the same and women have not experienced an increase in personal power. If anything, there has been more of an effort to keep women diminutive—physical appearance is symbolic of the lack of power women experience economically, legally, and even in being able to protect their bodies from being violated.

In the face of this dilemma, many women have found a paradoxical solution in anorexia nervosa and bulimia. By losing weight in a way that so grotesquely changes their bodies, anorexic women are both conforming in the ultimate manner to the standard for a diminutive presence and rebelling in an ultimate manner: "You want me to act like a man? Well, here's my no-longer-female body. You want me to be little and childlike at the same time? Well, I'll be so little and childlike that it will be intolerable to you." The bulimic statement is similar: "You are asking me to live many contradictions. Well, here is the ultimate one: I can eat and not eat at the same time—I can accept and reject sustenance and nurturance. You have demanded that I not be the one in charge of my body through your attempts at limiting choices about abortion and birth control, as well as through more direct violations such as battering and rape. Well, my body is out of my control—isn't that what you want?" These statements are not made directly and verbally: assertion and instrumentality in women are discouraged, and often meet with disapproval. The statements are expressed through their bodies, and it is a powerful rebellion at a tremendous cost.

The emaciated bodies of anorexics are both the ultimate capitulation to the unrealistic societal expectations for women's bodies and the ultimate parody of those expectations. By such absolute conformity to the value placed on thinness and on denial of female needs, these women are also rebelling against the standard, and exposing the oppression inherent in that standard. Ohrbach (1986) and Steiner-Adair (1986) both view anorexia as a hunger strike, as the use of the body to make a political statement about a public policy. Until the voices of these women are heard, and until the meaning of their voices is valued, the protest will continue.

REFORMULATION

The next section proposes a reformulation of structural family therapy concepts within a framework that attempts to be more compatible with and sensitive to the struggles and goals of eating-disordered women and their families.

Enmeshment and Connection

As Bograd (in press) and Hare-Mustin (1978) have written, basic family systems terms reflect prototypically male attributes, and often define those as the requisites for healthy family functioning. Intense relatedness, according to Bograd, therefore is termed "enmeshment," and carries a negative connotation. Instead, if one returns to the basic premise that women need to develop within the context of relationships, enmeshment with a child can be seen as the mother's cry for a relationship. The eating-disordered daughter, given her own female socialization, knows the terrifying cost of isolation. Therefore, she is willing to remain with her mother until she feels certain that both she and her mother have other meaningful relationships. Only then can she try to negotiate the waters of adulthood.

One frequently mentioned goal of family therapy with eating-disordered patients is to modify enmeshment and thus help the patient to separate from her family. However, this contradicts the basic tenet of female development, and misunderstands the needs of the eating-disordered patient and her mother. Thus, another way of viewing the goal of family therapy is to help families connect and develop differentiated relationships. The assumption is that many eating-disordered families who apear "too close" are desperately and unsuccessfully trying to find ways of being close, failing in their efforts, using the same methods more frantically and dramatically, and failing again.

Whereas family therapy often assumes that men and women constitute systems that display complementary relationships and circular influence, feminist family therapists (cf. Libow, et al, 1982) have discussed the power differential between men and women that systemic patterns in the family reproduce. The one arena where women have some power is with their children. The anorexic family is often a poignant example of this power differential: mothers often feel so powerless that they reaffirm their very being by an intense focus on their daughters. It can take the form of shopping for a teenager, not permitting closed doors, pushing the daughter toward accomplishments in a number of areas, and in other ways blurring the boundaries between mother and daughter. When a mother gives up this very intense relationship with her daughter—the only arena in which she has some power—she must replace it with something. If she cannot, the result at best might be a cured anorexic daughter and a severely depressed mother (or, more likely, an anorexic daughter plus a depressed mother).

One common structural (and strategic) intervention with eating-disordered families is to suggest that the parents spend more time together, to allow their daughter to "separate" or to "prove" to their daughter that they will survive without her so that she is freed up to enter the next developmental stage. Often, when this occurs, the daughter no longer manifests anorexic symptoms. Perhaps, however, an alternative to the interpretation that when the parents make such a shift, they have allowed the daughter to separate is that they have modeled the possibility of relationship, of connectedness in adulthood, of an alternative to isolation. A daughter who equated growing up with loss of relationships can now see the possibility of gaining a relationship in adulthood, and becomes less fearful of growing up.

In an effort to foster the development of relationships, families of inpatient eating-disordered adolescents with whom I worked also participated in a multiple-family group. In that forum, they met other families of hospitalized adolescents. Often, such a patient would express relief, and even joy, when her mother established a friendship with another mother in the group, or when her parents went out with another couple in the group. Another level of connection had been demonstrated: not only could the daughter hope to gain a relationship with a spouse when she entered adulthood, but the possibility of adult friendships also emerged.

Finally, several mothers with whom I have worked have moved from isolated jobs or no careers to careers in which they interact with others. This models to their eating-disordered daughter the possibility of connection in the work world.

Thus, although traditional structural techniques may involve placing a boundary around the spouse subsystem and forming more flexible boundaries between the family and outside world, the critical element in overcoming eating disorders may be that this restructuring models the formation of relationships.

The reader may respond by recalling how overinvolved these families appear, and thus the therapist's concern that separation is necessary in order for the eating-disordered patient to avoid engulfment. I believe that it is an error to equate "overinvolvement" with "too much relationship." Although the issue of language in family therapy cannot be addressed here (see Chap. 4), the point is that some families have not learned to connect or relate in ways nurturant and supportive of female development, and in their misguided efforts to do so, they have developed a destructive pattern that undermines such development. Our job becomes helping them to find more mutually enhancing and growth-facilitating relationships. An example may clarify this idea. Most eating-disordered families with whom I work have been labeled "overinvolved" or "enmeshed." They have been told that they have to have some distance in order to help their eating-disordered daughter, and are often labelled resistant as they cling to their old patterns. These families assume that distance means a loss of whatever fragile connection they have with one another. Thus, I view these families' primary difficulty as a problem in relating, and I asked them to participate in the following exercise. I ask them to come to the center of the room, stand as close as possible to each other, and hug each other as closely as they can. When they finally agree that they are standing "close enough," I ask them such questions as, "What color shoes is Susan wearing?" or "Is John smiling right now?" Of course, they do not know, as they are standing too close to see anybody clearly. After some time in this position, they become sweaty and uncomfortable, but stay in that position. I then ask them to take a few steps back. Each member can now see the others, touch one another and speak without a muffled voice. It is a much more comfortable position for everyone, and they can now interact. The movement away did not separate them. In fact, the opposite occurred: the possibility for connection and relationship opened up. "Close enough" means being in the position that maximizes their relatedness. This exercise can be used symbolically with anorexic women who feel that they are betraying their family by any movement away, and parents who worry about losing their daughters as they move into the next developmental stage. Boundaries are thus drawn—within the individual, between individuals, among the family members—in an effort to create the best space for developing relationships that are responsive to the needs of women as well as other family members, and thus empower women in the family.

In summary, the interventions of structural family therapy can be powerful with eating-disordered patients if they represent a formation of more meaningful husband-wife, parent-child, and family-member-outside-the-family relationships.

Rigidity

A similar argument can be made about the family's "rigidity." Why have the flexibility to change and move to a new stage of development, when that new stage is seen by the mother and daughter to be more isolated and less fulfilling, and by the father to be more demanding and intrusive (he could be in the position of "filling in" for what daughter once did if she were no longer present).

The childhood phase of family development allows the young daughter to be nurtured, the mother to be useful and connected, and the father to be autonomous. Anorexia is an attempt to return the family to that earlier stage of development: the daughter looks younger and needs caretaking. She may even need to be fed in much the same way as one would feed a young baby! Mothers report that they watch their bulimic daughters with a vigilance that reminds them of a return to toddlerhood. Parents report that they are just as afraid for the physical safety of their bulimic daughter when she enters a bathroom alone as they were for their toddlers. The rigidity can be countered with the same interventions as the overinvolvement/underrelationship: by helping the family to lay a richer and less isolating foundation for the next developmental stage.

Conflict Avoidance

Eating-disordered families have a difficult time recognizing and negotiating conflicts. This conflict avoidance may be viewed as yet another desperate but ineffectual effort to maintain some relationship in a society that prohibits women's anger. It is difficult to separate the issue of conflict from the feeling of anger. Often, anger generates conflict, and vice versa, and the successful resolution of conflict defuses anger. However, as Miller (1983) has written, the expression of anger is constrained in our society, although differentially for women and men. Miller goes on to explain that in a patriarchal society, women are economically, socially, and politically dependent on men. This subordinate position generates anger, but the societal message is that women have no cause for or right to anger. In addition, women are socialized with the belief that their activities should be for the benefit of others, and that their task is to develop and maintain relationships. Although there is much that is positive about that task, this socialization makes anger more difficult for women since women perceive anger as a disruption in relationship.

Eating-disordered adults and mothers of anorexic adolescents often feel extremely dependent on husbands for economic and social support. These mothers are so isolated from friends and other relationships that their need to maintain a conflict-free shelter at home is exacerbated. There is a great fear that arguments and expression of anger will disrupt their haven, and lead to the disintegration of the only context for relationships that the woman is now experiencing and prizing.

Miller also discusses how men have difficulty with appropriate expression of anger, given that boys are encouraged to act aggressively rather than to sustain and express a range of emotions. In anorexic families, this sex-role constraint leads to two roles frequently taken by fathers. The first is a father who inappropriately and dictatorially expresses anger that goes unchallenged by his wife and children. For example, Mr. J. was furious each time his daughters brought home grades of less than A, and grounded them until their grades went up. Nobody challenged or argued with Mr. J. until the family therapy reached a point where there was an ability to take the risk of opening the conflict. At that point, Mr. J. raised the concern that if he did not respond to his daughter's grades, neither would his wife, and their education would go down the drain.

The second is a father who is so distanced that he reports never feeling angry. For example, Mr. B. described his daughter as "perfectly behaved" and his wife as an "ideal wife." He said that he never was given cause to get angry. Mrs. B., who felt that she subordinated all of her own interests and goals to maintain that relationship, was not in touch with her anger until therapy reached the point where open conflict could be risked. Mr. B. was genuinely surprised at the anger directed toward him, and had assumed that his wife was as content, if not fulfilled, in the marriage as he was. Although many fathers of bulimics have also taken on the above roles, a third, disturbing type of behavior is more and more often being reported by bulimics, and that is male aggression directed toward the bulimic patient. This seems to take the form of sexual abuse of the bulimic (at times, but not always, by her father).

When questioned about anger, anorexics tend to say that they have no right or cause to be angry, and further, that they are "bad" when they are angry. Amanda, a 45-year-old woman, reported being told by her father that she was "sinning" when she disagreed with him. A religious woman, Amanda grew up feeling that when she was angry, she had evil feelings that had to be driven out of her, rather than angry feelings. Part of her anorexic fasting came from the religious belief that she needed to fast to purge her body of its badness. Her bulimic cycles could be seen as symbolic of the efforts to drive the evil out of her body. A recommended goal of therapy was to help Amanda view her anger as a healthy rather than sinful response to a difficult situation.

Jane also had difficulty with conflict. After seeing her parents' marriage fail, she made a supreme effort to make her own marriage work. Jane felt that if she expressed anger, she would lose the already tenuous hold she had on her relationship. In a supreme effort, she had to distance herself emotionally in order to avoid the angry feelings that would sometimes arise in her. The relationship was one in which Jane would carry out all her caretaking and sexual "wifely duties," but remain emotionally detached. Her husband, who also had difficulty with identifying and expressing feelings, was in part comfortable with the lack of intensity in the relationship, but was also disturbed by the diminishing affection displayed by his wife. Jane also felt a void in the relationship, but feared addressing it. The marriage was maintained in this manner, and Jane developed anorexia. As Miller (1983) wrote, when anger is not conveyed openly, it is often expressed via the remaining route, psychological or physical symptoms. Jane's anorexia was a way of rebelling against an empty relationship in which she felt both overwhelmed by and detached from feelings that she was prohibited against expressing. Through anorexia, she exaggerated the distance between herself and her husband (after all, she almost disappeared), and yet maintained the exterior of the gentle, caring wife whose outbursts were caused by her illness, not by her feelings.

In summary, the descriptive labels enmeshment, rigidity, and conflict avoidance are value-laden terms, implying fault and blame. The patterns observed in eating-disordered families can be seen instead as ways of handling the roles and limitations imposed on women in our society, and, at the same time, as efforts toward maintaining fragile relationships within the family. These dynamics can be understood only within the context of a society with unequal power arrangements, a prohibition against expression of anger by women, and a devaluation of the meaningfulness of relationships.

Power and Hierarchy

Because of the unequal distribution of power between men and women, many feminists oppose utilizing power and hierarchy in any family context, even between parents and teenagers. However, one of the most effective interventions of structural family therapy with eating-disordered adolescents has been to put parents in charge of the adolescent. Because expectations were unspoken, the preanorexic child was placed in the position of figuring out what parents wanted of her and complying. Failure to do so meant disappointing the parents. The child thus became expert at "mind reading," and also at setting her own limits. As many adolescents have reported to me, this is a scary and difficult position for a child who feels most cared for, protected, and most free when limits and consequences are clear. Also, as children do not have the ability to provide their own controls, many eating-disordered patients reported feeling out of control as children, although they appeared to be functioning well. Many bulimic patients reported that the rules in their families were inconsistent—they did not know what, if any, rules there were and whether breaking them would be ignored, rewarded, or punished.

The advent of the eating disorder brings to everyone's attention how out of control the adolescent really is. Initially, parents view the problem solely as an illness, ignoring any of its rebellious implications. Reframing can help parents see that this is the adolescent's avenue for rebelling. The critical point then becomes to help the adolescent move the rebellion away from food and into more age-appropriate and less self-destructive areas. Parents often report that they never had to set limits with this child before, and so are novices at disciplining their child. Parents need a great deal of support to come up with realistic and age-appropriate rules, explicitly state the rules, and enforce them. It sometimes helps parents to observe how well their adolescent responds to the consistent set of rules at the hospital, and also how the adolescent tests the hospital rules before settling down.

The difficult issue to resolve is how parents can be placed in charge of the adolescent without recreating the societal sex roles in which the husband has more authority than the wife. The therapist must pay particular attention to the process of how the rules are decided upon, and work with the mother and father so that both take active roles in making and negotiating decisions. In this way, the mother can be a role model for her daughter and demonstrate that women can be assertive and decisive, while maintaining sensitivity and ability to negotiate.

The Role of the Therapist

Modeling is an important therapeutic tool for family therapists as well as feminist therapists (Libow, et al., 1982). Structural family therapy requires that therapists taken on an active role in the therapy that allows them to serve as role models for their patients. When a female therapist models instrumentality in combination with warmth and nurturance, she can be a powerful role model for an eating-disordered patient. Through the therapist, the young woman can begin to imagine having an active, powerful role in a situation while maintaining connections. As the therapist faces conflicts, the eating-disordered patient can see that although conflict is uncomfortable, it can often be resolved without loss of the relationship. The therapist also models the type of conflict resolution where negotiation is emphasized. The therapist can demonstrate that respect for the other person and his or her opinion is maintained without compromising one's own belief system, and that one's own opinion can be modified or changed without losing oneself in that process. Both of these ideas are new to most eating-disordered patients, and very important in the recovery process.

Through her behavior and interventions, the therapist also models appropriate boundaries. Many of the areas that are difficult for eating-disordered families—acknowledging and respecting privacy, dyadic relationships, parental limit setting—can be demonstrated by the therapist.

Unfortunately, the therapist can also support the status quo, and transmit the message that women must continue in a subordinate position. If a therapist is directive and powerful, he or she runs the risk of obtaining compliance from women only because women are trained to comply with authority. An eating-disordered woman has already carried compliance to an extreme—she feels that she has spent her entire life obeying other people, and accepting their definitions of her personality, her likes, and her dislikes. The therapist can offer more of the same, and this can lead to several outcomes. First, the person can comply with each therapeutic task but still not eat. Second, she can begin eating to please the therapist, but stop again when treatment ends. Finally, she can resume eating but remain depressed and lack the belief that she can have any mastery or control.

The therapist, therefore, walks a conceptual tightrope, trying to maintain a balance between modelling mastery and control and not wanting the family to feel externally controlled. The balance rests in how the therapist communicates instrumentality to the family: the therapist needs to form a team with the family, so that the therapy system is working together toward solving the problem of the eating disorder. In the case of an adolescent, the therapist works with the parents so that they establish stage-appropriate authority over their adolescent, as well as an ability to hear their daughter without assuming that they know what she is thinking and feeling. The eating-disordered patient can then feel comfortable with her therapist, knowing that the therapist understands her need to be parented as well as her loyalty to her family. As the therapist does this work, she needs to communicate through her behavior and words that although there is an unequal distribution of power in our society that is reflected in families, there is also an opportunity within families for couples to work together in a more equitable, supportive, and satisfying way—although this is certainly easier said than done, given the sex-role behaviors prescribed by society. How the family makes decisions and negotiates change becomes more critical than the content of the negotiation. The therapist needs to model negotiating with a father who may have been the sole decision maker in the family. She also needs to model a process of negotiation in which she can be caring and warm, but at the same time assertively communicate her beliefs; express conflict over an issue rather than attack the person who has the differing belief; and do all of this directly and not through flirtatious behavior or a one-down submissive stance with fathers. This is not an easy job, but it certainly enables the therapist to come face to come face to come face with the sexual politics of the family and the difficulties encountered by families trying to negotiate change!

An adolescent with an eating disorder feels as if she has no control or power, and must be supported in making age-appropriate decisions and negotiating for changes in the rules. She also feels that her parents have unrealistic and, at the same time, unstated expectations for her, so parents must be supported in concretizing their expectations, and setting and enforcing age-appropriate limits.

Finally, should therapists choose a cotherapy arrangement, they run the risk of recreating a sex-role stereotyped pattern (Raskin, 1984). If a male and female therapist are working together, they need to evaluate whether she is the expressive therapist and he is the instrumental one, whether she consistently complies with his wishes when they disagree, and whether they communicate that he is in charge and she subordinate. If this is the case, then the message to the eating-disordered patient is that even a therapist, who is supposed to help her overcome her problems, cannot have mastery over her situation. Flexible roles for both therapists, an ability to move from the nurturant to the active, from the leader to the follower, will model the alternatives available for the family.

CASE EXAMPLE: PORTRAIT OF AN ARTIST*

The following case study will attempt to offer the therapist a way of utilizing the structural model while still remaining faithful to a process that is respectful of women and takes into account the larger societal context. Rather than viewing the eating-disordered family as a unique, pathological unit, it is seen within the context of the society it reflects.

I first met Diana when she was a 17-year-old high school senior. She was an emaciated, silent young woman with straggly hair and tired, sunken eyes. Her parents reported that, only six months earlier, she was an attractive, popular, outgoing girl with a steady boyfriend. During the summer before her senior year of high school, Diana began to diet in order to have a better chance at becoming prom queen. Her initial goal of a 15-pound weight loss became 20, and then 25, pounds. By September, she was eating a cup of nonfat yogurt, a small bowl of salad, and a glass of water per day. She meticulously recorded the number of calories she consumed, being careful that they did not exceed her daily limit of 250. In December, when the five-foot, four-inch adolescent weighted 75 pounds. she fainted in school and was brought to a psychiatric hospital.

Upon admission, Diana was placed on a weight program similar to the ones proposed by Minuchin et al. (1978) and Mirkin (1983). I told her that she was the one who should have control over what entered her body, so nobody here

*The names and some of the details of the case have been changed in order to protect confidentiality.

would monitor what she ate, but we were concerned about her medical condition. Therefore, each morning at wake-up, she would be weighed and privileges at the hospital would be contingent upon weight gains of one-fourth pound. Bed rest was required for weight loss. Diana argued that the policy was unfair because normal weight fluctuations are more than one-quarter pound. She was told that she could choose to gain enough weight so that she would not have to worry about losing privileges over small fluctuations. Diana's anger about weigh-ins and her attempts to cheat at weigh-ins provided the first material over which the family could begin to deal with conflict.

I met Diana's parents the day after Diana's admission. They were an attractive couple, dressed with an artistically bohemian flair. Mr. C. is a famous artist who exhibits his paintings internationally and frequently travels. Mrs. C., also a painter, gives art lessons to children and teaches an occasional seminar at a local college. Diana's 20-year-old sister, Regina, was away at college with plans to become a lawyer, a field in which her father is deeply interested but was unable to pursue.

Mr. and Mrs. C. presented themselves as a happy, fulfilled couple, active in their careers and enjoying their family. They reported having no close friends, though Mrs. C. stated that she was very close to her three sisters, who live in another state and whom she can visit only occasionally.

They reported that much of their time is spent painting. On weekends, Diana and her mother frequently attend art exhibits. This information puzzled me, as Diana had privately informed me that she found art boring. The family spends its summers at an art festival where Mr. C. exhibits his paintings. Although the parents said they enjoy the festival, Diana had so little interest in attending and begged so to stay home that Mrs. C. was considering staying home with her in the coming summer.

During individual meetings, Diana told me that the previous year, she had considered marrying her boyfriend, and also planned to attend college after high school graduation. She now had no interest, either emotionally or sexually, in her boyfriend, and had no idea what to pursue in college. She had neither Regina's academic interests nor the artistic talents of her parents. Her one interest was fashion, but she did not consider herself attractive enough to pursue a career in the fashion industry. Further, she knew that this particular interest would be denigrated by her mother as too sex-role stereotyped and by her father as not sufficiently academic, and she wanted her parents' approval. Her secure world of high school was falling apart, and her confusion and uncertainty about the future were evident.

Diana also confided that she was concerned about her mother. She felt that her mother was depressed, but denied her depression. Diana questioned her own perceptions, but remained concerned. She described her mother as someone who once had a promising career, and gave it up for a family. She blamed herself for interfering with her mother's career. Alternatively, she reported that her mother spent more time painting than attending to the day-to-day business of her growing daughter. She reported never feeling close to or accepted by her mother. She said that they had nothing in common. Regina, on the other hand, shared her parents' deep interest in painting. In the past, Regina accompanied her mother to exhibits, and they would spend time over dinner discussing the nuances of painting. This bored Diana, but she assumed that being a painter was a prerequisite for acceptance into her family. When Regina left for college, Mrs. C. stopped attending exhibits. Concerned about her mother's isolation, and wanting her mother's acceptance, Diana began to give up her own social engagements to go to exhibits with her mother.

Diana graphically described the loneliness she experienced in her house: "Everyone lives in their own rooms, works quietly, and each room is too dark."

Diana also had happy memories, primarily from when she was a young child and her family would go to zoos and parks. She also had warm memories of the way her mother ministered to her and Regina when they were ill.

She had few memories of her parents' setting limits with her. She described her confusion as she tried to ascertain what was expected of her, obey the unspoken rules and meet the unspoken expectations.

Therapist's Assessment

From Diana's description of her life, her concerns about womanhood became obvious. I felt that there could be several precipitants for, or events correlated with, Diana's anorexia. First, she was approaching her senior year at high school, which was a secure place for her—she was popular, did well, and a routine was in motion. The future was much more frightening for her. She decided to go to college more to meet her parents' unspoken expectations than because she wanted a college education. Yet, she had no idea what to do once she entered college, and her interest in the fashion industry was fraught with conflict and ambivalence.

Not only was she reaching a career crisis, she was also approaching a crisis in relationships. Adulthood seemed very empty to Diana. Her mother, once happy with her own parents and sisters, was depressed. There were many clues, from Diana's perspective, that her parents were not emotionally connected at this time. The clue I took most seriously was Diana's need to go to art exhibits with her mother, because nobody else would go with her.

The meeting of the relationship and career crises is highlighted by Diana's view of her mother's choices: mother attempted to juggle career and family, and so Diana felt that she was able to do neither well. The family did not recognize, as evidenced by their statements, that it is unrealistic to expect a woman to spend her days with her children, and, at the same time, become a famous painter. This dilemma was not acknowledged by anyone but Diana, and only in the context that her mother was not capable of doing both, not that she should not be expected to do both.

Diana was able to have a relationship with her mother when she was sick. This concerned me, as the primary goal of therapy was for Diana to give up the anorexia, and so, there had to be a different way for mother and daughter to connect.

Thus far, the father was an enigma to me. He was warm and concerned in the sessions, appeared to be sensitive, asked questions, and attempted to respond to questions from others. I was not sure what he would be willing to do when it came time for me to introduce tasks, nor did I have a sense of why he and his wife withdrew from each other as he seemed fond of her.

Therefore, I decided to set the following goals for the sessions:

1. Draw a boundary around the spouse subsystem. In this way, Diana would no longer be her mother's "husband," nor would her mother be as isolated.

2. Redefine the parent-child relationship so that Diana could feel connected to her mother without needing to pursue a career in painting, and so that she could feel approved of by her father without having to become a lawyer.

3. Support each individual subsystem, so that each family member could develop friendships outside of the family and become less isolated.

4. Help the family to acknowledge the conflicts within the family, including Diana's concerns about her career, the relationship between Mr. and Mrs. B., and the larger societal dilemmas of being a woman in a society that expects the impossible from women.

5. Help parents verbalize their expectations of Diana, and form realistic expectations. Help them enforce the limits they had set.

6. Have Diana take control over her own body as well as other areas that are appropriate for her to control at her age. The weight program would be continued, and discharge contingent upon maintaining her goal weight (set at the low end of normal for her height) for five days.

My hope was that the family could reorganize so that Diana could witness the positive aspects of growing up: close relationships and career enjoyment, in particular. Related to this, I wanted the family to see their dilemma as both personal and societal: that women in our society struggle with juggling career and family and struggle to attain the intimacy that they long for, and that the power differential between men and women makes the woman feel that she is compromising more than she would want to. As these are unspoken, powerful expectations for a woman, she receives little or no appreciation for her attempts at caretaking, compromising, and juggling—and in fact, the feedback is that she should do more and do better.

Treatment

Although Diana brought up her concern about her mother's depression during the next family meeting, Mrs. C. denied feeling depressed. When Diana told her mother that she went to art museums and exhibits with her because she did not feel that her mother could go alone or find someone else to go with, Mrs. C. looked surprised and upset. She guaranteed Diana that there was no need to accompany her. I asked her whether anyone else could be her partner at the museum. Mrs. C. said she did not feel that a partner was necessary. I then quipped, looking at Mr. C. "What is this? She doesn't even want to ask you as a last resort!"

"Yes," Mr. C. responded, "What is this? I guess I'm not good enough to go with you to museums." He smiled. I jumped on his invitation, and told the parents that somehow they needed to convince Diana that Mrs. C. would do just fine without her vigilant caretaking. Their marriage had held up for 22 years, and they could prove to Diana that they could continue their relationship without her being a stand-in for her father. Although Mrs. C. sat quietly and icily, Mr. C. responded warmly to the effect that he would do things with his wife and prove to Diana that they were capable of supporting each other. I pointed out that Mrs. C. and Diana did not look convinced, and, much to their amusement, Mr. C. spent the remainder of the session trying to convince Mrs. C. to date him. Mrs. C. was finally able to express her concern that he would go to one or two exhibits with her, and then back out. He responded that he had not known she wanted his company, and that he had felt left out of the "women's circle." They set a date for that Saturday. Diana gained some more weight.

The subject of mother's depression came up again during the next session. Since Mrs. C. felt more comfortable speaking about herself in the context of how she could help her daughter, I told her that we all needed confidantes, and that right now Diana did not have one. With whom, I asked, did Mrs. C. speak when she felt blue or needed to confide in someone? She immediately named Gina, one of her three sisters, then a friend who had moved away two years earlier, then another sister, and finally, after a pause, her husband. Mr. C. picked up on that immediately. This opened up a discussion of how Mrs. C. did not feel able to talk to her husband, because he was either concentrating on his painting or on tour, and also because he had a quick temper and she valued calm and quiet discussion. The tip of the conflict was out in the open, and the parents could begin to negotiate their concerns.

Once this small opening was made, Mrs. C. was able to acknowledge that she did indeed feel depressed. She said that she never wanted to admit it aloud, because she did not think a parent should share her problems with her children. Yet, as Diana quickly interjected, she knew about the depression and questioned her own reality testing as mother continued to deny it. Diana was relieved when Mrs. C. ackowledged those feelings, because it confirmed her view of the world, it gave Mrs. C. a chance to get some help, and it gave permission for Diana to talk about her own sadness. Diana also felt that she now had a chance to get closer to her mother—that her mother's honesty made her a real person instead of a "perfect but unreachable lady."

Diana's former efforts to protect her mother, as well as the difficulties her mother was facing as a woman in this society, were highlighted as the sessions continued. Mrs. C., who originally talked about looking forward to summers at the festival, now discussed the darker side of her feelings. She felt that she once had great promise as an artist. When she married, she was expected by her family of origin and her husband, as well as by her internalized view of her role, to make her career secondary to her job as a mother and housewife. By the time the girls were old enough for her to pursue her career, she felt that she was too rusty and had missed too much to ever become a "great" artist. Every summer, she felt that she was reminded of that fact as she watched artists painting and exhibiting, and knew that she could never be one of them. She resented her husband for the ease with which he was able to move through his career, without any of these pressures and mixed expectations. Diana's push to spend summers at home was in part motivated by her own distaste for art, and in part to get her mother out of that situation. The latter goal became evident when Mrs. C. recalled that she did leave Diana alone in their house for one weekend because she had visitors at their summer home. Diana took a bus and joined her parents at the festival, and helped her mother prepare for the visitors. Mrs. C.'s struggle, so poignantly communicated to Diana, created the perfect opening to discuss the contradictory expectations placed on women, and the universality of their family's struggle.

The flip side of that coin was Mrs. C.'s concern that she was not a good enough mother because she was not happy to stay home and completely forfeit her career. Further, in an effort to raise girls who would be more independent and less guilt-ridden than she, she had set few limits. The girls could sleep until noon, need not do chores, and did not have a curfew. Diana construed this as evidence that her mother was not concerned about her, and expected her to "know" what was correct behavior without guidance. Mr. C. felt that this lack of maternal limit setting placed him in the "bad guy" role because he would explode after trying to be patient and understanding with the girls for an extended time. Mrs. C. felt that she had to counter his verbal explosions by being even gentler and less demanding with the girls. Parents were helped to set realistic limits for Diana.

As the career and home issues were discussed, Mr. C. supported his wife's decision to become more involved in her career. Risking his anger, she retorted, "And who is going to take care of the house? Or do the nitty-gritty everyday things?" Regina was at this session, and both she and Diana started laughing when the father said, "I will." Although he did agree to share the cooking and cleaning, by the end of therapy it was clear that he was "helping" his wife rather than sharing the household responsibilities. However, Mrs. C. seized on this opportunity to start exhibiting her work more and to rent a studio with several other women instead of working in isolation at home.

Therapy (individual and family) continued on an outpatient basis. Diana began college, still too concerned about her parents' disapproval to change her plans. Midway through the semester, she was able to tell her parents that she wanted to be a hairdresser. Mr. C. was disappointed that his daughter was dropping out of school and Mrs. C. was disappointed that she was doing something as sex-role stereotyped and "inconsequential" as hairdressing. I reframed it as Diana's artistic endeavor, pointing out that everyone in the family had mistakenly labeled Diana as not artistic, but now she was receiving training to further her artistic abilities. Although her parents were disappointed, they were able to talk about their feelings and support Diana's decision.

By the time therapy ended, Diana had maintained her weight for ten months. She had graduated from high school, left college, entered hairdressing school, and made new friends. She and her parents were able to connect not over art, but over honest discussion of thoughts and feelings. Mr. and Mrs. C. continued to spend time together, and Mrs. C. spent more time with her art group and exhibiting her work.

Follow-up

Five years later, Diana is still maintaining her weight. She is doing well as a hairdresser, and is specializing in a new type of technique. She is engaged to be married to a young man supportive of her career, and she has several close friends. She reports that her sister is now a lawyer, that her mother has been exhibiting her work regularly, and that her father frequently attends her mother's exhibitions. Diana says that she felt the most valuable part of therapy was getting to know her mother better. She also commented on how important it was to her to watch her mother blossom during and after therapy, and how relieved and hopeful she felt as she observed those changes. In addition, she recalled the weight program at the hospital and said that it helped her to realize that she did have some control over what was happening to her; she felt more in charge of her body, and she felt that she could not have recovered without the experience. Finally, she continues to view her appearance as an ongoing problem. Although she maintains her weight, she still does not like the way she looks, and she hopes that one day she will be able to accept herself and her body without this self-criticism.

In summary, the ability to form a more meaningful relationship with her parents, in conjunction with a larger systems perspective of the problem, enabled Diana to move on to the next stage of her development and to leave the anorexia behind. This goal was accomplished by utilizing structural techniques from a perspective that is compatible with the developmental needs of women.

CONCLUSION

This chapter is just a beginning. For all the issues raised, more still loom ahead: Are eating disorders a response to the broken dreams of mothers and their daughters' feelings of guilt and responsibility if they surpass their mothers (Chernin, 1985)? Is the rejection of full, round bodies yet another expression of mother hating, in which pregnancy is symbolically denigrated whereas maleness, as represented by gaunt bodies, is applauded (Chernin, 1981, 1985; Libow, 1987)? The questions, symbolism, and metaphors are just beginning to be explored. Yet, whatever the metaphor, the desperate cry of eating-disordered women relates to the meaning of being a woman in this particular society at this particular time (Chernin, 1985; Ohrbach, 1978; Steiner-Adair, 1986; Surrey, 1984).

This chapter was an initial attempt to integrate feminist and structural family therapy perspectives of eating disorders by asking the questions, "Why women? Why now? How can we intervene in a respectful and effective manner?" Eating disorders are viewed as one understandable, albeit tragic, response to the unrealistic and contradictory expectations placed on women by a society that devalues women's desire for connection and mutually enhancing relationships. Being an adult woman is viewed grimly by women and girls with eating disorders: it is equated with losing relationships, feeling isolated, and being unable to adequately meet the many contradictory demands placed on women.

Structural family therapy has the potential for being a useful modality with eating-disordered patients since it has the capability of respecting women's growth in the context of relationships, establishing connections within the family and outside the family, facilitating the surfacing of conflict without concomitant family disintegration, and modeling mastery and instrumentality as well as nurturance. However, in order for that potential to be realized, family therapy needs to broaden its boundaries to include and emphasize the larger context of what it means to be a woman in contemporary society:

> The radical protest she might utter, if she correctly understood the source of her despair and depression, has been directed toward herself and away from her culture and society. Now, she will not seek to change her culture so that it might accept her body; instead, she will spend the rest of her life in anguished failure at the effort to change her body so that it will be acceptable to her culture. (Chernin, 1981, p. 106)

In therapy, there is a tremendous opportunity to help women and families to understand their situation within our society, to use words and action instead of one's body to respond to that situation, and to emerge with a stronger sense of self, family, and relationship.

REFERENCES

American Psychiatric Association (1980). *Diagnostic and statistical manual of mental disorders (3rd ed.).* Washington, D.C.: Author.

Bograd, M. (in press). Feminist perspectives on family systems theory: power, gender, and the family. In Maryann Douglass and Lenore Walters (Eds.), *Feminist psychotherapies: integration of therapeutic and feminist systems.* New York: Ablex Press.

Boskind-White, M. (1985). Bulimerexia: A sociocultural perspective. In S. W. Emmett (Ed.), *Theory and treatment of anorexia nervosa and bulimia.* New York: Bruner/Mazel.

Broverman, I., Broverman, D., Clarkson, F., Rosenkrantz, P., & Vogel, S. (1970). Sex role stereotypes and clinical judgments of mental health. *Journal of Consulting and Clinical Psychology,* 23, 1–7.

Bruch, H. (1973). *Eating disorders: Obesity, anorexia nervosa, and the person within.* New York: Basic Books.

Cash, T., Winstead, B., & Janda, L. (1986). The great American shape-up. *Psychology Today,* Apr. 30–37.

Chernin, K. (1985). *The hungry self: Women, eating, and identity.* New York: Times Books.

Chernin, K. (1981). *The obsession: Reflections on the tyranny of slenderness.* New York: Harper & Row.

Chodorow, N. (1978). *The reproduction of mothering.* Berkeley, Calif.: University of California Press.

Clausen, J. A. (1975). The social meaning of differential physical and sexual maturation. In S. E. Dragastur & G. H. Elder, Jr., (Eds.), *Adolescence in the life cycle,* New York: Halstead Press.

Crisp, A. H., Palmer, R. L., & Kalucy, R. S. (1976). How common is anorexia nervosa? A prevalence study. *British Journal of Psychiatry,* 128, 549–554.

Emmett, S. W. (1985)l. *Theory and treatment of anorexia nervosa and bulimia.* New York: Bruner/Mazel.

Fisher, S. A. (1975). *Body consciousness.* New York: Jason Aronson.

Garner, D., & Garfinkel, P. (1985). *Handbook of psychotherapy for anorexia nervosa and bulimia.* New York: Guilford Press.

Garner, D. M., Garfinkel, P. E., Schwartz, D., & Thompson, M. (1980). Cultural expectation of thinness in women. *Psychological Reports,* 47, 483–491.

Gilligan, C. (1982). *In a different voice.* Cambridge, Mass.: Harvard University Press.

Glamour Magazine (1984). *Feeling fat in a thin society,* Feb., 1984.

Glass, A. (1980). *Facts and figures: A man alive*. London: BBC-TV.

Guttman, H. (1986). Family therapy of anorexia nervosa and bulimia: A feminist perspective. In M. Ault-Riche (Ed.), *Women and family therapy*. Rockville, Md.: Aspen Systems Corp.

Halmi, K.A., Falk, J. R., & Schwartz, E. (1981). Binge eating and vomitting: A survey of the college population. *Psychological Medicine, 11,* 697–706.

Hare-Mustin, R. (1978). A feminist approach to family therapy. *Family Process,* 17, 181–194.

Hudson, J., Hope, H., Jonas, J. & Yurgelson-Todd, D. (1983). Phenomenologic relationship of eating disorders to major affective disorder. *Psychiatry Research* 9, 345–354.

Imber-Black, E. (1986). Women, families, and larger systems. In M. Aulte-Riche (Ed.), *Women and family therapy*. Rockville, Md.: Aspen.

Jordan, J. (1986). The meaning of mutuality. Stone Center for Developmental Services and Studies, *Work in Progress*, no. 23.

Kohlberg, L. (1976). Moral stages and moralization: The cognitive-developmental approach. In: T. Lickona (Ed.), *Moral development and behavior*. New York: Holt, Rinehart, & Winston.

Libow, J. (1987). Personal communication.

Libow, J., Raskin, P., & Caust, B. (1982). Feminism and family systems therapy: are they irreconcilable? *American Journal of Family Therapy,* 10, 3–12.

Miller, J. (1983). The construction of anger in women and men. Stone Center for Developmental Services and Studies, *Work in Progress,* no. 83–01.

Miller, J. (1976). *Toward a new psychology of women*. Boston: Beacon Press.

Millman, M. (1980). *Such a pretty face: Being fat in America*. New York: W. W. Norton.

Minuchin, S., Rosman, B., & Baker, L. (1978). *Psychosomatic families: Anorexia nervosa in context*. Cambridge, Mass.: Harvard University Press.

Mirkin, M. P. (1983). The Peter Pan syndrome: Systemic approaches to short term inpatient treatment of anorexia nervosa. *International Journal of Family Therapy,* 5(3), 289–295.

Nielsen, A. C. (1979). *Who's dieting and why?* Chicago: A. C. Nielsen.

Nylander, I. (1971). The feeling of being fat and dieting in a school population: Epidemilogical interview and investigation. *Acta Sociomedica Scandinavica,* 3, 17–26.

Ohrbach, S. (1986). *Hunger strike: The anorexic's struggle as a metaphor for our age*. London: W. W. Norton.

Ohrbach, S. (1978). *Fat is a feminist issue*. New York: Paddington Press.

Raskin, P. A. (1984). "The woman question" and family therapy. Keynote address for *Symposium on Feminism and Family Therapy*. Vancouver, B.C.: Feminist Counseling Association of Vancouver and Pacific Coast Family Therapy Training Association.

Root, M., Fallon, P., & Friedrich, W. (1986). *Bulimia: A systems approach to treatment*. New York: W. W. Norton.

Rosenbaum, M. (1979). The changing body image of the adolescent girl. In: M. Sugar (Ed.), *Female adolescent development*. New York: Brunner/Mazel.

Schwartz, R., Barrett, M. J., & Saba, G. (1985). Family therapy for bulimia. In D. Garner and P. Garfinkel (Eds.), *Handbook of psychotherapy for anorexia nervosa and bulimia*. New York: Guilford Press.

Stangler, R. S., & Printz, A. M. (1980). DSM-III: Psychiatric diagnosis in a university population. *American Journal of Psychiatry,* 137, 937–940.

Steiner-Adair, C. (1986). The body politic: Normal female adolescent development and the development of eating disorders. *Journal of the American Academy of Psychoanalysis,* 14(1), 95–114.

Steiner-Adair, C. (1987). Personal communication.

Surrey, J. (1984). Eating patterns as a reflection of women's development. Stone Center for Developmental Services and Studies, *Work in Progress,* no. 83–06.

Theander, S. (1970). Anorexia nervosa: A psychiatric investigation of 94 female patients. *Acta Psychiatrica Scandinavica Supplementum,* 214, 1–194.

Thompson, J. K. (1986). Larger than life. *Psychology Today,* Apr., 39–44.

Todd, T. (1985). Anorexia nervosa and bulimia: Expanding the structural model. In M. P. Mirkin and S. Koman (Eds.), *Handbook of adolescents and family therapy*. New York: Gardner Press.

6

THE CONTEXT FOR COUPLES TREATMENT OF WIFE ABUSE

Dennis A. Balcom, M.S.W.,
and Donna Healey, Ph.D.

INTRODUCTION

This chapter began as an extended conversation between the authors. The conversation led into territory we had not planned to enter. We are both systems-oriented family therapists, with a strong loyalty to this orientation. Yet in approaching the issue of wife abuse, we quickly became aware of the inadequacies of a family systems model in confronting and dealing with this problem. The more we read and talked, the more convinced we became that wife abuse is not just a personal or family problem; it is a societal problem. In fact, there are structural properties in society that account, in large part, for wife abuse.

As we continued to think critically about the problem of how systems theory deals with wife abuse, our analysis expanded to include a number of flaws in the way systems theory approaches families in general. Our effort to understand the problem of wife abuse led us to a critique of several of the basic assumptions of family therapy. This is where we did not intend to go.

We first review the family therapy literature on wife abuse and critique it. We then present an alternate theoretical understanding of the origins and maintenance of wife abuse and use this understanding to raise questions about the utility of the concepts of equality, mutuality, reciprocity, and coevolution.

Finally, we deal with the clinical implications of such a critique. Even if family systems theory is lacking in its ability to provide a comprehensive model of wife abuse, we are still family therapists with an interest in and an obligation to treat couples in which wife abuse occurs. Although we will argue that the origins of wife abuse are primarily outside and the maintenance is both outside and within any particular family, we still need to provide treatment to families.

Finally, a word about terminology. Violence between men and women has been variously termed marital violence, domestic violence, spouse abuse, couples violence, and wife battering. We have chosen the term "wife abuse" because we believe it is an accurate description of the inequality between women and men.

SYSTEMS THEORY APPROACHES TO WIFE ABUSE

We believe that family therapists' explanation of wife abuse is part of a culture that expects and sanctions violence in the family.
Murray Straus (1976) cites a popular British joke:

> First Woman: I'm worried my husband doesn't love me anymore.
> Second Woman: Why not?
> First Woman: He hasn't hit me in a fortnight. (p. 546)

Straus cites the joke to emphasize the acceptance, and even valuation, of violence directed toward wives in the popular culture. The following review of the literature will show that, in many ways, family therapists, who are also culture bound, have developed understandings tha fail to challenge these cultural biases toward violence.

The major contribution of family systems theory is that it contextualizes behavior. Systems theory is concerned with the ways in which individuals play a part in the family system. It seeks, as well, to understand the function of behavior in terms of the system as a whole. The family is seen as a system of interlocking parts and as the primary context for understanding the individual (Hoffman, 1981).

The focus on the family system as the unit of intervention underlies the therapeutic stance of neutrality (Selvini-Palazzoli, Boscolo, Cecchin, & Prata, 1980). According to this view, the therapist needs to take a stance of neutrality toward the different parts of the system in order to facilitate change in the system as a whole. As the premise is that causality is circular rather than linear, each person in the system is assumed to have equal responsibility for how the system operates, and for whether the system stays the same or changes. Our position is that, in many cases, but in particular in the case of wife abuse, participants do not have equal responsibility because they do not have equal power.

To provide a fuller understanding of the family systems approach to wife abuse, we briefly review the literature on this topic. The authors cited have in common a belief that wife abuse can be viewed in terms of the ways in which it fits into or maintains the family system. One approach is concerned primarily with the location of the problem of abuse in the individual, the couple, the larger family, or the family of origin. A second approach views violence an nonnormative and pathological and attempts to delineate a typology of families that produce violence.

The Individual or Couple as Problem Locus

A number of writers have assigned wife abuse a homeostatic function within the family. Violence has been conceptualized as a way for the couple to experience closeness (Cook & Frantz-Cook, 1984) and as a way to maintain equilibrium (Elbow, 1982). The assumption here is that the basis of the violence is in the relationship.

Margolin (1979) characterizes abusive relationships as having three components: abusiveness is learned, abusiveness is mutual, and abusiveness is related to poor problem-solving skills. Behaviorally oriented, Margolin maintains that each coercive behavior elicits a similar or equally coercive counter response. Willi (1984) contends that couples bond in conscious and unconscious ways and that it is in this bonding that the predominant collusive themes for the relationship are established. In other words, couples agree either consciously or unconsciously what the rules of the relationship will be, including whether or how much violence is tolerable.

Weitzman and Dreen (1982) hypothesize that violence is bilateral and symmetrical, which is to say, both partners are responsible for the violence. Neidig, Friedman, & Collins (1985) assume that violence is primarily a function of specific skill deficits in each member of the couple: Both partners participate in an abusive relationship, although not necessarily equally. Their treatment goal, however, is for each partner to come to understand how each of them is "abuser and victim, both sinner and sinned against" (p. 196). Taylor (1984) locates the source of the violence in the individual but the maintenance in the couple. He posits that the abuser has an anger-control disorder that eventually develops into an abusive system that is dangerous to both partners.

What these authors have in common is that they locate the deficit in either the individual or the couple and ignore the cultural prescriptions and proscriptions about violence.

More recently, there has been an attempt to apply the Milan systemic model to abusive relationships. Lane and Russell (1987) suggest that therapists approach spouse abuse from a position of neutrality. They give as an example of a neutral question: If one of you is dead and the other is in prison, and your children grow up without you, who will they blame for not having parents?

The problem with this approach is one of undercontextualization. The seemingly neutral question can be neutral only if one ignores the likelihood that it is the wife who will be dead and the husband who may or may not be in prison. The supposed neutrality supports the status quo by not confronting the reality that women are seriously physically assaulted and killed by men much more frequently than the converse.

Typologies of Violent Families

Another approach in the family literature seeks to identify typologies that characterize violent families. Families in which there is violence have been described as enmeshed, rigid, and socially isolated (Nichols, 1986). Both abusers and victims often come from abusive families themselves, and often have either been victims of or witnesses to violence in their families of origin (Hilberman, 1984; Kalmus, 1984). These efforts at catagorizing seek to identify the particular pathology or dysfunction that characterizes these families.

In sum, family systems theorists have begun with the assumption that wife abuse serves some system-maintaining function. One approach has emphasized an investigation into the location of the problem. A second approach defines violence as pathological and nonnormative and seeks to define the type of family that produces violence.

LIMITATIONS OF SYSTEMS THEORY

Our fundamental criticism of the family therapy literature is that it under-contextualizes wife abuse. It seeks to locate the problem in the couple or in the individual and ignores the crucial structural contributions of the larger society. The enormity of the problem itself indicates that we need to look beyond individual families for the origins of the problem. Nearly one out of every four murder victims in the United States is killed by a family member. One of every three couples experience a violent incident each year and, over time, such incidents occur at least once in two-thirds of American marriages (Straus, 1974). These numbers alone indicate a need for a shift in conceptual focus.

There are other criticisms of family therapy approaches to wife abuse. Bograd (1984) has cogently criticized the systemic literature for its treatment of the subject. She states that interpretations of violence as symptomatic of other, deeper problems, such as diffuse boundaries, rigid structures, or runaway feedback loops, minimize the importance of the violence.

The Boundary Problem

Although Minuchin (1974) defines the family as an open system in transformation, until recently the family therapy field has not seriously considered how the family is structured in this particular historical period. Most of us took the idea of the family as an open system to mean that a particular family was more or less open to its particular environment (school, laws, community values). As a group, most family therapists have stopped short of a serious analysis of how the family in this period is structured by the social, political, and economic contexts in which it exists. Family therapy has drawn the boundary around the family as tightly as the early psychoanalysts drew it around the individual.

Recently, several writers have challenged the way we have drawn this boundary, and have pointed out serious problems attendant on ignoring the social context. Goldner (1985) points out that families do not just accommodate to intrafamilial needs, but are profoundly regulated by social forces outside of their awareness. Only recently (Bograd, Chap. 4; Goldner, 1985; James & McIntyre, 1983) have there been efforts to delineate the ways in which the social, political, and economic contexts produce patterns of dysfunction in families.

Both Goldner (1985) and James and McIntyre (1983) use the clinical example of the overinvolved mother and peripheral father to illustrate this point. As clinicians, we see all too many families that fit this description, but few of us consider that this clinical problem is socially produced. It derives from the unequal economic positions of men and women in which labor is divided so that men's primary commitment is outside the home and women's place is inside the home, and also from sex-role socialization, which teaches and promotes nurturing capacities in women and stunts these same capacities in men.

These same factors act to produce wife abuse. A woman, dependent on her husband for her financial and social status, believes that the well-being of the relationship and the family is her responsibility. A man, believing himself to be the rightful head of the household, trained not in feelings but in the concept that might makes right and backed by a social, legal, and economic system, views his wife as property to do with as he wishes. This setup is perfect for wife abuse.

Rather than consider this larger picture, family therapists 'particularize' each family's responsibility for the origins and treatment of problems that are, in fact, largely socially constructed (Bograd, 1984; James & McIntyre, 1983).

This insistence on the family as the primary unit of diagnosis and treatment has led to a further distortion. By seeing the family as only a "special case of a system" (Taggart, 1985, p. 115), we fail to attend to the real differences in position, power, resources, and experience between men and women. By treating family members merely as players within a nuclear system and ignoring the social context, women's issues disappear (Taggart, 1985).

In the case of wife abuse, for example, one of the things that disappears is the way that the legal system's failure to protect women operates to sanction wife abuse, and even murder. In two well-publicized cases in Boston in 1987, women were murdered— One by her husband, the other by her lover—after repeated requests for police and court protection had been denied. Men and women are not merely interchangeable players in a system. In all spheres, men have greater power than women. To deny or minimize this indisputable aspect of reality is to ignore the foundation of the problem.

If we are to place violence behavior in its proper social and political contexts (Dobash & Dobash, 1979), we must discuss the important social forces that define the differences between men and women.

BEYOND THE FAMILY

Once we move to the larger social context, we need not belabor the point that women's position is one of socially structured inequality (MacKinnon & Miller, 1987, p. 140). This structured inequality has a long history. What Alexis de Toqueville (1969) wrote in 1840 is largely true today.

In America a woman loses her independence forever in the bonds of matrimony. While there is less constraint on girls there than anywhere else; a wife submits to stricter obligations. (p. 592)

Nor have the Americans ever supposed that democratic principles should undermine the husbands authority and make it doubtful who is in charge of the family. In their view, every association, to be effective must have a head, and the natural head of the conjugal association is the husband. (p. 601)

Women have less power then men economically, legally, and sociopolitically.

The Economic System and the Family

Women earn less money than men and suffer a greater drop in their standard of living upon divorce than men do (Goldner, 1985). Some progress has been made, but women still suffer economic discrimination.

Although these facts are well known, we have hardly attended to them when working with the problem of wife abuse, let alone focused on their centrality. Consider the following: A 1985 study (Aguire, 1985) revealed that a wife's economic dependence on her husband was the most powerful predictor of whether she would return to an abusive relationship. Money, not masochism or systems regulation, seems to be the crucial variable. Observe the obstacles to leaving a marriage on which one is economically dependent. The woman must enter a whole new sphere. She must join the paid labor force, receive public assistance, or try to increase her marketable skills so as to increase her income. If she has not worked previously, she is faced with finding child care, which is often both inadequate in terms of quality and time and extremely expensive.

Straus and Gelles (1986) found a drop in the rate of wife abuse between 1975 and 1985. On considering possible reasons for this decline, they hypothesized that a trend toward more economically egalitarian marriges over the past ten years (as more wives have entered the work force) is an important contributor to the decline in wife abuse. Straus (1974) cites his previous research showing that husband-dominant marriages have the highest level of violence and that egalitarian marriages have the lowest.

Here is the essence of the problem. By failing to attend to the clear evidence that women have less economic power than men and that a woman's economic position relative to her husband's is a crucial determinant both in the occurrence of wife abuse and as to whether she then leaves or stays, family therapists omitted a crucial factor from both theorizing and treatment.

The Legal System and the Family

When women are battered by their husbands, they receive little protection from the legal system. Historically, the police and the courts have viewed domestic violence as a private problem and are reluctant to intervene. Even when women reach the point of seeking legal protection, they are largely unable to obtain it. The failure of the legal system to offer protection to women is a power proscriptive sanction for male dominance and male violence.

A study by Sherman and Berk (1984) in Minneapolis underscores this point. Police randomly selected three tactics in response to "moderate" domestic violence—arrest, advice or mediation, or ordering the violent spouse to leave for eight hours. Outcome was measured by the numbers of new official reports of violence during the next six months. The results were dramatic: Of those arrested, 10 percent were reported for new offenses during the trial time. For advice or mediation, the number was 16 percent, and for ordering the violent spouse to leave for eight hours, the repeat rate was 22 percent.

Other studies, from Canada (Jaffe, Wolfe, Teford, & Austin, 1986), California (Berk & Newton, 1985), and New Zealand (Fergusson, Horwood, Kershaw, & Shannon, 1986), confirm the result that arrest is best as an initial intervention in stopping wife abuse.

Clearly, the police and the courts as social control agents have the power to send the message that domestic violence is societally unacceptable and that this message acts as a powerful deterrent. They do not routinely do so.

Sex-Role Socialization and the Family

Sex-role socialization is a crucial area that has not been emphasized in the family therapy literature. A theory that talks about neutrality, feedback loops, and coevolution has not found room to incorporate the powerful role gender plays in socialization and experience (Goldner, 1985, James & McIntyre, 1983, McKinnon & Miller, 1987, Taggart, 1985).

Differences in socialization alone between men and women go far in accounting for the prevalence of wife abuse. Men are socialized to be emotionally constricted and to value autonomy, isolated achievement, and power (male activities), and to devalue emotional connection and feelings (female activities). Violence as an ultimate resource is legitimized as an appropriate male behavior (Adams & Penn, 1981). We have only to turn on the television set to see abundant evidence for the last statement. Men are identified with work and the world outside of the home. What happens inside the home is not their responsibility. They are socialized to expect to be taken care of and nurtured by women.

Women are socialized to be accommodating, emotionally expressive, and nurturing; to put themselves second; to internalize blame; and to value male activities and perogatives and to devalue female activities and rights. Women are identified with the home and wife roles. What happens in the home is their responsibility. This identification has given rise to such culture-inspired adages as, "Behind every successful man is a good woman."

The descriptions of wife abusers are, for the most part, enlargements of normative sex role socialization in which men learn that they are both to be taken care of by women and to be dominant over them. Men who are physically and psychologically violent with their wives have been found to be childlike, remorseful, yearning for nurturance, jealous, possessive, and sexually promiscuous (i.e., emotionally immature). They have also been found to be more violent when wives are pregnant (and presumably less available and more helpless) and when they do not get their way (Hilberman, 1984). Straus has reported more violence in husband-dominant homes—that is, where husbands have more power and believe in the ideology that husbands should dominate wives (Straus & Gelles, 1985). Given sex-role socialization, wife abuse can be viewed not as deviant behavior but as an example of prescriptive norms.

Wives who are abused by their husbands have been described as coming from families where they either saw abuse, were themselves physically or sexually abused, or both (Hilberman, 1984). Wives are more likely to be in abusive marriages, if, during their adolescence, they witnessed marital violence in their homes (Kalmuss, 1984). Star (1982) has characterized abused wives as raised in emotionally restrictive home environments where they were encouraged to be passive and socially isolated. They, therefore, became wives who internalize and assume blame for husbands' violence. They are compliant with their husband's demands to the best of their abilities. Thus, the ways in which abusive men and abused women embody exaggerations of general sex-role socialization produce a situation ripe for wife abuse.

We could continue to ask ourselves, "What's wrong with these people, or the families in which abuse occurs?" Instead, let us suggest that we begin seriously to ask ourselves and each other what is wrong with a society that continues to support male dominance and to legitimize wife abuse.

Family therapists will not have much change of really being useful to women who are beaten or to the men who beat them until they understand the full nature of the relationships between men and women. Understanding the larger social context brings into question some of the basic assumptions of family therapy.

CHALLENGING BASIC CONCEPTS

Equality, reciprocity, mutuality, and coevolution are central to a systemic understanding of couples. For the most part, family therapists have been unwilling to question the effect of these beliefs. As Goldner (1985) writes:

> Family treatment ideology would oppose the suggestion that social forces could differentially regulate the nature and distribution of power within the family, such that *some family members would be more equal than others* [italics added]. (p. 33)

Nevertheless, it is impossible adequately to understand wife abuse without questioning family therapy ideology.

Equality can be conceptualized in several ways. One is in terms of equality of resources. Do men and women have equal access to economic, legal, social, and political resources? The answer is clearly No. Another way to think about equality is to consider whether women and men benefit equally from marriage. Here, again, the answer is clearly No.

The mental health patterns of married and unmarried adults have received much attention. In *The Future of Marriage*, Bernard (1972) argues persuasively that marriage as an institution is generally detrimental to the mental health and happiness of wives but beneficial to that of husbands. Citing a number of studies, Bernard notes that:

> More wives than husbands report marital frustration and dissatisfaction; more report negative feelings; more wives than husbands report marital problems; more

wives than husbands consider their marriage unhappy, have considered separation or divorce, have regretted their marriages, and fewer have reported positive companionship. (p. 28)

This would indicate that wives experience less satisfaction in marriage than husbands.

There is also evidence that wives have poorer mental health than do husbands (Gurin, Veroff, & Feld, 1960). Gove (1972), in an extensive review of the literature on community surveys of mental health, first admission to mental hospitals, and public and private outpatient care, found that women are more likely to be mentally ill than men. Moreover, it is the relatively high rate of mental illness among married women (not single, widowed, or divorced women) that accounts for these rates.

The evidence shows that wives function at a lower level of psychological adjustment than do husbands. These findings might be attributed to sex differences rather than to the differential effects of the traditional husband and wife roles. The evidence, however, shows that it is marriage and not sex that accounts for the difference. For example, it has been found that divorced and widowed men have higher rates of mental illness than divorced and widowed women (Gove, 1972). Comparison of the rates of mental illness of married men and women with those of single men and women again points to marriage, rather than sex, as the differentiating factor.

Gove (1972) cited 1960 census data showing that although married women are more likely to be residents of mental hospitals than married men, men who are single, divorced, or widowed are more likely to be residents of mental hospitals than are women. Gove (1972) concluded:

At least in terms of mental illness, being married is considerably more advantageous to men than it is to women, while being single, if anything, is slightly more disadvantageous to men than to women. (p. 430)

Here are convincing empirical data that men and women do not benefit equally from marriage. Men benefit more from marriage than do women in terms of mental health and happiness. The data do not support the assertion that couples relationships are characterized by equality.

Yet family therapy's assumption of equality among members of a family is a dearly held one. According to Goldner (1985):

To question the idea that work or suffering or pleasure might be distributed unequally between marital partners would clearly complicate and perhaps compromise the circular presumption that family members are eternally involved in a balancing operation in which all positions are psychopolitically interchangeable—that anyone can play any part in the service of system maintenance. (p. 33)

Equality, mutuality, reciprocity, and coevolution are inextricably linked. Mutuality implies participation by both parties in working toward common goals. The concept of reciprocity posits that participants are both mutually and equally involved in systems creation and maintenance (MacKinnon & Miller, 1987). Further, coevolution is based on the belief that both parties participate in the outcome of interactions and in the maintenance of the system as a whole. These beliefs can only be held by ignoring the systematic structurally produced differences in power held and exercised by men and women.

These four concepts are based on a set of romantic and politically conservative values that simply do not fit the facts. Few relationships between men and women are equal, mutual, or reciprocal. Why should marriage be any different?

These assumptions are particularly damaging when applied to the problem of wife abuse. In considering the capacity to inflict physical damage, men and women are seldom equal. Men have more power to be violent than women have to stop them from being so. Failing to stop the violence of men, women have few options for leaving the marriage because of both their socialization in the wife role and economic discrimination.

Wife abuse is not a mutual interaction. The man's goal is to inflict physical or psychological pain and the woman's goal is to protect herself. Wife abuse is not reciprocal. There is nothing a person can do that makes physical abuse an appropriate response. Therefore, to talk about the coevolution of violence maintains the larger cultural system's sanctions of male violence and fails to disrupt the foundations of the violence within the couple. Coevolution is a damaging concept when referring to this problem, given the difference in physical strength, economic dependency, and the priority of relationship between the partners.

Instead, this view further victimizes women in that it assigns coresponsibility in causation and, therefore, coresponsibility for maintenance and cessation of the abuse.

TREATMENT

In couple relationships, family therapy is only one point of intervention, and not necessarily the most powerful point. Critical societal changes are needed in order to eliminate wife abuse, including changes in the economic system so that women will have more economic power and independence; changes in socialization that will increase men's identification with the home and women's identification with the public sphere; changes in the criminal justice system; changes in the cultural norms that legitimize violence by men; more resources in the form of shelters, economic support, and counseling for battered women; and treatment programs for abusive men.

Despite our emphasis on the need for societal change, we affirm that there are ways that family therapists can be instrumental in helping to stop wife abuse.

Here, we deal only with couples voluntarily seeking treatment, and do not include the involuntary treatment of couples, treatment of individuals, or group therapy.

Our philosophy regarding conjoint treatment is based on the premise that although both partners are part of a couple system, and so, descriptively, both play a part, they possess unequal resources, and the inequality inherent in the relationship is the primary determinant of the outcome. Therefore, our initial step is to take a stance that the man must stop being violent. Our concern for the safety of the woman outweighs any concerns for the continuation of the couple relationship.

How Couples Enter Treatment

Couples may or may not identify wife abuse as their presenting problem when they enter treatment. As much wife abuse is not publically identified, it is essential in all couples interviews to ask about fighting style in general, and about physical violence in particular. One is more likely to receive an accurate response by asking how much, what types of, and when violence occurs rather than by asking if there ever is violence. To ask about fighting or arguing without seeking specific details of violence is insufficient and can be collusive in denying this problem. If therapists do not get the violence out into the open, women may be coerced by continued threats of violence into sabotaging the treatment and it will fail (Willi, 1984).

When violence has already been identified as a problem, couples typically come in crisis, after a violent episode, frequently following a physical separation, an arrest of the man, or a shelter stay by the wife and children. In this situation, the therapist needs to take the violence seriously and to discuss the possibility of a structured separation, with either the wife in a shelter, or the husband or wife leaving the home for separate housing. Legal options need to be discussed, such as vacate and/or restraint orders, legal separations or divorce. One of the actions therapists can take to become more effective in stopping wife abuse is to educate themselves about resources available to women, including shelters and legal and social services.

It is important to note that the agendas of the husband, wife, and therapist may all be different. The man's agenda is often the continuation of the relationship and the preservation of his superior position. The woman's agenda is most often to preserve the relationship with more safety for herself. The therapist's agenda needs to prioritize the woman's safety, whether by stopping the violence or by helping her leave the relationship. As with other life-threatening situations (i.e., homicidal and suicidal clients), physical safety must be the absolute central focus in the formation phase of treatment.

Obviously, we will not always be successful in either stopping the violence or helping the woman to leave the relationship. However, we can increase our chances of success by understanding the problem correctly, by knowing about and utilizing available resources, and by, in other areas of our lives, advocating for womens' rights.

Therapist's Stance

The first step in treating couples in which the wives are abused is to say that the man must stop being violent, even though almost as many wives as husbands are violent (Kalmuss, 1984). Husbands inflict greater damage than wives even when the violence is mutual. This is true for a number of reasons, including mens' greater strength and their greater knowledge of and comfort with ways to inflict damage.

Why is it so important to say to the man, "You must stop?" On a systemic level, both the husband and the wife believe that male violence is legitimate. Saying No to that belief is a powerful intervention in itself, and sets the stage for future interventions. Saying "you must stop" to the man also puts the responsibility where it belongs, with the perpetrator, not in the couple interaction.

One of the concerns that sometimes stops therapists from labeling a particular behavior as bad or destructive is a concern for the alliance. However, Grunebaum and Chasin (1978) point out that telling the truth diagnostically can actually enhance the alliance. Speaking to the couple about the ways a behavior such as male violence dominates family life confirms reality for the entire family.

The establishment of a no-violence contract is the next move. The intention and word of the couple in these situations as demonstrated by a verbal or written agreement will establish a good-faith therapeutic contract. Can we be assured that this will suffice? In the majority of cases, absolutely not. The no-violence contract is merely the beginning of the work. The body of the work revolves around enabling the men to become nonviolent by enacting a variety of interventions.

Interventions

In effect, men need to learn that they can be in control of themselves in healthier ways. A question we often ask a man who says that he is out of control is, "Why didn't you stab her?" His usually horrified response that he would not do that shows that the use and extent of violence are in his control and opens a discussion about his exercise of choice as to whether or not to use violence and in what amounts.

Men need further help in identifying the behavioral antecedents of their violence and specific alternative plans to detour or deescalate their pattern. This behavioral strategy is useful as it gives men the message that their violent behavior (which is unacceptable) is learned and within their control, and that they can succeed in correcting it by learning new self-management skills.

One important skill for the couple to learn is time-out. Each spouse learns to identify his or her own bodily experience signaling that a danger point is being reached. Either person calls for a time-out, each person having previously agreed that he or she will honor time-out requests. For example, the man might identify his bodily signals that he is about to become abusive as shortness of breath, queasy stomach, and clenched fists. The woman might identify her signals of fear as dizziness or headache. When these signals are noted, either party calls for a time-out. The length of the time out varies—it can be for 20 minutes or two days. During the time out, they do not discuss the disagreement that led up to the body signals.

Men always need to learn to recognize the signs of their impending violence, and to implement alternative behaviors. Women need to identify their fears as a signal to utilize escape strategies. As part of the initial contract, the woman needs to identify a plan to escape if the man should become violent. She needs to know in advance whether she will call the police or leave the home (to go where?), and ensure that funds are available to do so.

Each spouse can employ self-reward statements for succeeding in time-out behaviors, such as, "I did a good job that time staying out of a fight." Any similar statement in the couple's own language is appropriate.

Other techniques to deescalate the violence cycle may also be employed by the man. Some useful interventions include actual physical separations for specific periods of time, and the use of physical exercise to detour violent behavior. Writing a journal or log about the current emotional and behavior experience and calling for help from the therapist, friends, relatives, or self-help group members are useful techniques.

In the couples session, circular questions can be used to diminish isolation and privacy. Circular questioning does this by enlarging the psychological field (Penn, 1982). The couple can begin to imagine other people's responses to the situation. This enlargement of psychological space helps to diminish violence because abusive behavior is more likely to occur when it is kept secret or hidden. In the beginning phases, we ask who of their friends and relatives would be most surprised, outraged, indifferent, helpful, or concerned about the violence. As the couple makes positive changes, we continue to ask who would be most supportive, disappointed, helpful, or pleased by the diminution of violence. Circular questioning can also be used to address larger social issues in a therapeutic manner. "Who would have the most to lose financially if the relationship were to end? Who would have the most to lose emotionally? Which one of you would gain most by the cessation or continuation of violence?" These questions enlarge the psychological field, and loosen the tight boundary around the couple, thereby helping to diminish violence.

In this phase, the reasons for the escalation are noted for future reference but are not addressed in any detail. The capacity to deescalate is most important. The goal here is not to eradicate anger (Novaco, 1976) or argument from the relationship, but to establish a nonviolent, noncoercive foundation so that in later stages the couple can learn to resolve its differences without harm taking place.

One of the ways therapist can minimize the possibility that couples are not telling the truth about the continuance of violence in the relationship is to ask very specific questions about recent disagreements. If previously violent partners maintain that they have had no disagreements, or are unable to provide the details of how the disagreements have been resolved, there is a good chance that the violence is continuing unreported. In this case, the therapist needs to probe the areas of disagreement and not be put off by the couple's sparse responses.

We contend that the cycle of escalation can be stopped at any point by the conscious and deliberate use of these and other strategies. The conscious nonuse of these interventions constitutes a violation of the no-violence contract and consequences must ensue. Abusive men often claim that they did not know what they were doing, citing the use of alcohol or drugs, or amnesia, or of forgetting whole episodes. This 'unconscious' acting out also needs to be prevented by confronting the man's denial and minimizing. No-drinking contracts can also be employed to block this strategy on the part of the man. Alcoholics Anonymous and Alanon are crucial resources. Larger network interventions, including family, friends, and employers, that focus on the substance abuse, the violence, or both, are helpful strategies.

Our experience is that these strategies are powerful interventions. Yet, sometimes, they may not be successful, and in that case, we determine that the man is currently unable to keep a no-violence contract. In such a situation, couples treatment is not the treatment of choice. We then work toward a structured separation, using vacate and restraint orders or arrest if necessary, and refer both spouses to individual and/or group treatments.

As in many family therapies, the importance of alliance building or joining is crucial in this initial stage. The unacceptable, bad, violent behavior on the part of the man must be labeled. His violence needs to be clearly stated as the single most detrimental block to the continued life of the relationship and to the usefulness of the couples therapy. The woman needs to be assured that she did not provoke or cause her husband's violent behavior. At the same time, the distinction between bad behavior and "bad person" needs to be acknowledged. We can be neutral in alliance building while being opposed to the violent behavior.

Accomplishing this joining with both is essential. We do not see it as contradictory to alliance building to label the man's abusive behavior as the primary focus of the treatment. To do otherwise puts the therapist in a collusive position that, subtly or directly, gives permission for violence to continue.

In cases where men are intimidating to a female therapist, a male-female cotherapy team is helpful, as is a team behind a one-way mirror.

After the violence stops, the couple is often uninterested in continuing treatment. Once the crisis is over, the man appears remorseful, the woman appears forgiving of him, and he promises not to hit her again, yet changes in the relationship rules are only the beginning. This is similar to the dry-drunk phenomena seen in alcoholic couples—substance abuse is not occurring, yet the same associated behaviors, and the underlying dynamics, continue unabated. It is crucial at this point for the therapist to warn the couple about the likelihood of the recurrence of violence unless they continue in treatment to learn how to have a relationship without violence, much as an alcoholic family needs to learn how to function without alcohol.

Two criteria mark the close of this first phase of treatment for the couple. First is the cessation of violence, and the appropriate use of the techniques employed to maintain a safe environment. The second criterion is the willingness of the couple to enter into a new marital relationship or to end the relationship. The close of the first phase may be premature when it includes only the cessation of violence and not the motivation to renegotiate other aspects of the relationship.

If the couple terminates because the therapist takes a strong limit-setting stance here, it is obvious that marital therapy is contraindicated. Couples therapy can be resumed after both spouses have participated successfully in individual or group therapies.

Ongoing Treatment

At this point, the couple is considered to be violence-free and seeking a better marital relationship. The nature of this phase of treatment is to maintain the safety and the lack of violence, and to enhance the relationship. Further positive problem-solving and communication skills are developed. A more historical approach is utilized in tracking the family or origin and earlier relationships for the origins of violent behavior. A cognitive restructuring of the beliefs both have about violence is combined with a fuller understanding of the societal forces that established and maintained the violence. Relapses are addressed by a resumption of earlier contracts and interventions being repeated as needed. This phase of treatment resembles the treatment of nonviolent couples.

CONCLUSIONS

The difficulty of treating wife abuse using systemic family theory has been discussed to illustrate the ways in which core concepts are inapplicable. By utilizing information from other fields, we have reconceptualized the issue of wife abuse in a broader social and political context and allowed the inclusion of a greater range of interventions. We have replaced the systemic concepts of equality, mutuality, reciprocity, and coevolution with an understanding of the inequality between men and women and its effects on marriage.

A nontraditional therapist stance of limit setting is prescribed in the beginning phase of treatment, and appropriate consequences in the legal arena are recommended, if needed. Marital therapy should be discontinued and other interventions utilized if violence continues in the relationship because, unless safety is the priority, couples treatment is unlikely to succeed in eliminating violent behavior.

Although a clear therapeutic strategy is available, the essential education of therapists on the social context of wife abuse and the normative aspects of violence in our society needs to be developed. Violence in marriages and in society will only cease when gender-based inequalities are addressed and changed, and when clearly set prohibitions and consequences are enforced.

REFERENCES

Adams, D., & Penn, I. (1981). *Men in groups: The socialization and resocialization of men who batter.* Paper presented at the annual meeting of the American Orthopsychiatric Association.

Aguire, B. (1985). Why do they return? Abused wives in shelters. *Social Work, 30,* 350–354.

Berk, R., & Newton, P. (1985). Does arrest deter wife battery? An effort to replicate the findings of the Minneapolis spouse abuse experiment. *American Sociological Review, 50,* 253–262.

Bernard, J. (1972). *The future of marriage.* New York: Bantam.

Bograd, M. (1984). Family systems approaches to wife battering: A feminist critique. *American Journal of Orthopsychiatry, 54,* 558–568.

de Toqueville, A. (1969). *Democracy in America.* J. P. Mayer (translator). New York: Doubleday.

Dobash, R.R., & Dobash, R. (1979). *Violence against wives: A case against the patriarchy.* New York: Free Press.

Elbow, M. (1977). Theoretical considerations of violent marriages. *Social Casework, 58,* 54–65.

Fergusson, C., Horwood, L.J., Kershaw, K., & Shannon, F. (1986). Factors associated with reports of wife assault in New Zealand. *Journal of Marriage and the Family, 48,* 407–412.

Goldner, V. (1985). Feminism and family therapy. *Family Process, 24,* 31–47.

Gove, W. (1972). The relationship between sex roles, marital status, and mental illness. *Social Forces, 51,* 38–44.

Grunebaum, H., & Chasin, R. (1978). Relabeling and reframing reconsidered: The beneficial effects of a pathological label. *Family Proceess, 17,* 449–455.

Gurin, G., Veroff, J. & Feld, S. (1960). *Americans view their mental health.* New York: Basic Books.

Hilberman, E. (1984). Overview: The "wife beater's wife: reconsidered. In P.R. Rileker & E. (Hilberman) Carman (Eds.), *The gender gap in psychotherapy, social realities and psychological processes.* (pp. 213–236). New York: Plenum Press.

Hoffman, L. (1981). *Foundations of family therapy: A conceptual framework for systems change.* New York: Basic Books.

Jaffe, P., Wolfe, D., Teford, A., & Austin, G. (1986). The impact of police charges in incidents of wife abuse. *Journal of Family Violence, 12,* 37–286.

James, K., & McIntyre, D. (1983). The reproduction of families: The social role of family therapy? *Journal of Marital and Family Therapy, 9,* 119–129.

Kalmuss, D. (1984). The intergenerational transmission of marital violence. *Journal of Marriage and the Family, 146,* 11–19.

Lane, G., & Russell, T. (1987). Neutrality vs. social control. *The Family Therapy Networker, 11,* 52–56.

MacKinnon, L., & Miller, D. (1987). The new epistemology and the Milan approach: Feminist and sociopolitical considerations. *Journal of Marital and Family Therapy, 13,* 139–155.

Margolin, G. (1979). Conjoint marital therapy to enhance anger management and reduce spouse abuse. *The American Journal of Family Therapy, 7,* 13–23.

Minuchin, S. (1974). *Families and family therapy.* Cambridge, Mass.: Harvard University Press.

Neidig, P., Friedman, D., & Collins, B. (1985). Domestic conflict containment: A spouse abuse treatment program. *Social Casework, 66,* 195–204.

Nichols, W. (1986). Understanding family violence: An orientation for family therapists. *Contemporary Family Therapy, 8,* 188–207.

Novaco, R. (1976). The functions and regulation of the arousal of anger. *American Journal of Psychiatry, 133,* 1124–1128.

Penn, P. (1982). Circular questioning. *Family Process, 21,* 267–280.

Selvini-Palazzoli, M., Boscolo, L., Cecchin, G., & Prata, G. (1980). Hypothesizing-circularity-neutrality: Three guidelines for the conductor of the session, *Family Process, 19,* 3–12.

Sherman, L., & Berk, R. (1984). The specific deterrent effects of arrest for domestic assault. *American Sociological Review, 49,* 261–272.

Star, B. (1982). Characteristics of family violence. In J. Flanzer, (Ed.). *The many faces of family violence.* (pp. 14–23). Springfield, Ill.: Charles C. Thomas.

Straus, M. (1974). Leveling, civility, and violence in the family. *Journal of Marriage and the Family, 35,* 13–29.

Straus, M. (1976). Sexual inequity, cultural norms, and wife beating. *Victimology, 1,* 54–76.

Straus, M., & Gelles, R. (1986). Societal change and change in family violence from 1975 to 1985 as revealed by two national surveys. *Journal of Marriage and the Family, 48,* 465–479.

Taggart, M. (1985). The feminist critique in epistemological perspective: Questions of context in family therapy. *Journal of Marital and Family Therapy, 11,* 113–126.

Taylor, J. (1984). Structured conjoint therapy for spouse abuse cases. *Social Casework, 60,* 11–18.

Weitzman, J., & Dreen, K. (1982). Wife beating: A view of the marital dyad. *Social Casework, 63,* 259–265.

Willi, J. (1984). The concept of collusion: A combined systemic-psychodynamic approach to marital therapy. *Family Process, 23,* 177–185.

7

FATHER-DAUGHTER INCEST: CONSIDERATIONS FOR THE FAMILY THERAPIST

Dorothy Wheeler, Ph.D.

Within the field of family therapy very little attention is given to the problem of intrafamilial child sexual abuse. This absence may be taken as an endorsement that sexual abuse within the family is, more or less, like any other family problem and may be effectively treated within any one of several existing models of family therapy. That is, the emergence of abuse signals some dysfunction in the system as a whole, thus necessitating theoretical formulations and clinical interventions focused almost solely upon the problematic intrafamilial interactional patterns within which the abuse appears to be embedded. This chapter will suggest that the ethical and effective treatment of incest is possible only when clinicians consider the ways in which individual, family system, and larger system dynamics interact to establish and maintain the abuse. When we rely on systems theory as the primary explanatory framework, we leave ourselves vulnerable either to failing to stop the abuse or to block its reoccurrence.

Although certain family structures can be understood as rendering a family more vulnerable to tolerating the abusive behavior of the offender, the responsibility for the abuse needs to be seen as belonging to the individual who offends. He brings the tendency to offend with him to the family, where it may or may not emerge. Systemic formulations typically do not adequately address issues of individual responsibility and move too quickly to spread accountability throughout the system. Incest is a problem in which one person's abuse of power violates and victimizes others whose accesses to power are simply not comparable. Part of this inequity can be explained because the victim and the offender are of different generations. Standard family therapy generational explanations cannot begin to explain, however, why more than 90 percent of offenders are male. To understand this reality, we need to explore gender politics and, as suggested by David Finkelhor (1984), begin to understand sexual abuse as a problem of masculine socialization (p. 12).

Working from this view, this chapter will describe treatment considerations effective in (1) stopping the incest, (2) counteracting the tendency to blame the victim and/or the mother for the abuse itself and (3) holding the offender in treatment while adopting a confrontative and respectful position toward him. Father-daughter incest will be the focus of this chapter because it is one of the most prevalent and well-documented forms of abuse and is believed by some to be the most traumatic (Russell, 1986).

DEFINING INCEST

For purposes of this presentation, incest, or intrafamilial sexual abuse, encompasses any form of sexual activity between a child and a family or extended-family member, including adults in surrogate parent roles, such as live-in boyfriends. This activity is, by definition, exploitative and nonconsensual, as it describes sexual acts imposed by a more powerful and dominant adult or older adolescent on a child who lacks the emotional, physical, and cognitive maturity to protect himself or herself.

When a male in a caretaking position pulls a young child up into his generational realm or steps down into hers by coercing her to engage in sexual touching, individual, family, and cultural factors interact in a particularly damaging way. Men who commit sexual assaults against children are clearly not one-dimensional villains, but the particular adjustment they make to their own victimization or rigid socialization—that is, to offend their daughter or stepdaughter—results in a victimization of women that is devastating.

The offender is claiming ownership of the daughter's body and her experience, and teaching her about submissiveness and disassociation. He is dividing her from her mother, and teaching both of them about isolation and competition among women. He will convince her that either she or her mother is responsible for the abuse, and will, therefore, teach them both about hating themselves and blaming women. His insistence that the victim care for him at her expense will school her in self-denial and nonreciprocal caretaking.

Father-daughter incest can be conceptualized as the selfish, exploitative, and assaultive behavior of an immature, emotionally depleted male. This male has been placed in an authoritative and caretaking position while being severely handicapped by social injunctions against connecting in an empathetic, nonsexual, and "feminine" way. His female partner has been placed centrally in a devalued role where she has too much responsibility and not enough power. The family is itself weakened to the point of tolerating or being unable to repel the powerful organizing force of his abusive behavior. The primary point of weakness is in the adult spousal-parental relationship. This relationship tends to be socially prescribed as an intragenerational hierarchy with positions disproportionately determined by gender or, more accurately, the prescriptions attached to being male or female.

THREE LEVELS OF EXPLANATION

Denial, minimization, rationalization, and secrecy are qualities characteristic of incest and crucial to maintaining the abusive dynamics. Family therapists may be more vulnerable than other helping professionals to colluding in these dynamics if one relies exclusively on systemic formulations to describe sexual abuse. In attempts to be consistent with nonpathological, nonblaming, circular conceptualizations, therapists may inadvertently find themselves working within a frame that is so neutral, abstract, and contentless that the coercive behavior of the offender and the resultant damage to the victim and to the family's interactional life are almost impossible to comment upon and challenge.

Family therapists make a serious error when they treat sexual abuse as simply a symptom of a typical interactional problem or as peripheral to a more serious problem, such as the lack of an intimate connection between the offender and his partner. Therapists cannot afford to convey neutrality with respect to how they think about the abuse or where they place the responsibility for the abuse itself. To do so is to risk participating in the process of minimization and to contribute to a further invalidation of the victim's experience. It is necessary, therefore, to decide upon a definition of sexual abuse that includes the individual and cultural contributions along with the family systems aspects.

The Individual Contribution of the Offender

Family therapists have been criticized by experts in the field of sexual abuse for viewing incest as *primarily* a reflection of a disordered system and ignoring the powerful organizing impact an individual can have on the family system (Conte, 1986; Finkelhor, 1986; Herman, 1981; Sgroi, 1982). The position taken by these critics is that while certain organizational or interactional patterns may render a family at risk for the emergence of incest, the key element is the individual offender and what he brings into the family system. The family of origin may be mentioned by these authors as a causal antecedent, and although current dynamics of the nuclear family may also be noted, they are seen more as a contextual backdrop against which an individual's disordered behavior is viewed.

David Finkelhor (1986), one of the most thought-provoking and prolific researchers in the field of child sexual assault, argues that systemic formulations obscure the finding that incestuous fathers have a "rather autonomous proclivity to abuse" and that "incestuous abusers would be inclined to abuse independent of family dynamics" (p. 56). Finkelhor (1984, 1986) suggests that offenders enter the family with a motivation to abuse children. For example, as a result of the father's own damaging childhood sexual experiences or because of inappropriate modeling, he may experience sexual arousal to children. Also, because of his own victimization or the ways in which his adjustment to being victimized interact with the more general masculine requirement to be dominant, he may use the sexual coercion of children to meet his needs for mastery, control, and competence. He may be blocked from obtaining adult sources of gratification because of deficient relational skills. Nicholas Groth, in his earlier work on offenders (1978), describes this man as a fixated child offender, a man who has a rather permanent compulsion to interact sexually with children and that these interests "have become a part of his nature" (p. 7).

According to Finkelhor, the offender must also overcome internal inhibitions to assault children sexually. Frequently, this results from disinhibition attributable to substance abuse. He may also be experiencing extreme stress as a result of illness, marital difficulties, or job-related difficulties and so revert to a highly irresponsible position with respect to children under his care. Sexual abuse as a response to stress also closely fits Groth's (1978) description of the regressed child offender who has a history of relatively normal interactional and sexual functioning, but in periods of heightened stress regresses, demonstrates highly dysfunctional behaviors in order to regain his sense of competence as a man. Offenses are also frequently common in men who exhibit general problems with impulse control or, less frequently, symptoms associated with psychosis.

With this perspective on individual pathology, changing the system alone is clearly not sufficient to stop the abusive process. The offender's attraction to children and his ability to influence the system in order to meet his needs to overpower must not be underestimated. Therapists working with incestuous dynamics must include the individual contribution of the perpetrator as part of their definition of the problem. When they minimize the role of the individual and restrict their treatment to changing the system, they may unintentionally collude with the offender in minimizing his contribution to the maintenance of the problem.

The Family Contribution

Families in which abuse occurs are frequently disorganized, rigid, and socially isolated. The parent figures have themselves, more often than not, come from extremely dysfunctional families where they were neglected and abused physically and/or sexually. They, therefore, exit their families of origin profoundly handicapped. Their ability to develop and maintain a positive sense of themselves is quite damaged and their ability to trust others is tentative at best. It is difficult for them to believe that they could be valued or respected by another. These deficits become crucial limitations in their attempts to set up healthy marital or family relationships (and become central issues in building a therapeutic relationship).

It appears that the early phase of a marriage or intimate relationship between these fragile partners may proceed smoothly enough. The delicate relationship complementarity is rocked and then fractured when children arrive and naturally need parental care. The woman in such families was usually a parentified child in her own family of origin (and often a victim of sexual abuse herself), is unfamiliar with either recognizing her own needs or having them met, and is attracted to men who need caretaking. Her own experience of parentification interacts with the normal socialization of females, leaving her doubly deficient in asserting her own needs or views. With the arrival of dependent children, she becomes even more depleted, and her partner does not move in to take care of her or assume his fair share of the parental responsibility. Instead, his own neediness and sense of being neglected are exacerbated. That is, both parents begin to disengage. They may continue to be sexual with each other, but they avoid emotional closeness and conflict resolution. Denise Gelinas (1986) has called this process "bilateral parental estrangement," emphasizing that it is not just that the mother is unavailable, but that her male partner also disconnects. The consequences are a family constellation that looks like an almost internally boundaryless system in which there are no spouses and no parents, just a group of needy children struggling to access a very impoverished pool of resources.

Not receiving support from her male partner and not taught to expect it, the mother may turn to her daughter as an agemate and as a helpmate. In this way, and before her daughter has had the experience of having her own needs validated and met, the mother passes on to her the devastating pattern of non-reciprocal caretaking. That is, the daughter's sense of self begins to be constructed around this dynamic.

Because he has been taught, as a man, that he has a right to expect caretaking from a female and that females are obliged to provide nurturance, the father begins to turn to his daughter for comfort and companionship. Men are also directed by their socialization to sexualize females and to get emotional needs met through sexualized interactions. If he himself has been a victim of neglect or incest, is disinhibited by substance abuse, is under heightened economic or personal stress, and/or has inadequate impulse control, he is extraordinarily vulnerable to progressing gradually to more sexually explicit and exploitive behaviors with his daughter. When the marital partners are estranged and avoid each other and the father has begun to set up a competitive relationship between the mother and the daughter, the children will be receiving minimal nurturance or protection. Because of the child's need for affection and her parentification, she will be more vulnerable to being exploited by her father. The system will be highly at risk for the emergence of sexual abuse.

Sociocultural Contributions

Sexual abuse is committed primarily by men. According to Finkelhor and Russell (1984) men constitute about 95 percent of the perpetrators in cases of abuse of girls and 80 percent in cases of abuse of boys. Such facts clearly incriminate men, or, more accurately, the process by which our culture turns male infants and children into masculine adolescents and men. The process by which sex-role conditioning constricts the ways in which men are allowed to define their masculinity and express caring has been identified as leaving men more vulnerable to abusing children (Finkelhor, 1984; Sanford, 1980).

Males are narrowly tracked into associating connection and the exchange of affection and nurturance with sexuality. Their sense of themselves and their sexuality is strengthened by social mandates against being feminine or dependent. Prescriptions for masculinity are loaded in favor of independence, dominance, and prowess. Missing from this formula is cultural support or cultural insistence that a man develop empathy or a sense of responsive connectedness to others as part of his masculinity. As a culture, we fail to hold men accountable for balancing their considerable authority with a sensitivity to the needs of those over whom they wield their power. The failure of empathy and the exploitative use of power characteristic of the man who offends has been defined as an extension of generally accepted patriarchal norms (Brickman, 1984; Herman, 1981).

In addition, social norms converge around the expectation that men have an obligation to be authoritative, and to control and be taken care of by females. To complement this expectation, women are defined as the caretakers of emotional life and the gatekeepers of human connection. It is antagonistic to a woman's sense of herself as feminine to assert her own emotional needs or her autonomy. How passivity and self-deprecation are woven into the social definition of womanhood is a basic variable that contributes to a female's difficulty in protecting herself from various forms of victimization (Sanford, 1980).

Experts in the field of child sexual assault indicate that it is relatively rare for women to offend children and that only a small percentage of women "collude" with their partners (Gelinas, 1986; Russell, 1986). Despite this fact, for many family members, as well as clinicians, the mother's inactivity becomes far more interesting, provocative, and problematic than the active and clearly damaging exploitation of the child by the man who commits the assault. For example, clinicians who have not questioned the cultural expectation that it is *primarily* a woman's obligation to be the guardian of the family's relational life assume that the mother knew of the abuse, should have anticipated her partner's deviance, or had at her command a wide range of resources (economic, social, and personal) with which to combat it if she had known or suspected its occurrence.

The continued failure to place cultural factors at the heart of analysis and treatment leads to blaming mothers and victims, and simultaneously robs men of the opportunity to achieve a position of respect and mature masculinity by taking responsibility for their behavior. When therapists ignore the social pressures on men to sexualize affection and exercise their power coercively, they miss the opportunity to help prevent them from initiating abusive interactions. Successful treatment of child sexual assault requires that clinicians insist that a more complex definition of male identity is both possible and preferable, a definition that includes more empathic, caretaking, and cooperative elements.

GENERAL TREATMENT GOALS

Treatment should be organized around stopping the individual and systemic dynamics that maintain the incest and transmitting an alternative meaning system to all family members. The meaning system, which includes a multilayered description of what incest is and how the offender must be held accountable, alters the family's understanding of the individual, interpersonal, and social factors that maintain the incest. Of particular importance is helping the family understand the crucial distinctions between the incest itself and other dysfunctional family dynamics.

Treatment for the offender must go beyond simply stopping the overtly physical aspects of the sexual abuse. The therapist must be committed to naming and stopping the abusive, nonempathic, exploitive, and intimidating behaviors in the whole family, but particularly in the offender. The offender must eventually become responsible for modeling a different kind of power and caring. At the same time, the therapist must be prepared to support the offender as he enters into a period of mourning for the loss of his abusive power. Offenders frequently reexperience the early rage and helplessness they felt when their own developing mastery was interrupted and coopted by experiences of abuse and neglect. Under the best of circumstances, these reexperiences will eventually become the basis for an offender's building a sense of empathy for his victim and the pain and loss of mastery she suffered because of him.

The mother must be helped to function and feel more active and competent. The therapist can enlist her as a cotherapist and seek her advice regarding what she thinks is best for her family. She will need help in identifying her needs and much support to enable her to feel deserving of having those needs met. She will need to learn how to negotiate on an equal basis with her partner and other adults. The therapist can, in this regard, help her plan and navigate meetings with numerous helping professionals, taking care not to placate or infantalize her. In couple or family work, her competence as a mother and a wife become central themes. Her tendency to blame herself for the sexual assault must be countered. Frequently, her own sexual victimization as a child is revealed in tandem with her daughter's disclosure and the resulting symptoms must be addressed.

The victim will need assistance in establishing a positive sense of self and in changing the destructive affective, cognitive, and behavioral patterns that result from the victimization process. Freeing her from being a victim entails helping her discover and name her own experience of loss and betrayal, which includes learning to identify and assert her own needs. An important and related focus is to assist her in understanding that it is her choice, not her obligation, to care for others.

Siblings and extended-family members will need help in not feeling polarized and forced to choose between the victim or the offender. Siblings who have not experienced abuse often suffer from "survivor's guilt," which the clinician can help them anticipate and resolve.

The family must be helped to reorganize its role structure and belief system so that power and caring are more evenly distributed, clear boundaries between the adult and child subsystems are established, and threats and secrecy cease to be the predominant communicational currency. All members of the family can be educated to understand better the links between their private family experience and the ways in which that experience is invaded and distorted by cultural ideas that link notions of intimacy with power, sexuality with aggression, and love with possession.

INITIAL TREATMENT CONSIDERATIONS

Helping professionals usually make contact with these families after the disclosure of sexual assault. In many cases, protective services or state attorneys will have previously intervened (often against a family's will), mandated treatment, and insisted on the separation of the victim and the offender. This move, although in the best interests of the victim, is usually experienced by the family more as an abduction than as a protective move. The family then enters treatment under pressure from uninvited helping professionals and shortly after having suffered a major, unexpected, and unwanted loss. This means that the therapist will frequently be dealing with a family in shock and in the early stages of mourning. The family's structure will have been dramatically altered. Alliances and coalitions formed by the secrecy surrounding the abuse will be broken. Various family members may be removed and relocated by social service agencies. Legal, social service, and clinical personnel will be added. This explains, to some degree, why such intense denial and anger are encountered. An understanding of these losses and additions is crucial in anticipating the family's reaction and in setting up treatment.

Understanding What Has Been Lost—The Family in Mourning

Once the secret of incest has been broken, the experience of loss will be felt throughout the family. The family may feel a severe loss of pride, autonomy, and legitimacy at having been defined as an incestuous family—a label that carries with it not only shame but also serious social and legal consequences. If the offender has left the home, the family has lost a father figure, a spouse, and, in the majority of cases, vital economic support. If the daughter has left the home, there is the loss of a child or sibling, and the parental and spousal functions, both instrumental and emotional, she was performing.

The offender will have lost his access to the victim and the satisfaction of the vital relational and dominance needs provided by his sexual abuse of her. His control over the family is also threatened, and with it his sense of mastery. The public knowledge of his crime will raise his fears of loss of status and reputation. His spouse may leave him and he may be asked to vacate his home. Such losses may bring on a serious depression and ideas of suicide.

Removing the victim from the home protects her from further sexual exploitation, but causes her to lose her special status and her parental role in the family. Such a removal is frequently experienced as blame and robs the victim of having her pain validated and cared for. In spite of the abuse, she may have a deep attachment and sense of loyalty to the offender. Helping professionals will often move in too quickly and insist that she give these emotions up. She usually feels responsible, and may be held responsible by family members for the losses resulting from the disclosure. She may, as a result, lose the affection of her entire family. She is in a particularly poignant position and highly at risk to be scapegoated, as the dynamics of abuse have often put her in competition with her mother and in a position of unappreciated authority over her siblings. If she is removed from the home, she may lose all that is familiar to her.

The siblings will lose their sister or their father and, in a sense, their innocence as they learn about the abuse. They may be pressured to take sides regarding who is the villain and who the victim.

In most cases, the mother is in an extraordinarily difficult (and often un-appreciated) position. She is frequently put in charge of dismembering the family when she is asked to choose whether her male partner or her daughter should leave the home, and is pressured to align with her daughter rather than being given the option of attempting to maintain her connections with both. Because of the cultural definitions of the "good mother," she will also be held responsible for the losses the other family members suffer. She often will have to choose between economic deprivation and the loss of her status as wife or the loss of a child and her status as a mother. Given her definition of self as wife and/or mother, she is at great risk for losing her most basic sense of self. Given her female socialization and its mandate to tend to connectedness and the emotional well-being of everyone in her family, she cannot move without suffering de-bilitating losses and/or social condemnation.

Understanding What Has Been Added—The Helping Entourage

In addition to these serious losses and organizational changes, the disclosure of incest usually means that families will be entered by a stream of helping professionals, which minimally include protective services, law enforcement and legal services, foster parents, medical professionals, school counselors/teachers, and various clinical professionals who will evaluate and treat various members or groupings of the family. All of these helping professionals may have different views of the problem, different ideas of where the responsibility for the abuse lies, and, therefore, different allegiances to different family members, different ideas regarding disposition and treatment, and different degrees of authority with which to enforce their views. In only the most ideal of situations will all these helpers communicate in any consistent or coordinated way among them-selves. This can lead to the development of dysfunctional patterns that replicate preexisting family patterns.

New alliances between protective services and the victim will be formed, frequently exacerbating the distance and competition between her and her mother and replacing one incongruous hierarchy with another. Whereas the abuse aligned the powerless daughter with the offender and over the mother, now she is aligned with the protective worker and over her parents. It is not uncommon for child protective workers to be quite hostile to offenders and "nonprotective" mothers. The protective service worker or the victim's therapist can unintentionally become the perfect mother for the one or two hours per week when he or she works with the victim. This structure is disturbingly isomorphic with the ways in which the offender seduces the victim by being more present and more attentive than the mother, thus undermining the mother's power and eroding the mother-daughter alliance.

In cases in which the offender and the victim each has legal representation, the relationship between the attorneys is often adversarial, and this conflict is passed on to family members through the attorneys' counsel. Although clini-cally, treatment for sexual offenders must be grounded in an admission of the facts, legally, it endangers the offender and raises the risk of imprisonment. It is, therefore, not uncommon for the offender's attorney to encourage him both to deny his offense and to avoid entering treatment until litigation is completed. In some states, this may take well over a year. Such a position supports the mechanism of denial and thus undermines the possibility of change in the offender and in the family. Because child sexual abuse is a crime, the therapist and his or her records can be called into court. Even the youngest of family members is aware of the legal ramifications of the information they hold and, out of fear and loyalty, will be painfully ambivalent about breaking their silence.

Prohibiting Splitting Among Helpers

Part of the initial treatment considerations should be an understanding of how one prevalent family dynamic—splitting—can hinder both the management of the case and the course of treatment. Splitting is, by definition, a divisive mechanism and is a central defensive dynamic found in these families. Perhaps the most basic form of splitting is that which results from the secrecy that accompanies the incest. This secrecy splits the family into highly dysfunctional alliances and coalitions made up of those who know and those who do not know about the assault. Various other forms of splitting are, however, very characteristic in these families and serve important homeostatic functions, especially in the family's relationship with helpers.

For example, these families tend to define people as either good or bad, trustworthy or suspicious, helpful or hurtful, for them or against them. A closer look shows that this is the way these families have learned to handle their difficulties with trust and their inability to tolerate differences. Anyone who holds a view that is different from or critical of the prevalent family view may be split away from the family. This kind of splitting is very pronounced around the time of disclosure and in the early stages of treatment. Frequently, a victim who has told the secret will be defined as cruel, crazy, bad, or selfish, and will be banished from the family. In other families, the offender is defined as malevolent and is expelled.

It is not unusual for families, often under the direction of the offender, to try to protect their boundaries and to repel helpers who are uninvited intruders and who threaten the family's structure and challenge the family's meaning system. One offender made phone calls from prison commanding his wife and family to withdraw from therapy as his therapist had challenged him during a previous visit to the jail. He also wrote to his daughter in an attempt to seduce her to go to the District Attorney's office to retract her statement. Missed appointments, threats against the therapist, and warnings about the inability of a fragile family member to withstand treatment are all attempted. If these moves are not effective, the family may attempt to split the various social service, clinical, and legal helpers into factions. As previously mentioned, helpers may be very vulnerable to this process because of their different views and because communication between them is often poorly coordinated. The family may adroitly shift its negative and positive attributions from one helper to another in such a way that the helping professionals begin, in a process that mirrors the family's, to distrust and compete with one another. They are thus induced into a divisiveness that renders them ineffectual in stopping the abuse.

Helpers, even on the same treatment team, must be particularly careful as family members will often portray one helper as "good" and the other as "bad," and attempt to enlist the good helper in disempowering the bad helper. This dichotomy frequently is set up by a family member sharing some important information with one helper (who is defined as more sensitive and understanding than the other helper), with an attendant request not to tell the other (who is defined as incompetent and hurtful). To tell the bad helper is to betray the trust and confidence of the confiding family member and to undermine the trust between the family and the good helper. A relationship particularly vulnerable to splitting is that between the protective services case manager and the therapist(s). It is quite common for a family member to complain about one to the other, and, for example, to elicit the help of the case manager in "firing" the therapist. Whether it is the "unfortunate offender," the "helpless victim," the "oppressed mother," or the "beleaguered family system" that evokes a response, even the most experienced helper may be tempted to join a coalition.

All professionals involved with the family must be apprised of this almost inevitable process and have a strategy for dealing with it. One of the most effective strategies is to make it explicit to the family early in treatment that all information will be shared among helpers and that conflicts between family members and helpers will be addressed directly. Regular meetings with helpers, often with family members present, are crucial. This will keep the control of the treatment in the hands of the helpers, and will also to begin to model a very different way of communicating and organizing within a system. When this does not occur, the family will organize the helpers in ways that are consistent with their need to protect themselves from change.

ESTABLISHING THE THERAPIST'S POSITION AND SETTING THE TONE OF TREATMENT

In working with child sexual abuse, the therapist must find a way to position herself or himself so that she/he can be supportive and expand the competencies of the family, and, at the same time, take a strong, active, and critical stand against the sexual assault and the abuse of power that perpetuates it.

Individuals and families who enter treatment for sexual abuse will frequently have been through a legal and/or protective service investigative process before reaching the treatment setting. They will have been prodded and scanned for their pathology. Their sensitivity and hesitancy to reveal that pathology will have been defined as denial and resistance. They will arrive having been scolded or blatantly attacked for their defensiveness. If the therapist continues in a hard-line investigative approach as the primary therapeutic stance, they will devote themselves to defeating the therapist, and frequently succeed. Many helpers, either because of their commitment to a highly confrontational model of treatment for sexual abuse or because of their moral repugnance, will adopt this treatment stance. However, a more overtly confrontational style in which the therapist seizes authority and explicitly attacks the sexual assault often results in all or part of the family fleeing from treatment. In cases where the family is held in treatment by a court mandate, its members may internally split into warring factions or join together and assume a highly defensive, adversarial position vis-à-vis the therapist, thus rendering treatment difficult at best.

If one soft-peddles the abuse, one aligns oneself with the family's tendency to remain the same by minimizing. Neutral and curious questioning or positive reframes, although successful in eliciting dialogue and avoiding a head-on collision with a family, can invalidate the victim's experience of being terrorized and violated, and can too easily be coopted by the dynamics of minimization or rationalization so prevalent in these families. A more neutral position is attractive to clinicians who have a distaste for the more coercive and controlling tone of the previous approach. However, because these approaches neither accurately take into account the tenacity with which this problem persists nor name the incest as violent and unacceptable, it will often continue unchallenged.

Because sexual abuse is such a difficult problem to dislodge and, as discussed earlier, a pathological extension of generally accepted norms regarding men's dominance, the therapist must take a very strong and socially controlling position with the family. However, because the offender, the mother, and the daughter are typically very depleted and often highly reactive to criticism or rejection, the therapist must also find a way to be nurturant and delicate with them.

The Stroke-Kick Rhythm of Treatment

Paradoxically, the therapist can move back and forth between supporting (stroke) and challenging (kick) the family by taking advantage of one of its prevalent interactional patterns. Building upon the individual and systemic tendencies in these famliles to split reality into opposing factions, the therapist adopts a position that is isomorphic with the splitting. That is, she or he shifts back and forth between strongly positive and strongly negative frames, making the stroke-kick rhythm the major therapeutic gait.

The Kick: Uncovering the Violence

Child sexual abuse tends to be part of a larger pattern of violent and controlling behaviors to which people within the family have become habituated or never had a language for, thus rendering the behaviors invisible and inaccessible for critical examination. Once the hurdle of disclosure has been negotiated, the therapist is often met with more subtle and enduring forms of avoidance and denial.

Typically, because the offender needs to protect his access to the daughter, the devastating impact of the incest will be minimized. As the abuser is, in many cases, in charge of defining reality for the family, the abuse will not be presented or named as a coercive, selfish, or oppressive process. The sexual assault of the child may be described as having no cause or not really being anyone's responsibility. In spite of considerable evidence that sexual abuse is a planned, patterned, and progressive phenomenon (Sgroi, 1982), the offender will typically absent himself from any intent or responsibility, as in, "It just happened," "I was asleep," or "I guess I was drunk, because I don't remember anything." Or in another move to displace responsibility for his violence to his victim(s), the sexual assault will be described as having been provoked by the victim's behavior, as in: "She sat on my lap and wiggled around," or "She liked it." Another variation of this displacement is shifting the responsibility to his spouse, who, he claims, drove him to abuse by her depriving and inattentive stance, as in: "I never would have done it if my wife had been around more," or "She should have known what was happening and stopped it."

One of the most insidious forms of minimization and/or denial used by family members and therapists alike is the adaptation of a language or descriptive frame that is either vague ("it"), sanitized ("I touched her"), full of pseudoscientific jargon ("loosened sexual boundaries"), or misrepresented as consensual and loving ("our special relationship"). It is thus stripped of its sexual and violent flavor, becoming almost tolerable.

Effective treatment should include a commitment to framing child sexual abuse in terms that are strong enough, critical enough, and graphic enough so as to be unforgettable and intolerable to therapists and to the family. The therapist insists on repeatedly using and teaching the family a sharply etched and decidedly negative frame for the abusive dynamics. For example, in working with the offender in individual, family, and group meetings, his beliefs about women, about sexuality, and about power are explored and challenged when they contain exploitative and nonempathic themes. The ways in which he attempts to seduce or coerce the therapist are tracked and commented upon. If the victim or the mother refers to the abuse in vague or contentless terms, the therapist corrects the language. For example, if a victim refers to the abuse as "being touched," the therapist can acknowledge the offender's need to be close and nurtured, but suggest that the touch was, in fact, a coercive and nonconsensual betrayal of the daughter's dependence. When conducting couple or family sessions, the therapist carefully watches for, explicitly labels as violent, and redirects those interactional sequences that contain abuses of power and caring.

The kick serves two important functions. First, a strong definition is necessary in order to break through the protective invisibility that is frequently drawn around this phenomenon and to provide a direction for therapeutic change. Second, it is meant to repulse each member of the family and seem so discordant with the members' view of themselves and their family that they become activated and motivated enough to mobilize themselves for positive change. In those cases, however, where deeply violent and sadistic behaviors have occurred as an integral part of the sexual assault, serious consideration must be given to the question of whether outpatient treatment is appropriate. In some cases, institutional or prison settings are more effective and more protective than outpatient clinical settings.

The Stroke: Holding Up the Competence

It is extremely useful to approach both the individual and the more systemic aspects of treatment with a commitment to sifting through the emotional and interactional rubble to find and hold up what is healthy and resourceful. As indicated earlier, pervasive individual and systemic weaknesses are characteristic in these families. After disclosure, family members are further exhausted and burdened with the threat of imprisonment, the dismemberment of their family, demanding schedules of therapy, and being shamed for the breaches in their moral conduct. Much of the therapeutic work, in tandem with the more controlling confrontational tone, becomes lifting out what is competent in the beliefs, behaviors, or hopes of these families in order to expand the healthy influence and make it more accessible for use in the service of healing the damage. In the spirit of setting a more hopeful and anticipatory tone to therapy, family members are informed early in treatment that they will be working to discover the strong and caring parts of themselves and their family from which they have become disconnected, or whose influence has been diminished. Generally, this beginning, which precedes the kick, is surprising and elicits both optimism and curiosity in the family and, as importantly, in the therapist.

For example, the therapist can connote the abusive behavior of the offender as an attempt to engage and establish a caretaking and intimate relationship, talking about how vital those experiences are and how so many men are disconnected from these basic needs—the stroke. If he wants to return to the family and fights against visitation restrictions, his commitment to maintaining connections can be emphasized. But then it is imperative that the therapist immediately link this intervention with a firm, hard, and critical stance with regard to how the offender went about getting those needs met—the kick. He must be helped to see how his self-centeredness and his betrayal of the victim's loyalty and trust represent a distortion of tenderness and an abdication of caring. He must be challenged to acknowledge his responsibility for the damage it caused the victim and the family. The work then becomes one of exploring and confronting his aberrant and violent patterns of connection and mastery while bolstering his resources so that they can be applied toward less damaging alternatives. The therapy always moves to explore the ways in which the offender should take the primary responsibility for repairing the damage of the abuse, even when it includes spending time in prison.

The mother is typically faulted for not acting to stop the abuse, for not believing her daughter's disclosure, and/or for choosing her spouse over the victim after disclosure. That is, these mothers present as exhausted, helpless, and incompetent parents, or as rigidly rejecting and selfish, for example, vis-à-vis the victim and her needs for protection and validation. A useful reframe at this juncture is to begin to hold up the mother's so-called selfishness as her beginning recognition that she has her own needs to attend to. Direct educational interventions or less direct circular questioning can then focus on the ways in which women do not learn enough about meeting their own needs and the problems this causes. It is done both individually and in the presence of the offender and the victim. It relabels the mother as more daring and competent, thus shoring her up, counteracting the blame directed at her, and suggesting an alternative role for both her and her daughter. Her so-called inability to protect can be labeled as her trust in her spouse and her expectation that he had a responsibility to provide appropriate nurturance and caretaking as a legitimate part of his parenting role. This reframe can become the basis for suggesting that the mother demonstrates an unusual courage in questioning the stereotypical peripheral father role.

Again, as with the work with the offender, the therapist must couple this frame with a challenge. The mother must begin to understand how she contributed to a distant and disengaged marital relationship and a nonnurturing parent-child relationship. When this is done in the context of emphasizing the offender's responsibility for the abuse and his contribution to marital and parental difficulties, therapy does not become just one more source of depletion for her. While acknowledging the inherent difficulty and even unjustness, the therapist must also help the mother take up the responsibility of protecting her children and repairing the damage of the incest. When this approach is carried out in the context of also supporting her meeting her own needs, therapy does not become one more vehicle for leveling blame at her or holding her entirely responsible for reparation.

EXPANDING THE NOTION OF PROTECTION: COUNTERACTING MOTHER BLAMING

Most treatment protocols for child sexual abuse are built around a commitment to protecting the victim from further abuse and repairing the physical, psychological, and more interactionally based damage she suffered as a result of the abuse. The most basic and most immediate moves toward protection of the original victim are active and structural ones. They involve finding a protective adult ally for the victim, blocking the offender's access to the victim and other children for a period of time, individual and group treatment for all family members, and, in the later stages of treatment, providing highly structured family meetings such as confrontational sessions (James & Nasjleti, 1983) or apology sessions (Trepper & Barrett, 1986) involving the victim, the offender, and other family members.

In one of the best articles to date that describes the characteristic problems with which incest victims must struggle, Denise Gelinas (1983) suggests that attention to three underlying negative effects must be the focus of treatment. These are:

1. Chronic traumatic neurosis with affective, cognitive, and behavioral components such as depression, problems with self-esteem, and self-destructive behaviors.
2. Relational imbalances that continue after the abuse has stopped and that frequently replicate the significant parentification that underlay the abuse.
3. Intergenerational risk for the recurrence of sexual abuse, particularly that the victim will become the mother of a victim and/or the wife of an offender.

Therapists and other helping professionals rarely view mothers, who are themselves frequently the unrecognized adult survivors of child sexual assault, as being revictimized by their daughter's abuse or by the treatment prescribed to heal its negative effects. While still in the shock of disclosure, mothers are expected, by the professional community, to choose their daughter, now labeled a victim, over their partner, now labeled an offender. The overiding assumption is that the mother knew or should have known of the abuse. A more basic, but hidden, assumption held by clinicians, family members, and even the mother herself, is that it was the mother's job to prevent abuse from occurring in the first place. In essence, the fact of the abuse itself proves her collusion or irresponsibility. She has failed in her socially prescribed duty as the watchful guardian of family life. If she was ill, pregnant, a substance abuser, working outside the home, disengaged from her mate, or perhaps characterologically dependent or passive, she is asked to face up to these failures, which are now defined as evidence of her part in the abuse itself.

If a mother should choose to remain with the offender, she will be treated unsympathetically. She has abdicated her role as mother. She is highly at risk to be labeled as selfish, narcissistic, and unable to protect. The children will probably be removed from the home and, although she is not the offender, she may be allowed to see them only under supervised conditions. In a movement as quick as a magician's sleight of hand, a team of helpers appears and offers these mothers the opportunity to work through their failure to protect and their guilt and denial at not having anticipated, prevented, or stopped the assault. If she resists these efforts, that is only further evidence of her inadequacy and unwillingness to look at her culpability.

Most clinical treatment in the area of sexual abuse is individual and peer group work. It is often the case that clinicians who work with mothers and children will not work directly with offenders. Left with treating only the mother and the children, it is not unusual that accountability for the abuse is unintentionally shifted to the mother. Nor are family therapists with their systemic formulations free from inadvertently scapegoating mothers, as has been documented and reviewed elsewhere in Chapter 4 by Bograd. There have been few articles in the family therapy literature dealng explicitly with a family systems approach to child sexual abuse, although an early article by Machotka, Pittman, and Flomenhaft (1967) demonstrates some of the more blatant errors raised by Bograd. Boldly stating that the appropriate focus for therapy should be "the family dynamics rather than the current or historical fact of sexual activity," they then examine the crucial role of the nonparticipating member, the diversity of motives for that member's collusion, and how the colluding member's denial of the fact of the incest freezes the role relations and preserves them from required change (p. 115). The sexual abuse itself is made invisible, as is the organizing role of the offender himself. Under the guise of systems thinking, the view is shifted away from the sex, the violence, and the offender to the family ship frozen at sea, with the mother at the helm.

Clinicians trained in sexual abuse work are cautioned to anticipate, respect, and support the victim's loyalty to the offender, as to do otherwise is to cause pain and elicit resistance from the victim. This may make good clinical sense, but rarely is as strong a parallel concern voiced regarding the need to safeguard, support, or restore her damaged loyalty toward her mother. Instead, victims and their siblings are assisted in getting angry at their mothers for failing them. Clinically, it appears that it is much easier for family members to identify and express anger at their mothers than it is for them to do the same toward the more powerful offender. Clinicians, unavoidably part of a sexist culture, have less difficulty working with mother-directed anger than with going against the grain to raise anger at a father figure who let his children down by using them to serve his own needs.

The offender's maintenance of the ongoing incest acted out in harmony with the culture's ideology about women sets up the mother, more than the offender, as the betrayer of the child. Bograd (1989) points out generally accepted cultural descriptions of motherhood portray mothers as larger-than-life perfect and naturally nurturant beings, responsible for the well-being of intimate others, and all-powerful destructive beings who are the locus of blame. It is, therefore, frequently the mother whom the child feels most betrayed and abandoned by because it is her role, not the offender's, that appears most compromised by the sexual assault.

Clearly, clinicians are faced with a complex dilemma. As Betty Carter (1985) comments:

> How shall we deal with the central role that mothers play in family emotional life? If we ignore or dispose of her, we are failing to acknowledge her efforts and importance; if we overfocus on her, we are blaming her for the problem and/or holding her responsible for change. (p. 78)

If, while working to undo her parentification and self-blaming, the victim senses that her mother is being blamed and held exclusively responsible for reparation, she will be caught in a puzzling paradox. As Byrne and McCarthy (1986) point out, the daughter's disclosure releases her from her parentified role in the family and disperses "her mission" of protecting others at her own expense. The therapist must be careful, however, not simply to hand that mission back over to the mother, giving both mother and daughter a message about the appropriate place of women in the family. To participate in the mother and daughter's induction into this stereotypical role not only limits their options but, more tragically, because of their history of abuse, increases the possibility that this pattern will continue down through the generations.

Ironically, not protesting the offender's failure at caretaking as a primary treatment goal further pushes men toward the isolated periphery of family life while capturing women in an exclusive and lonely role at the family's center. Biased formulations that place the mother too actively and too centrally within the abusive dynamics must be recognized not only as a distortion of the abusive transaction, but also as a misrepresentation of her power and her ability to influence family functioning. Continued adherence to these formulations perpetuates conditions that further deplete and incapacitate her. When she is relieved of the burdens of adhering perfectly to the cultural dictates of the good mother, her self-esteem can be strengthened and the relational imbalances in which she habitually participates can be restructured. When the mother's victimization by the current abuse is more clearly highlighted and worked with, she will be more able, in the later, less crisis-oriented stages of treatment, to explore the ways in which she failed to face and resolve her part in the various marital and parental dysfunctions that contributed to the family's tolerance of the abuse.

CONCLUDING COMMENTS

This chapter has raised a series of considerations that family therapists may integrate into their treatment of sexual abuse. Because their attitudes and beliefs will shape their clinical interventions, this chapter has focused primarily on a way to think about sexual abuse and its treatment. It is hoped that clinicians will consider a more complex definition of the problem and the forces that perpetuate it. This definition, while inclusive of systemic dynamics, also points to the offender's power to dominate and victimize his family and, as tragically, to be dominated by a cultural ideology hostile to women and supportive of male violence.

By drawing a clear distinction between the abuse itself and the dysfunctional family context that tolerates it, a more useful discrimination of responsibility and a more ethical distribution of accountability are possible. In particular, because sexual abuse is primarily committed by men, their individual contribution has been emphasized. It is hoped that family therapists will respect men enough to feel bold and unapologetic about challenging the offender's misuse of power and encouraging in him a more cooperative, generative, and tender way of making connections.

This discussion has emphasized various ways in which systemic formulations may, by their very neutrality or circularity, be misinterpreted as suggesting that the mother of the victim, and even the victim herself, should share in shouldering some of the blame for the abuse. Because the dominant cultural ideology, from which categories of analysis are drawn, contains such pervasive mother-blaming themes, therapists are particularly vulnerable to imposing them on families. The most dangerous consequence of this error is that the abuse of power exerted by the offender may be mislabeled as less serious or less relevant than the depletion of the mother whose exhaustion becomes labeled as nonprotective mothering. It has been arued that mother-blaming descriptions will yield interventions that recapitulate the pattern of significant parentification she may have suffered in her family of origin. In this way, treatment inadvertently contributes to her emotional depletion and self-sacrifice. Rather than foster her competence and her participation as a self-responsible ally in her daughter's treatment, the therapist further victimize her. Although, clearly, it is the children who are the primary victims, a case has been made for considering the ways in which mothers may be victimized by the abuse, and by the treatment that follows.

REFERENCES

Bograd, M. Scapegoating mothers: Conceptual errors in systems formulations. In M. P. Mirkin (Ed.), *The social and political contexts of family therapy*. New York: Gardner Press.

Byrne, N. O., & McCarthy, I. C. (1986). Caring and abusing: A systemic perspective on incest. Guest workshop at the Family Institute of Cambridge.

Brickman, J. (1984). Feminist, nonsexist, and traditional models of therapy: Implications for working with incest. *Women and Therapy, 3,* 49–67.

Carter, B. (1985). Ms. intervention's guide to "correct" feminist family therapy. *Family Therapy Networker,* Nov.-Dec., *9*(6), 78–79.

Conte, J. (1986). Sexual abuse and the family: A critical analysis. In T. S. Trepper & M. J. Barrett (Eds.), *Treating incest: A multimodal systems perspective* (pp. 113–126). New York: Haworth Press.

Finkelhor, D. (1984). *Child sexual abuse: New theory and research.* New York: Free Press.

Finkelhor, D. (1986). Sexual abuse: Beyond the family systems approach. In T. S. Trepper & M. J. Barrett (Eds.), *Treating incest: A multimodal systems perspective* (pp. 53–65). New York: Haworth Press.

Gelinas, D.J. (1983). The persisting negative effects of incest. *Psychiatry, 46,* 312–331.

Gelinas, D. J. (1986). Unexpected resources in treating incest families. In M. A. Karpel (Ed.), *Family resources: The hidden partner in family therapy* (pp. 327–358). New York: Guilford Press.

Groth, N. (1978). Patterns of sexual assault against children and adolescents. In A. W. Burgess, A. N. Groth, L. L. Holstrom, & S. M. Sgroi (Eds.), *Sexual assault of children and adolescents* (pp. 3–24). Lexington, Mass.: Lexington Books.

Herman, J. (1981). *Father-daughter incest.* Cambridge, Mass.: Harvard University Press.

James, B., & Nasjleti, M. (1983). *Treating sexually abused children and their families.* Palo Alto, Calif.: Consulting Psychologists Press.

Machotka, P., Pittman, F. S., & Flomenhaft, K. (1967). Incest as a family affair. *Family Process, 6,* 98–116.

Russell, D.E.H. (1986). *The secret trauma: Incest in the lives of girls and women.* New York: Basic Books.

Sanford, L.T. (1980). *The silent children: A parent's guide to the prevention of child sexual abuse.* New York: McGraw-Hill.

Sgroi, S.M. (1982). *Handbook of clinical intervention in child sexual abuse.* Lexington, Mass.: Lexington Books.

Trepper, T.S. (1986). The apology session. In T. S. Trepper & M. J. Barrett (Eds.), *Treating incest: A multimodal systems perspective.* New York: Haworth Press.

8

THE LESBIAN COUPLE

Thelma Jean Goodrich, Ph.D.,

Barbara Ellman, M.S.W.,

Cheryl Rampage, Ph.D.,

and Kris Halstead, M.S.Ed.

> The rules break like a thermometer,
> quicksilver spills across the charted systems,
> we're out in a country that has no language
> no laws, we're chasing the raven and the wren
> through gorges unexplored since dawn
> whatever we do together is pure invention
> the maps they gave us were out of date
> by years.
>
> —Adrienne Rich (1978)

They could be recognized as brave women, spirited women, loving women, but instead they are said to be perverted, criminal, ill, insane, sinful, deviant, depraved, deprived. They are called old maid, witch, butch, dyke. The homophobia and hatred reflected in these words permeate not only personal belief and cultural values, but professional theory as well. The literature of family therapy, for example, makes lesbians* invisible by what must be regarded as malevolent neglect. Two recent articles are welcome exceptions to the general pattern of ignoring lesbian existence (Krestan & Bepko, 1980; Roth, 1985). Equally troubling is the fact that some of the most widely used theoretical concepts in family therapy would pathologize a lesbian couple by fiat if we applied them.

In contrast to a pathologizing points of view, some lesbian feminist writers offer a highly idealized version of the love relationship between two women (Lewis, 1979). They describe the lesbian couple as attempting, though admittedly not always succeeding, to respect the individual needs of the partners even when these needs seem potentially threatening to the relationship. The aim of each partner is to rise above the jealousy, possessiveness, and dependency that

---

*We use the term lesbian in this chapter to refer to women who have adopted that term for themselves.

This chapter is reprinted from Goodrich, T.J., Rampage, C., Ellman, B., & Halstead, K. (1988). *Feminist family therapy: A casebook.* New York: Norton.

those writers believe are prevalent in heterosexual couples as a result of the assumption of male ownership over women. Thus removed from the dictates of romantic love that engender passive swooning heroines and active rescuing heroes, lesbian love claims to be born of friendship and mutuality.

Idealized versions of the dynamics that bind partners to one another are no more useful for therapeutic work than pathologized versions but, as an opposite pole, they do point up the long distance therapists have to travel to reach a balanced view. Family therapists—feminist or not, lesbian or not—must know themselves and their therapy to be profoundly influenced by attitudes of aversion toward women loving women. Their own struggle against these attitudes is the prerequisite to any salutary work with lesbian couples.

We will elaborate upon these and other issues by presenting two lesbian couples in therapy with us. In our practice, one of us works in a case as primary therapist and the other three serve as consultants. We meet weekly to provide consultation to one another, and in a single meeting, each of us might serve as therapist on one case and consultant to several others.

We introduce the case here by describing the early meetings with one of us as primary therapist, showing the line of reasoning that led to a stuck point and how the therapist posed her problem to the consultation group. We report the consultation in two sections, although we consulted at least six times. We later develop a feminist analysis of various points that arose for us in the consultation process, including our critique of family therapy. Feminism must be thorough precisely because everything that is not feminist is sexist.

Following our analysis, we set forth the goals that guide our work, and then the therapy. The description is, at best, an approximation, much like writing a story of any personal experience, so to read it as a literal account leads off in the wrong direction. We need to acknowledge that therapy is often mysterious, an encounter where more happens than we know, more than we can tell. We think we know what helped, and this is what we report. We think we know what did not help, and we report that, too. Our account does not convey what brought tears to our eyes or made us laugh out loud, nor does it capture the relationship between therapist and client, which is critical. To do so, we would need to sing a song, write a poem, paint a picture.

We close with the pitfalls that await a feminist family therapist in approaching the issues raised in the case. These were identified during our consultations with one another. Some we discovered because we had fallen in; others, because we had chanced to look before we leaped.

JOY AND KATHY; LOUISE AND ANNE

Kathy and Joy had been live-in lovers for more than 15 years. They were both employed as administrators in separate departments of a large insurance company. For the last five years of their relationship, they had been in and out of therapy, working on issues of finances, professional dilemmas, and, most often, sexual infrequency and/or disinterest. Their most recent request for help concerned their mutual desire to reevaulate the entire relationship. They came in shaken and fearful that "this time, the relationship is really in trouble." Their questions and doubts were related to new romantic attractions they were both feeling toward another couple, Louise and Anne, who had been their long-time friends.

Louise and Anne had been live-in partners for eight years. Louise had recently become a Certified Public Accountant and was working for a middle-size public accounting firm. Anne had supported Louise through graduate school by working as a secretary and was currently a full-time student pursuing a degree in medical technology. The two couples had a common network of friends in their community, and over the years they had offered support and nurturing to one another in various personal and professional dilemmas. Besides spending a good deal of time in each other's homes, they shared parties, business ventures, and political causes.

By the time Kathy and Joy came in to evaluate their relationship, Kathy had started a sexual relationship with Anne. Joy and Louise were attracted to one another, but most of their emotional energy seemed to be going into grieving over the losses in their primary relationships. There were no secrets among these women and so all four had information about one another's attractions and behavior. Soon after Kathy and Joy came in to talk, Anne and Louise called for therapy, also wanting to evaluate their relationship.

In my sessions with Kathy and Joy and with Anne and Louise, I heard how these women were reaching out emotionally to one another as well as to women outside the foursome, looking for comfort regarding their distress over troubles in their original relationships. Some of these comforting relationships became sexual and upsetting to other intimates. I heard how the women's community rallied around with support and advice. My reaction was a mixed one, as it had often been with lesbian couples in therapy. It was clear to me that the sexually open relationships were problematic and a source of pain for all four clients. I was drawn to focus on what seemed a serious disregard for boundaries: boundaries around self, relationships, homes, and information. I began to think in terms of triangled and fused. However, I also admired the active and loving concern these women demonstrated toward one another and honored the courage that enabled them to "go that hard way together. . . ." (Rich, 1979, p. 188). Pulled between a pathologizing perspective and an admiring one, I presented my perplexity to the consulting team.

FIRST CONSULTATION

As feminist family therapists, we know that women are often labeled as pathological simply because their behavior, values, or feelings do not conform to the expectations of male theorists and clinicians. Because we are committed to an understanding of our clients that is free from such sexist bias, it concerned us to realize that the therapist's assessment of these women as triangled, fused, and disrespectful of boundaries made sense to us. We thus began the consulting process by posing a question for ourselves and the therapist. What assumptions about relationships and sex were producing our opinions about these clients' situations? A brief discussion brought out several specific assumptions: that stable relationships are dyadic and have clearly defined boundaries around them, that friendship should be asexual and distinct from a primary relationship, and that monogamy is preferable to any of its alternatives. We thought it possible that such assumptions emanate from heterosexism, a view that holds heterosexuality as the only legitimate form of sexual identification. A different view might create a different set of assumptions about primary relationships. We wanted to leave that possibility open for our consideration rather than have it closed arbitrarily by prejudice. Heterosexism has informed the development of cultural and individual value systems as well as family therapy theory; we intended to stay alert to signs of that bias in our thinking.

After further discussion together, we decided that working with these relationships as one system would offer additional options for therapeutic leverage and we planned the next steps: (1) invite all four women to participate in conjoint sessions; (2) use a member of the consulting team as a cotherapist; (3) gather information about the nature of the boundaries and rules of this system; (4) inform the clients of this interest and share observations with them; and (5) consider nonpathological understandings of the way this system functions.

KATHY, JOY, ANNE, LOUISE

All four women agreed to attend a conjoint session. Kathy and Joy were still living together, as were Louise and Anne, although in neither case were the house mates still intimate or sexual. Anne was contemplating finding her own apartment; Kathy was doing the same. Kathy and Anne said that they had gravitated toward each other for mutual support and then evolved into lovers. Louise and Joy said they felt abandoned.

We listened to the content that these women brought into the session: sexual disinterest, ambiguous loyalties, financial disagreements, feelings of being unloved and misunderstood. The flow of details and the descriptions of all the alliances—present, past, and potential—caused us to parallel the very process of feeling confused and being overwhelmed that we observed in our clients. We had to remind ourselves to be open to observing this system as it presented itself and to avoid judgments about the changing connections.

What made that openness especially difficult was the way that these women presented their concerns to us. They appeared to have absorbed society's lesson that their lives were pathological and they came to tell us about the pathology. We told our clients that we admired the commitment and courage they were demonstrating by agreeing to work together in therapy. We said that they seemed to be experimenting with different ways of organizing relationships and asked them to tell us about their experience of themselves. Acknowledging to them that there was value in what they were doing seemed to shift their thinking. They began to talk about their behavior with more respect and described themselves as striving to make choices that were for the good of themselves and one another.

We commended the women for their continuing interest in and support of each other, and pointed out that such a thing could not occur where couples are more isolated from others. At our request, all four women agreed to return in two weeks in order to see where things appeared to be heading and to discuss their individual reactions. Both of the original couples stated that the relationships they had been in were extremely important to them and they wanted to understand what had happened to them.

At the next session and in several succeeding sessions, we observed behavior that demonstrated the difficulties the group was having with conflict resolution, sexual coupling, decision making, and caretaking. Anne and Kathy decided to move out of their respective homes and move in together. Telling about this change had little observable emotional impact on the four women involved. Louise expressed some sadness at the loss of Anne, but the others spoke of the change as if it were a temporary readjustment of alignments rather than a permanent separation.

We asked about feelings of abandonment and proposed that some "leaving" had been happening for a while in the form of one person's disappointing the other, rejecting the other, ignoring the other's concerns, and so on. At this suggestion, Anne and Kathy became tearful. Joy appeared unmoved. We encouraged the four women to talk about their reactions, suggesting that the session could be used as a supportive and structured place to speak about thoughts and feelings that were probably even more difficult to discuss outside the session. There was little response, and we said that perhaps more time was needed for each to examine her own response before sharing it with others.

At the next session, Joy, Kathy, and Anne reported that they had slept together. Joy said she had liked sleeping in the same bed with Anne and Kathy, but had become very upset by their sexual advances, which she had refused. She was unable to articulate what most upset her. She did not think the idea itself was the problem, as she had been a part of a sexual threesome from time to time and still maintained an interest in group sex. All members of the group told of experimenting with multiple sexual partners, describing these instances as attempts to keep from losing anyone or leaving anyone out of their lives. After remarking upon the continual fluidity of the women's relationships, we asked the women to consider for the next session what advantages, in addition to what they had already mentioned, were available to them in threesomes that were absent in their previous grouping into dyads. In this way, we stayed with our plan to avoid judgmental statements. Once the clients gathered more information for themselves, we could suggest a discussion about the gains and losses of relating in various configurations.

SECOND CONSULTATION

With the information obtained in the group sessions, the therapists returned to us to discuss their current assessment and to plan further treatment. The therapists reported that in answer to the query about threesomes, each of the women had described herself as terrified of exclusion. Each woman said that she wanted to do what was best for herself but not hurt another; if another should express hurt or disapproval, then the aim would be to redo the original decision until mutual accommodation could be found.

Again, we, as well as the therapists, struggled with the fundamental challenge to our usual ways of thinking—both personally and clinically. As we looked to family therapy for help, we realized that our training would lead us to see inadequate boundaries in this system, and to apply the term "fused" to these women. Yet we know that theory determines what can be seen, and if we adopted a different theory, we would see something quite different. For example, boundaries might recede in importance and relatedness emerge more prominently.

We faced a similar question about theory when we tried applying the concept of triangles to these relationships. According to the common usage in family therapy, triangles represent the effort of a dyad to avoid direct conflict by involving a third person to take sides or become a scapegoat. It was certainly true that members of this system did not resolve conflict well, but was that *because* they involved more than two people in their struggles?

The therapists were presented with a situation that afforded them the opportunity to pursue these issues. Immediately before the consultation, Kathy and Louise independently called the therapists requesting individual sessions. We debated whether this request represented progress toward recognizing individual needs or an effort to draw in a third party (the therapist) to alleviate a conflict with another member of the group. As we had no evidence that the clients were making gains in dealing with conflict directly, we decided on the second interpretation. For the present, we advised the therapists to insist that issues relevant to relationships within the group continue to be dealt with in the group.

As we moved toward making the treatment plan for subsequent sessions, the therapists' assessment was that the best thing they had done up to now was to maintain a stance of noninterference in the system long enough to allow some patterns to emerge. It had been a difficult stance because the therapists did see so much behavior and individual history that are ordinarily called pathological. The therapists had resisted temptations to pull individuals prematurely out of the group for family-of-origin work, or to draw boundaries arbitrarily around dyads and engage them in couple counseling. The therapists agreed that the stance would have been altogether impossible were it not for working as cotherapists, each keeping the other from becoming too involved with any one member of the group.

We discussed two issues as priorities at this stage of therapy: finding effective ways to resolve conflict, and addressing individual needs—identifying them, speaking of them, and managing the consequences. The team discussed these issues as being particularly loaded for women. We know the enormous cost to women of their typical adaptation in these areas. We also want to remember that there are distinctive aspects about living as lesbians that shape the way women's issues and human issues are experienced and incorporated.

ANALYSIS

There are many dimensions to consider in working with lesbian couples. We recommend instructive references (Gartrell, 1984; Krestan & Bepko, 1980; Rich, 1980; Roth, 1985; Vida, 1978). Also, we urge special care in selecting supervisors and consultants. Here we discuss only those aspects particularly relevant to our work with the presented case. There are four.

Heterosexism/Homophobia

American culture is heterosexist. Discussion regarding universal bisexuality, hormonal determinism, or nature versus nurture obscures this fundamental point: Heterosexuality serves as the linchpin in the patriarchal structure and functioning of our society. That is to say, heterosexuality has been "imposed, managed, organized, propagandized, and maintained by force. . . ." to ensure that women are physically, emotionally, and economically dependent on men (Rich, 1980, p. 649). Women who remove themselves from the ranks of the available are met with all the diagnostic, medical, legal, religious, and social power at the disposal of those who suffer their loss and resent their nerve. Widespread homophobia is a grim tribute to the success of the campaign and to the threat of reprisal that accompanies it.

Heterosexist bias is a major problem for the therapist working with lesbian clients. So pervasive is the bias, so automatically does it guide thinking and with such familiarity, that the therapist continually risks projecting it into the therapy or becoming paralyzed into inaction for fear of doing so. To complicate matters further, our homophobia may match the clients' own. Then we will miss it entirely. We may think that we are successfully offering our clients our empathy and understanding when we are actually and unknowingly supporting their own self-hatred.

For example, it is homophobia that leads a therapist and her lesbian clients to attribute disturbances in a relationship to lesbianism rather than to the often-disabling effect of prejudice. Such was evident when Joy and Kathy first presented their sexual problems in therapy. Joy wondered if women could really remain sexually interesting to her over time. The revulsion toward sex between women that Kathy and Joy and the therapist had been taught should have been considered as the possible source of the problem.

Problems in Daily Living

Lesbian couples have conflicts over the same issues as do heterosexual couples: money, closeness, sex, and tasks. Louise and Anne, for example, frequently argued about finances, and they, as well as Kathy and Joy, had difficulty with closeness. Sex was the salient issue between Kathy and Joy. Kathy wished for more frequent and passionate lovemaking, whereas Joy demonstrated little interest, except to oblige Kathy. Allocation of household tasks was somewhat less troublesome for these couples than for other lesbian couples we have seen, primarily because they had been together long enough to have reached a workable agreement.

In each of these traditionally conflictual areas, the lesbian couple must establish its own creative solution. Roth discusses distinguishing features of that effort and we recommend her paper for its descriptions of the patterns and pressures in each conflictual area (Roth, 1985). Here we want to hold up two factors that complicate the process of finding solutions in general for lesbian couples.

One complicating factor has to do with models. Whereas the heterosexual couple can call upon families of origin in memory or in fact, this resource is rarely useful to the lesbian couple because heterosexual couples typically base their arrangements on gender-role stereotypes. (A small proportion of lesbian couples do adopt highly differentiated roles modeled on heterosexual gender-role stereotypes. The majority of lesbians, however, do not adhere to rigid role behavior.)

Other sources of models that give covert or overt lessons on managing a partnership for living—such as magazines, newspapers, self-help books, formal courses, and television programs—are based on assumptions about arrangements, outlooks, and supports that generally do not apply to lesbian couples. Although it may be an advantage to have the freedom to design one's own solutions, that freedom entails losing the sense of certainty and direction found by following tradition and receiving the attendant social validation.

The second factor complicating the lesbian couple's effort to resolve daily problems derives ironically from the very feature that can make the relationship so enjoyable. That is, the relationship consists of two women. Like other women in this culture, a lesbian has been socialized to be more concerned about the feelings of the other than about her own, more responsive to the needs of the other than to her own. Since in a lesbian relationship the other is also a woman, each partner finds herself receiving a degree of attention unknown in her relationships with men or family members, where women are expected to be the unilateral givers. The sensitivity to each other in a lesbian relationship can bring deep pleasure and well-being. At times, however, it has troublesome side effects. In her novel *Other Women,* Alther (1984) characterizes such an outcome in her description of the long-term relationship between Caroline and Diana:

> Their relationship wasn't working, they finally concluded, because each had an equivalent need to be needed. . . . (W)ith each other life was a constant struggle to outnurture. . . . Each put on ten pounds from the candies and pastries the other brought home, which were dutifully devoured to please the donor. During lovemaking each would wait for the other to climax first, until both lost interest altogether. They fought over who got the most burnt toast, or the lukewarm second shower. . . . Eventually they were compelled to address the issue of what to do about two people in whom thoughtfulness had become a disease. (p. 16)

How does such thoughtfulness make problem solving difficult? It impedes the capacity to be aware of one's own needs and, even if aware, to voice those needs in the clear terms that create conflict, but also make possible the explaining and negotiating that resolve conflict.

The Lesbian Community

Members of the lesbian community rather than legal kinship groups may well make up the primary interactional context for the lesbian couple. In therapy (and in hospital visitation, insurance policies, courts of law, funerals, banks, etc.), the relevance of these friends is usually disregarded. We point out their relevance because they serve not only as primary relationships, but also as sanctuary and identification.

The lesbian community often functions as a sanctuary by providing refuge and protection. Anywhere that lesbians congregate can become a sanctuary: a women's music concert, a political rally, a women's bookstore. Numbers create for the moment a sense of place where the heterosexual majority is not intruding, watching, ready to condemn and possibly persecute. As all oppressed people use their group affiliation to help them exist in a hostile world, lesbians, too, embrace their group identity as a way to survive hatred. They create a proud identity by drawing upon the characteristics that make them unique and strong, finding positive images in women's song and literature.

Lesbian women look to the lesbian community for companionship, sister-hood, family, and kindred spirits. Those women most connected to the community are aware of the norms that a particular lesbian community expects of its constituency. For example, some lesbian communities may expect couples to be monogamous, whereas other communities may hold monogamy to be oppressive. The most influential community for the four women discussed here shifted from a closed group of ten couples to an open group with couples, singles, and former lovers. This shift took place several months before the women sought therapy, and it is this context that also needs to be considered as part of the entire picture.

Traditional Concepts from Family Therapy

Several core concepts in family therapy, such as triangle, fusion, and boundary, might well describe and explain the distinct patterns and characteristic problems of lesbian relationships. These three concepts are imbued with heterosexist bias, and application of them to any relational system may yield a distorted view. In particular, application to lesbian relationships will inevitably result in a pathologized and impoverished description.

Triangles

In the lesbian system described here, the number of overlapping threesomes was certainty noteworthy and pulled the therapists toward analyzing interactions from the traditional view in family therapy that triangles are always perverse (Haley, 1971). Granted that drawing in a third person may sometimes create a perverse triangle, what grounds are there for saying that sometimes it might not? First, given the web of relationships lesbians tend to sustain, the primary unit relevant to a specific conflict which appears to be a dyadic problem, may well be three persons, or four, or more. Further, we may be looking at an expression of women's psychology. Gilligan (1982) proposed that, in contrast to men's way of applying an impartial principle to resolve a moral dilemma, women cast a wide net of relational concerns, giving attention to every affected party. Perhaps the same is true about women's way of resolving conflict.

Second, we know that managing conflict in a productive way is difficult for everyone, but especially for women. Because they have no power base in the real world, women, both lesbian and straight, are used to conducting conflict only in indirect ways (Miller, 1976). Pulling in a third person or several other persons does make confrontation less direct; however, doing so may make the confrontation become possible. The diluting of intensity so that anger can be managed without loss of the other person is the desired and facilitative effect.

Fusion

In family therapy, fusion figures prominently as an explanatory principle in the two major articles on working with lesbian couples (Krestan & Bepko, 1980; Roth, 1985). Thus, in conceptualizing our work with the clients presented in this case, we wanted to examine the meaning and usefulness of the concept of fusion. The difficulties that we found with the concept here led us to question it altogether.

In family therapy, fusion is most closely associated with the work of Bowen (1966), who uses the term to anchor the lower end of a continuum measuring the individual human being's capacity to act and feel as an independent self. People who suffer from ego fusion have poorly defined ego boundaries, are excessively dependent on the opinions and approval of others, and have great difficulty in speaking on their own behalf. At the upper end of the continuum are differentiated people who have a clearly defined self, think and feel independently of the needs and desires of those around them, and make decisions based on rational rather than emotional grounds. The term "fusion" is also applied to relationships. According to the theory, a person whose emotional and intellectual systems are fused will fuse into relationships, that is, will lose self (Kerr, 1981). We found that if we applied the concept of fusion to Louise, Anne, Kathy, and Joy, we did see some fit. These four women do seem excessively reactive to each other, are intensely close, and have difficulty taking positions that might incur disapproval.

Nevertheless, further thought led us to question fusion as a way of explaining clients' behavior. The term describes a person who places a higher priority on the maintenance of the relationship than on self-expression, self-development, and even self-health. For the fused person, the distinction between what is best for the self and what is best for the relationship becomes blurred or disappears altogether. The trouble with applying the concept to women is that women are routinely taught that ignoring the self-relationship distinction is the path to self-fulfillment. In fact, a woman's ability to ignore that distinction is regarded as a mark of her mature womanhood.

There is a second way that fusion is an implicitly gendered concept. Fused people are described by Bowen (1966) as living "in a 'feeling' world," and spending the majority of their "life energy . . . maintaining the relationship system about them. . . . They are incapable of using the differentiated 'I' . . . in their relationship with others" (p. 357). In this culture, the foregoing statements add up to an adequate description of a so-called healthy woman (Broverman, Vogel, Broverman, Clarkson, & Rosenkrantz, 1972). Women are trained to be relational, to take care of the relational aspects of all our lives, to respond to the feelings of others, and, specifically, to avoid saying "I want, I need." In contrast to fused people, differentiated people are "principle-oriented, goal-directed," not affected by "either praise or criticism from others," able to "assume total responsibility for self," and to "disengage from [intense emotional experiences] and proceed on a self-directed course at will" (p. 359). Correctly acculturated men are trained in just such skills.

The fused/differentiated dichotomy is mistaken in polarizing human capacities. The mistake is compounded by reflecting the culture's higher valuation of autonomy skills over relational skills, that is, the high valuation of manly skills over womanly skills. The effect is to polarize the sexes. Men, by their cultural training, will appear highly differentiated, and thus will be labeled normal and healthy. Women, by their cultural training, will appear less differentiated and will be labeled pathological for so being. We challenge the valuation that leads to such a result. This earth would be a safer, more habitable place if more than only the female members of the race were trained to nurture relationships, to respond to the feelings and opinions of others, and to foster the well-being of others.

The overlapping biases against women and relatedness inherent in Bowen's schema become even more apparent when the concept of fusion is extended to describe what happens in intense emotional experiences. Bowen claims that even the well-differentiated person "relax[es] ego boundaries for the pleasurable sharing of 'selfs,' " and then will need to disengage from this kind of "emotional fusion" to go on "about [his] business" (p. 359). The disengagement counteracts the feeling of "too much togetherness, with its accompanying sense of loss of self. . ." (Kerr, 1981, p. 236). This conceptualization of intimacy again represents the culture's view (which is men's view) that intimacy represents a danger; that it is life threatening rather than life giving, depleting rather than enhancing, and so best taken in small discrete doses. In contrast, women experience intimacy as enlarging the self, expanding the self, and defining the self, not obliterating the self. Obliteration of signs of self may occur for women, but not because of the experience of intimacy per se.

As the gender bias in this concept redoubles when viewing women in relationships with other women, we suggest that the therapist first consider alternative explanations for observed behavior in lesbian couples that they might otherwise describe as fusion. Following are examples.

1. A relationship between a man and a woman in which she is always pulling for more and putting out more while he moves near and far, tolerating intimacy for only brief periods, is usually seen as normal and typical. If, however, the relationship is comprised of two women, both of whom are trained and ready to engage for a prolonged period in intense relating, then it may look pathological by comparison. Therapists should consider that they may be viewing richness rather than fusion.

2. Lesbians have available to them a small community of kindred souls, surrounded by a society that is antipathetic or openly hostile to their existence.

Thus, the social context in which lesbians exist makes the penalties for losing a partner higher than would be the case with straight clients. Rather than an inadequate sense of self, it may be this fear that causes the panic and desperate holding on that therapists often identify as evidence of fusion.

3. Similarity, mirroring, or twinning, all phenomena that therapists have observed in lesbian couples, need not represent fusion, but rather a benign identification with each other, a protective response to a hostile surround.

4. A therapist may be led to the diagnosis of fusion because of an unexamined envy of the observed closeness or because of an ambivalence about intimacy.

5. The vocabulary and emotions women have been taught to associate with erotic attachment are laden with sacrifice and catastrophe. "Nothing matters to me but you." "I cannot live without you." When a woman describes herself to a man this way, the words sound normal and familiar. When a woman describes herself to a woman in this way, the words signal fusion. We recognize this reaction as homophobic.

6. A woman may be suffering from the consequences of a cognitive error that has given her to believe that she by herself is inadequate to meet the demands of her life. This cognitive error is common in women, as it is taught to them at an early age. It results in excessive dependency on a partner who is erroneously seen as having all those qualities that the woman herself lacks. The emotional component of this cognitive error is the panic the woman feels at any threat of the loss of such a profoundly important relationship, a reaction often exacerbated in lesbian relationships because of the conditions cited above, that is, limited choices, increased intimacy, and heightened identification. Still, this reaction is neither clarified nor adequately described by calling it fusion.

Boundary

Boundary is the "line" around a set of people formed by the rules governing membership and participation inside that set. The term facilitates discussion in family therapy about the responsibilities and privileges of one group in relation to another, one part of the family in relation to another, even one individual in relation to another. Whatever the original intent for the term, it has come to be commonly used in a way that moves it from making neutral distinctions—yours versus theirs—to being a philosophy of life, "Keep your boundaries clear." Whether said eloquently by theoreticians or instructively to clients, the emphasis is on ownership, possessiveness, protectiveness, separation, caution, vigilance. Much more is written on what must be kept out than on what must be let in; more on clarity and firmness than on fluidity and adaptability; more on what ought to be than on what might suit. Little is mentioned in the family therapy literature about ever loosening the grip on boundary, about times when it would be advantageous to lower the guard—in play, in crises, in transitions, in certain groupings. As we began our work with the women described here, we found no direction provided by family therapy theory telling us that we should examine the necessities and benefits that would lead some couples, in this case, lesbian couples, to avoid the tight boundary typically recommended. As a result, early in therapy, the women appeared to be either wrong or sick, even though other boundaries in their lives (regarding work and families of origin) seemed to function well.

We want to challenge the use of boundary as a prescriptive rather than descriptive term. Other than the incest taboo, the key purpose of prescribing boundaries appears to be to protect hierarchies in the family, which are also prescribed. Such a vision of family is in the service of patriarchy and its favored mode, domination. Other ways of managing family life are seldom explored in family therapy.

The emphasis on boundary indicates that family therapy views relationships in the family, and relationships in general, as battles for territory, as power struggles from first to last. Undoubtedly, there are people who experience relationships in precisely that way, but there are other ways to experience relationships. It is unnecessarily restrictive on the field to create no other metaphors and attend to no other models. Lesbian couples do intend a different vision: relationships based not on power politics, but on intimacy, mutuality, interdependence, and equality.

TREATMENT

Goals

Our goals with the group in treatment are:

1. To help each woman identify her individual needs.
2. To explore with each woman what it would mean for her to take care of her individual needs and the consequences that might follow from doing so.
3. To normalize conflict, increase tolerance for it, and expand resources for resolving it.
4. To encourage the women to negotiate explicit rules regarding the patterns of interaction that would suit them, especially with respect to defining the nature of primary relationships and the expectations about tasks, money, sex, and closeness.
5. To support the women in their reliance on the resources available in the lesbian community.

Plan

Individual Needs

An important way of helping the women recognize their needs is to identify something in what they are already saying and doing as an expression of an individual need. The expression may be described to them as overstated, understated, or disguised, but it will help validate direct expression if the therapists indicate that there already is some expression and show them that some expression is unavoidable. The therapists can request a direct statement of the identified need and work with the speaker's own reactions to making the statement more direct.

Consequences of Needs

Once some progress has been made in recognizing and stating individual needs, each woman will require assistance in reacting to the results of those needs for others. The therapists will help each woman articulate the consequences for herself, and coach the owner of the need to hear the discussion without invalidating her need, even if it has undesired consequences for others.

Conflict

Options for dealing with conflict can be expanded for the women by interrupting their efforts to palliate and by encouraging them to relate to each other as competent adults. The therapists can explain to them that when they are indirect and nonconfrontive, they infantilize each other and deprive each other of opportunities to demonstrate maturity and strength. By making explicit any implicit conflict in the group, the therapists can invite the women to talk through the issue during the therapy session and can act as a coach for each participant while the other group members observe. Instructions can be given on fair fighting techniques, such as using I statements, staying with single issues, and time limiting the argument.

Explicit Expectations

Related to the first goal, this goal requires that the women learn about their expectations in primary relationships and what each is inferring about the other's expectations. Differing expectations between partners can then be discussed and negotiated with the help of the therapists and the support of friends.

Resources

To legitimatize the importance the lesbian community plays as a resource in these women's lives, the therapists can acknowledge the friendship network, dinner club, women-centered musical events, and political activities that make up the community that supports and nurtures lesbian women.

Kathy, Joy, Anne, Louise

During the next few months, we encouraged Louise to express her grief and anger regarding the loss of Anne, both to Anne and to the group. Gradually, Louise became more settled about the end of her relationship with Anne, and started developing a new relationship. As is not unusual in the lesbian community, the other women in the group warmly included Louise's new lover in their dinners and outings. This move seemed to take care of Louise's desire to stay connected not only to Anne, but to Joy and Kathy as well. Soon, Louise decided that she no longer needed the sessions because she had completed what she needed to with Anne and trusted that her friendship with Anne and with the other members would continue. We concurred with Louise's assessment.

Kathy's display of empathy in every session was remarkable. She always sat near the one who was in the most pain. She wept as they told their stories, reached out to comfort them physically, and kept her own story inside so as not to take attention away from the one who she believed needed it more. We challenged Kathy with the fact that she was interfering with the development of a mutual and reciprocal empathy among the group members—not giving the others a chance to nurture her. We suggested to the others that whenever Kathy offered expressions of concern to them, they might ask her if she could be holding back a need for some attention. After this suggestion, group members began to watch for behaviors on the part of any of them that might mask individual need and to comment on the advantages of direct over indirect requests.

Kathy demonstrated confusion about whether she would prefer a primary relationship with Anne or Joy, weeping over the potential loss of either of them. We asked her to define her needs and to tell us how each woman seemed to fulfill them. Kathy's response led us to believe that the question of her own needs in a relationship had never occurred to her; she had believed that the only legitimate question was who needed her.

After a few thoughtful moments, she acknowledged that Anne's energy and enthusiasm fulfilled her need for shared history, security, and familiarity, all represented in the home they had created together and in her inclusion in Joy's loving family, a family quite different from her abusive alcoholic parents, both of whom were now dead. Our understanding of this response was that Joy had given Kathy her first real home; its value must surely have been increased by the sanctuary it provided from the hostile world. The thought of losing it terrified Kathy. This interpretation seemed to fit as she went on in tears, describing their shared life of 15 years.

Anne displayed an exaggerated selflessness in her unconditional regard for Kathy. She repeatedly stated that she would support Kathy in whatever decision she might come to, even though she thoroughly enjoyed their sexual and emotional intimacy and hoped it would continue. We suggested to Anne that she might be denying to herself how important Kathy had become. When we asked Anne how she was taking care of her own needs, she said that she spent as much time with Kathy as circumstances would allow while being prepared for Kathy to move back to Joy at any time. Given the extent of her attachment, we warned Anne that she might be overestimating her ability to accept whatever happened and encouraged her to speak up as her reactions surfaced during the course of the therapy. She promised to do so.

Throughout these months, Joy stayed firm in her desire to have Kathy move back to their house and try again to have a primary, sexually exclusive relationship. She expressed sadness that Kathy did not share in her resolve, but she hoped that when she returned from her long-planned trip to Greece over the summer, Kathy would be ready to move back with her. When we asked Joy what would motivate Kathy to make the move, she replied that the desire to be a couple again would be her motivation to try. When we pressed further, Joy admitted that all their attempts at being sexually intimate in the past year had been unsatisfying for both of them but she believed that time and the elimination of distractions might make for better success.

We asked if Kathy and Anne's relationship acted as a complication. Joy said that her requests of Kathy to stop seeing Anne led to such pain for Kathy that she always withdrew her requests. We wanted to assist Joy in going beyond her typical backing-off point, but she told us that she had no energy to do so. Because of their unclear and indirect style of communication, Kathy and Joy had not confronted each other effectively. It seemed to us that they were again operating out of the belief that the other was not strong enough to hear the truth, that they were unentitled to sexual satisfaction, that their desire to redefine their relationship was, in some way, disloyal.

Here was a good opportunity for us to help the women find better ways to deal with conflict. We asked each woman to describe her optimum desire and helped the group negotiate the resulting list. After some discussion, all agreed that Kathy would move back to the house but continue to see Anne while Joy was vacationing, a complicated solution but one that seemed to satisfy everyone. We outlined the possible consequences and how any one of the women could be the loser: Joy, after returning from vacation, might find herself without Kathy; Anne might become more involved and then be less able to extricate herself; Kathy might develop a greater attachment to the house and neighborhood, as well as to Anne, and so her choice might be even more painful to make.

While Joy was away, Kathy and Anne told us how enjoyable their days were and how difficult it would be to end their sexual connection once Joy returned. Anne said that Kathy seemed happier now that she was back in her home. With reluctance, Anne said she was coming to realize that she could not compete with the 15 years of history, family, and home that Joy and Kathy had shared. Kathy again emphasized how essential her home and neighborhood were to her, and how much she did not want to lose Joy as a friend and soul mate. She said that it was hard to think of her as a lover, however.

In a session several weeks later when Joy had returned, Kathy announced that she had decided to live on her own in the old neighborhood and date Anne as well as others. With much prompting from us, Joy told Kathy that she was sad and disappointed, but she spoke with very little affect. Anne also tried to disguise her feelings, again displaying total acceptance. We suggested to Anne that she seemed to want to portray for Kathy an idealized image of the all-giving lover, and that this image was to her own disservice. We encouraged her to honor whatever feelings might come and not conclude that merely by doing so, she would be turning away from her friend. Anne agreed to try. Kathy explained that her decision to create her own home arose from her awareness of the importance a home holds for her—the home rather than Joy, who had faded as a sexual partner long ago.

In the next session, we learned that despite the intentions expressed in the prior session, Kathy had not moved out of Joy's house and was still living with her. When asked about how she intended to satisfy her affectional/sexual needs, Kathy said she was not going to address that dimension for fear that Joy would not allow her to live with her while dating other women. In this way, she hoped to avoid conflict, at least until an actual situation necessitated it. When we asked Joy to clarify her own position, she stated that it was not acceptable for Kathy to live with her and be sexually involved elsewhere. She hoped that, through the experience of living together, Kathy would desire her again. We asked Joy how she envisioned that this change might take place. When pressed, she admitted that she really could not imagine it.

We offered the observation that the solution Kathy and Joy had come to did not seem likely to last long and wondered if it might be their way of postponing an inevitable loss. They agreed, and we encouraged them to spend time exploring ways of making a life together to see if they could incorporate what each wanted. In making this suggestion, we were aware that it would not be an easy task. Our visions of what we want in a relationship are easily clouded by heterosexist assumptions that block out other possibilities for structuring relationships. Despite the difficulty, we urged them to the task, explaining that failure to be explicit increases the risk of living lives driven by assumptions that do not really fit.

Two weeks later, Kathy reported that she was living in the house, Joy was living in the spare room of a friend's home, and Anne was moving into a smaller apartment. Kathy and Joy had agreed that the house held more meaning for Kathy than for Joy, so Kathy would continue living there while they discussed the possibility of selling. The physical moves denoted a significant shift for Kathy and Joy in their view of the relationship. They told us that they had spent long evenings analyzing whether their relationship met their individual needs. Their conclusion was that it no longer could.

Once they had ceased their efforts to make the relationship work, Kathy and Joy were able to talk about their long-standing sexual difficulties. Joy admitted that she had always been frightened by Kathy's sexual intensity and added, with some embarrassment, that sex had little importance for her. After stating that this issue did not need to be thoroughly examined in Kathy's and Anne's presence, we suggested to Joy that perhaps her own sexual interest might not be deficient in any sense, but just different from Kathy's. This way of seeing was an obvious comfort to Joy. Kathy acknowledged that she had eventually given up trying to get Joy interested in sex. We wondered aloud if this were simply an extension of their rule about conflict: "If you cannot get what you want from your partner, backing off is preferable to arguing about it." Both women agreed with our interpretation.

We pointed out to the three women that Anne had said nothing during the session, that it had not seemed germane for us to ask for her comments, and that neither Kathy nor Joy had made any requests of her. After they discussed their responses to our observation, they concluded that Kathy and Joy had some private business in therapy that was not relevant to Anne, Louise, or anyone else. We then arranged a session for Kathy and Joy alone to ritualize the ending of their sexual relationship.

At the scheduled session, Kathy and Joy started by declaring their unwillingness to say good-bye. We reminded them that it is the influence of heterosexism that would make good-bye seem necessary simply because they were ending their sexual relationship. They need not participate in that thinking, we noted. They said that, in many ways, they still felt as close to each other as they had when they were lovers, even though sex was not desired. With some specific guidance from us, they began to grieve over the loss of their sexual relationship, openly sharing the pain and sadness of their last years together. In time, they moved into talking more about the importance of the relationship both past and present, and insisting on continuing it in the future. We proposed that though not born of the same mother, they had found each other to be a good sister and were experiencing how precious and wonderful sisterhood can be. Kathy answered that, in fact, none of the women in the group had a sister and wondered if that was part of the reason that leaving each other was so painful. One of us pointed out that she did have a sister, and would also despair if she could not count on her for special times and long talks into the night for the rest of their lives.

Joy and Kathy seemed moved by the idea of looking at each other as sisters and enjoyed the shape it gave their future. Then they became worried that, as they were not biological sisters, outsiders might not understand or support the continuing desire of each to keep the other so central to her life. Joy said she had already experienced trouble, explaining that the women she had recently dated felt threatened and distrustful of her relationship with Kathy despite her telling them it was nonsexual. We sympathized with this problem and said that even with the biological tie to our own sisters, there was often trouble anyway; our husbands and lovers had been jealous of the bond. In the lesbian community, we noted, the problem would obviously be more complicated: as the community is so small and the risk of exposing one's self to a stranger is so high, women tend to date their friends, and the line between friend and lover is frequently crossed. We urged them, over the next week, to think of other difficulties they could envision. They suggested including Anne in the assignment and inviting her next time. We agreed.

All three women came to the next session. Each one described various difficulties envisioned for future relationships, and we noted that these difficulties had a common cause: ambiguity about expectations in relationships. Here was another version of the problem we had worked on throughout therapy. This time we phrased it as an ambiguity about commitment. In response, they started talking about the oppression of marriage. We asked for specifics, and they all spoke at once, completing each other's sentences as if they had discussed this topic many times. They spoke of the unequal power between partners, the lack of mutuality in tasks and care giving, and the requirement to find fulfillment of all needs within marriage. We pointed out that these had to do with heterosexism, not with commitment itself. We asked, "If you were free to spread your commitment among as many as you wished, to whom would you be willing to commit for what?" With sudden ease and enjoyment, they described commitments of various attentions and services to several different friends, and then moved on to the threesome in the room. Joy and Kathy committed themselves to protecting their sisterhood and to continuing to learn about it; Kathy and Anne committed themselves to a period of sexual exclusivity while they examined the potential between them; Joy and Anne committed themselves to a friendship marked by the occasional sharing of music and conversation. At our suggestion, all three recognized that whatever was unstated was outside the commitment and open to experimentation and negotiation.

Six weeks later, Anne, Joy, and Kathy came to a session. All three reported that they felt they had resolved the issues that had brought them to therapy. Anne was enjoying school and her relationship with Kathy. Kathy was enjoying her house, time with Anne, and her evolving relationship with Joy. Joy was enjoying dating and her evolving relationship with Kathy. They all periodically had dinner with Louise.

PITFALLS

There are a number of pitfalls that await the feminist family therapist.

Insisting that "Some of my best friends are lesbians." The central pitfall for the family therapist working with lesbian clients is the failure to recognize mutually shared homophobia. The fact that therapist and client seem to espouse the same values may simply reflect their common rearing in a culture with a long history of revulsion and fear of women who love women. Despite all efforts to be rid of prejudice, the therapist needs to stay keenly aware of the remaining homophobic and heterosexist bias or it will surely insinuate itself into the therapy.

Holding on to a hands-off policy. Out of her desire to respect the uniqueness of her lesbian clients' experience, the therapist may be reluctant to address issues that she would not hesitate to comment on if she were working with a heterosexual couple. It is sometimes wise for therapists to assume an anthropological stance with clients who present unfamiliar problems and situations, but this stance can be held too long. The therapist is thereby deskilled and the clients will not be well served.

Detecting only legends and visionaries. Although most family theories ignore or implicitly pathologize lesbian experience, feminist family therapists may err in the opposite direction by idealizing lesbian existence. The lesbian may be viewed as heroic for having escaped the bonds of heterosexual coupling and rejecting the oppression of possessiveness and inequality that too often characterize heterosexual relationships. To the extent that therapists idealize any clients, they limit their ability to be useful.

Overestimating identification, underestimating difference. The therapist may believe that sharing womanhood with her lesbian clients is so fundamental a similarity as to render insignificant any dissimilarity arising from the lesbian experience. Although this error is most frequently made in the interest of establishing empathy with the clients, it is inevitably a disservice because it results in a failure to appreciate the uniqueness of the clients' own lives. A related pitfall for therapists is to mistake their familiarity with feminist thought for an understanding of lesbian experience. Actually, much feminist writing does not address lesbian experience at all.

Assuming that if you have seen one, you have seen them all. In spite of a commitment not to see lesbianism as a form of pathology, the feminist family therapist may fall into the trap of classifying these clients by their sexual orientation rather than by the way they present themselves in therapy. Such an error will lead to the absurd conclusion that all lesbians are alike and have the same problems.

REFERENCES

Alther, L. (1984). *Other women.* New York: Alfred A. Knopf.
Bowen, M. (1966). The use of family theory in clinical practice. *Comprehensive Psychiatry,* 7(5), 345–374.

Broverman, I., Vogel, S.R., Broverman, D.M., Clarkson, F.E., & Rosenkrantz, P.S. (1972). Sex role steroetypes: A current appraisal. *Journal of Social Issues*, 28, 59–78.

Gartrell, N. (1984). Issues in psychotherapy with lesbian women. *Work in Progress*. (Available from Stone Center for Developmental Services and Studies, Wellesley, Mass.)

Gilligan, C. (1982). *In a different voice: Psychological theory and women's development*. Cambridge, Mass.: Harvard University Press.

Haley, J. (1971). Toward a theory of pathological systems. In G. H. Zuk & I. Boszormenyi-Nagy (Eds.), *Family therapy and disturbed families* (pp. 11–27). Palo Alto, Calif.: Science and Behavior Books.

Kerr, M.E. (1981). Family systems theory and therapy. In A. S. Gurman & D. P. Kniskern (Eds.), *Handbook of family therapy* (pp. 226–266). New York: Brunner/Mazel.

Krestan, J., & Bepko, C. (1980). The problem of fusion in the lesbian relationship. *Family Process*, 19(3), 277–290.

Lewis, S. (1979). *Sunday's women: Lesbian life today*. Boston: Beacon Press.

Miller, J.B. (1976). *Toward a new psychology of women*. Boston: Beacon Press.

Rich, A. (1980). Compulsory heterosexuality and lesbian existence. *Signs*, 5(4), 631–660.

Rich, A. (1979). *On lies, secrets, and silence: Selected prose, 1966-1978*. New York: Norton.

Rich, A. (1978). "XIII." *The dream of a common language: Poems 1974-1977*. New York: Norton.

Roth, S. (1985). Psychotherapy with lesbian couples: Individual issues, female socialization, and the social context. *Journal of Marital and Family Therapy*, 11(3), 273–286.

Vida, G. (Ed.) (1978). *Our right to love*. Englewood Cliffs, N.J.: Prentice-Hall.

9

WOMEN IN PAIN: SUBSTANCE ABUSE/SELF-MEDICATION

Dusty Miller, Ed.D.

> Before they do it for you, you silence your own voice—from "Leviathan" (Beaching of the Whale), song by feminist musician and writer Chris Williamson

How we describe a problem can determine who we include in the system requiring intervention. Our description of the female substance abuser may determine whether we locate the problem at the individual level, at the family level (nuclear or extended), or as a symptom in a larger societal context. It is useful in discussing the multitide of possible descriptions of female substance abuse to consider an ecological epistemology. This means that we see the world as one of "observing systems" (von Foerster, 1981), "in which the act of observation changes that which is observed" (Anderson, 1984, p. 4). In this framework, it is helpful to understand the concept of the problem-determined system (Anderson et al., 1986; Hoffman, 1985). The problem of a woman's substance abuse creates a system that can be defined as a collection of *ideas* about the problem, rather than as an aggregate of family members, professionals, Alcoholics Anonymous (AA) counselors, or whomever else may be attached to the behavior or problem of substance abuse.

In this chapter, the problem of women abusing alcohol, drugs, and medicine will be addressed from both a feminist and a systemic perspective. The description of the problem will be considered as a central influence in examining treatment issues. The observing system will be described in terms of a recursive pattern of multiple realities: descriptions offered by the client and by all those interacting with her.

HISTORY OF INVISIBILITY AND SHAME

For centuries, women have found ways to dull the pain of oppression through a variety of self-destructive addictions. The abuse of alcohol, drugs, and prescription medicines knows no class or ethnic bounds. It is not, of course, a problem owned by women exclusively. Men have been the recognized alcoholics and drug addicts for far longer than women, receiving the lion's share of both blame and researchers' attention.

Until quite recently, women were the invisible alcoholics (Sandmaier, 1980); they were not associated in the middle-class public's mind with abuse of street drugs, unless, of course, they were part of a Black and/or poor or otherwise ghettoized subculture. The abuse of prescription drugs, however, has long been a "women's problem."

In the 19th century and into the early 20th century, many women were addicted to medicines that contained impressive amounts of morphine, opium, alcohol, or other addictive substances. These medications were often referred to as "women's friend," a description indicative of how involved women patients actually were with their medicines. As these dangerously addictive medicines were discontinued, new possibilities in the domain of medical addiction were offered in abundance to female patients: tranquilizers of the 1950s and 1960s, such as Valium and Librium, are now being replaced by Zanex and other new, equally addictive medicines.

There has always been a double standard in public as well as clinical attitudes toward female substance abuse, including even the abuse of prescription drugs. Female intoxication or impairment seems to touch a depth of fear and disgust in both men and women. It is easy to infer that the woman who is not behaving in a competent, compliant, or dignified manner is frightening because she represents a violation of the sanctity of motherhood (Sandmaier, 1980).

Perhaps because of the intense discomfort permeating societal attitudes toward female substance abuse, for centuries there has been either a judgmental stance, viewing the substance-abusing woman as a failure as wife and mother, or else simply a refusal to address the problem. In some sense, the alcoholic or chemically dependent woman has always been viewed as "unnatural" or not representative of the female species.

The other side of the coin is that women have renounced or rejected their identity as good wife or mother, or even as an attractive female, by insulating themselves through chemical dependence. Thus, the abuse of substances must be seen on some level, frequently not a conscious one, as a women's rebellion against her lot as subordinate in a patriarchal culture. Whether she is sexually promiscuous or sexually withdrawn or homosexual, she is refusing, in some sense, to give up the control of her sexuality to men. If she is unable or unwilling, because of her addiction, to put the needs of her husband or her children before her own, she is stepping aside from her biological destiny as the nurturing center of family life.

Women have often become addicted to drugs or alcohol because they could find no other way to tolerate the drug/alcohol abuse of their male partners. Although this is another form of self-medication against the pain of powerlessness and frustration, it is viewed unsympathetically according to a societal standard that measures a woman by her ability, as wife and mother, to endure hardship.

Doctors and psychiatrists have participated in enabling the chemical addiction of women by ignoring the physical signs of alcoholism (not asking questions, for instance, that might reveal their personal revulsion) or by prescribing medications that either provide the source of addiction or add to the female patient's problem of chemical addiction. It is the women who are blamed for medical noncompliance when they do not "follow doctor's orders"; it is, once again, a male-dominated subculture (the medical establishment), which is reacting to the refusal of women to show appropriate subordinate behavior. Women who abuse prescription drugs are another group defying male control through self-abusive acts.

WOMEN IN THE FAMILY: OVERRESPONSIBILITY AND REBELLION

The responsibility trap (Bepko & Krestan, 1985) created by societal rules concerning women and their families is especially complex for female substance abusers to negotiate. Women are socialized, generally, to be overresponsible for others and underresponsible for themselves. In the family, this tendency is exaggerated. Men are socialized to be less central, to be less active in, and less concerned about family relationships. If the man in the family is drug involved or alcoholic, he becomes increasingly less responsible; thus, the wife and mother must increase her responsibilities.

If the wife and mother in this situation is the adult child of alcoholic parents, she has already been trained to be overresponsible and to put the needs of others first. She may simply accept a continuation of this role, tolerating the pattern of shame that is an expected rule of family life.

Another response to this trap is to become addicted herself. As female alcoholism is far less visible (and thus underreported) than that of men, it is impossible to estimate accurately how many substance-abusing women are in marriages or relationships with substance-abusing men. Most studies confirm the fact that a high percentage of female alcoholics are married to male alcoholics. In Corrigan's often-cited study (Corrigan, 1980), two out of five husbands of alcohol-abusing women had been treated for drinking problems.

One of Corrigan's most interesting findings was that 57 percent of her sample reported having difficulty in their role as wife, and an equal number reported that their mothering was negatively affected by their drinking. This finding could be construed as a confirmation of the function substance abuse serves in reaction to the responsibility trap of family life.

Although decreasing her family responsibilities through drug abuse can be viewed as a vehicle for rebellion against the traditional female role, the under-functioning alcoholic or drug-addicted woman usually experiences profound shame in her failure as wife and/or mother.

Single-parent families may suffer the greatest degree of shame when the parent is addicted to drugs of alcohol. In a 1985 report from the American Orthopsychiatric Association, it was noted that well over 50 percent of American children live in single-parent households. If the alcohol treatment community's generalization holds true that most women describe their problem drinking and drug abuse as reactive, caused by an affective state of loneliness, anxiety, or depression, then the woman carrying the burdens and stresses of single parenting is at very high risk. Single mothers must also cope with the double bind of being expected to seek help for family problems (as well as their own addiction problem) and being blamed or judged as incompetent, too needy, or dependent when they turn for help to social services or medical personnel (Imber-Black, 1986).

The descriptions of women who abuse drugs and alcohol are perjorative, and more so if the woman is a mother. Women who perceive blame and disgust in the attitudes of all who interact with them quickly internalize the experience. These women live with a constant and painful sense of shame and guilt.

The problem of female substance abuse seems to generate a collection of beliefs that are resoundingly negative and blameful. The following case offers a richly complicated series of descriptions, which, as a collective entity, can be called the problem-determined system.

CASE EXAMPLE

Mary is the 35-year-old single parent of Patricia, age 12, and Joey, age 10. Like many women who are choosing a chemical "release" in articulating their pain and defying the constraints of a more traditionally compliant female role, Mary appears to be asking the system for help and simultaneously rebelling against it.

One day she rides her bicycle (she has no other form of transportation) to the supermarket to do her food shopping. She asks politely if she can leave the bike inside the store against the wall so that it won't be stolen (she lives in an urban, high-crime-rate area). When she is denied permission, she proceeds to ride her bicycle through the aisles, selecting her groceries; she is escorted out of the store by security guards, who threaten to call the police. She tells her story with some mixture of pride, humor, and embarrassment. Helpers are dismayed by the story, but the children share their mother's mixed presentation of glee and shame.

When Mary's children were younger, they had been placed for approximately five years in foster care because of the violence in the home. (Their father was an alcoholic who was physically abusive to the children and to Mary.) Although Mary had a drinking problem herself, she was allowed to keep her children with her after she divorced their father. The state had legal custody, but Patricia and Joey had been living with their mother for three years when the family was referred for family therapy.

Mary embodies the characteristics of both the rebellion and the shame that characterize many substance-abusing women. She relates to her children in a playful, loving, but somewhat nonparental, nonhierarchical way. Family conflicts look like sibling feuds and there is little clarity about family rules or routines. Mary is careful to hide her current substance abuse, although she refers occasionally to her past "problem," especially in relation to her alcoholic ex-husband.

The secret of Mary's substance abuse is both dangerous and well protected.

She is in danger of losing her children again if professionals begin to see her as an alcoholic woman: it will be suspected that she is abusive to her children, or at least neglectful. It may also be thought that she is sexually promiscuous and, in general, she is likely to be viewed as self-defeating.

Mary's children, like many children of alcoholic parents, appear to be working hard to protect her secret. Patricia, especially, creates a continuous smoke screen of defiant, belligerent behavior that serves to distract teachers and social workers from focusing primary concern on her mother. At the same time, Patricia and Joey may also be seen as attempting to draw attention to their mother's need for help by continuing to defy all attempts by the involved professional network to "help (Mary) get them under control."

The language used in telling Mary's story might vary greatly, depending on both the position of the observer in the observing system and the context in which the story is told.[1]

Nonsystemic Descriptions of the Problem

The scant literature on women and substance abuse is more concerned with treatment issues than with explanations or descriptions of the function of drug abuse in a gender-aware systemic context. There are notable exceptions (Bepko & Krestan, 1986; Sandmaier, 1980); generally, however, few writers or clinicians have considered the function of substance abuse in the context of gender inequality. We now realize that women have been virtually ignored in all major theories conderning the diagnosis and treatment of substance abuse. Few writers have ventured to describe interactional systems involving female abusers, nor have there been studies of the use of self-medication by women at the larger societal level.

Traditional Descriptions

If Mary were to be described by various proponents of etiologic models of alcoholism, she would receive a wide variety of diagnostic labels.

Those who favor theories about alcoholic personality traits, might describe Mary as suffering from depression or as having a sociopathic personality. In evaluating Mary's children, Patricia would be expected to be at very high risk for adult alcoholism. Studies by "experts" in the field of alcoholism and personality disorders show that children from homes where the father was alcoholic and who were viewed as hyperactive, aggressive, or truant and problemmatic at school were more likely to become alcoholic adults (Donovan, 1986).

Mary's story could also be told from the heredity viewpoint. What has been generalized as commonly accepted lay dogma is the belief that alcoholism is genetically transmitted from generation to generation. Alcoholism is seen to be

[1]These descriptions are not meant to be thorough reviews but rather to alert the reader to the importance of including gender in the examples of substance abuse.

a disease, like diabetes, which is passed on through the genes. Children of alcoholic parents are seen as more at risk of becoming alcoholic.

It is interesting to ponder the question of why male offspring seem to inherit this disease significantly more often than female offspring. If one looks at the nurture side of the "nature versus nurture" argument, it seems that the social context determines, in part, which members of the family are more likely to inherit the disease; males, for example, are less stigmatized by excessive drinking than females.

AA/Al-Anon

Although the disease model sidesteps questions of social context, it is clearly a foundation for the belief system of AA/Al-Anon, the first systemic treatment model. As both clinical and societal awareness of addictions increases, there are more questions about how the abuse of chemicals is generated and maintained through family interactions. It is clear that long before family therapists began looking at the role of the family in creating and maintaining patterns of addiction, the philosophy of AA and Al-Anon had addressed the familial interrelations of alcoholic and co-alcoholic. It was Al-Anon that first offered an empathic, decidedly systemic explanation of how spouses and children were implicated in alcoholic relational patterns.

Unfortunately, the descriptions of female substance abuse offered by AA tend to be no more enlightening on the larger societal level than the genderless explanations of systemic patterns proposed by other alcoholism experts.

From both the AA model and a family systems model, the patterns of family addiction and coaddiction ignore the gender-specific role of the substance abuser. The alcoholic or addict is viewed as one piece of the system, which, as a whole, generates and maintains a repetitive cycle of predictable addiction-based behaviors.

Responsibilities for familial relationships are not viewed as gender linked in the descriptions offered by AA or family systems philosophy. In this genderblind view, someone in the family is enabled by someone else in the family to behave in an incompetent or irresponsible way; others in the family system may be described as showing symptoms related to the behaviors of the addict or as becoming overresponsible to compensate for the underresponsible alcoholic/addict. Although assumptions are made about the prevalence of addiction in the male members of the family, the description of the system remains curiously genderfree.

This limited use of circularity distorts the real differences between the experience of female and male substance abuse. Not only is the refusal to be responsible for family relationships a very different experience for the family of the female substance abuser than for the family of the male, but the experience of the individual female addict is also very different. When the addicted female refuses traditional responsibilities for family well-being and relationship nurturance, there is, potentially, a systemic catastrophe. Also, with few exceptions, the female who refuses her traditional role as central caretaker in the family experiences overwhelming shame and guilt.

Alcohol and drug abuse are often transmitted from generation to generation; entire families experience life in a chronic pattern of shame and pain, which gives impetus to turn to a release through substance abuse, followed by out-of-control behavior that leads back to shame and pain (Fossum & Mason, 1986). All members of the family play a role in maintaining this transgenerational cycle.

Although each family member's role may mutually maintain and perpetuate the shame-bound system, the mutuality does not mean equal participation. Those with less power and few choices to "leave the field" do not share equal responsibility for the abusive behavior (MacKinnon & Miller, 1987).

To describe the problem of female substance abuse accurately, it is necessary to include the larger societal context of gender inequality. The description may begin with the history of the problem as it has been transmitted from generation to generation within a particular family. The differences between the experiences of the men and the women in the family are a vital part of the description, however.

When a man's drinking or drug abuse becomes dangerous both to himself and to others, he can leave or be ejected from the family system; his children and his spouse can be partially protected from his destructive behavior. When a woman's substance abuse is out of control, she may not be able to leave the system in which she is embedded. Despite the reality that her family situation may be contributing to the chronic maintenance of her abuse problem, she seems not to have the freedom to leave because children, aging parents, and even husbands are dependent on her as the primary caretaker. This is especially true when her husband or boyfriend is also a substance abuser.

Feminist Description

The critique of existing treatment modalities suggests the need to develop a compassionate, gender-focused treatment model, borrowing from traditional addiction-model treatment as well as a feminist world view.

A feminist description of Mary would be informed by an awareness of Mary's subordinate position in a patriarchal culture. Mary is seen by the feminist observer as being a victim of her marriage to an abusive, alcoholic husband, and as oppressed on the larger socioeconomic level in her position as a welfare mother without a coparenting partner.

Like all other mothers, she is expected to fill the central caretaker role for her family. If she does not seek adequate support for herself and her children from the professional network, she is seen as neglectful or underfunctioning. If she seeks too much help from professionals, she is seen as being too dependent on helpers and too needy (Imber-Black, 1986). Thus, Mary is in a bind in relation to the helping system, walking a tightrope swaying in the unpredictable breezes of ever-changing social policy (and a cast of ever-changing social workers, as well).

Mary's story of the bicycle episode might seem to the feminist observer to be an act of misplaced defiance against the oppressive patriarchal system. (To the average professional unfortunately, it is a story of immature, underfunctioning behavior serving to remind the professional system that Mary is "primitive," or at least immature and dependent.)

Invasion and Control: A Systemic Description

The pattern of female substance abuse can be conceptualized as a recursive loop of invasion and control (Miller, in progress). Girls and women often experience invasion of both physical and psychological boundaries. This invasion may occur in the more tangible instance of sexual or physical abuse or in the less concrete experience of psychological violation through being disqualified or humiliated. These psychological violations may take place from childhood into maturity.

Examples of psychological invasions include intrusions of family members who insist that the girl or woman give up her own needs to accommodate theirs or deny her the right of mental privacy. The violation might take the form of disqualification; individual thoughts, desires, and needs are rendered invisible through this kind of violation.

The perceived invasion of the individual can be expanded to the societal level of the female experience. Women living in a patriarchal culture often experience the oppression common to all subordinates in a hierarchical society. As long as there is a dominant group for whom power is measured by greater access to resources and more freedom to leave the field, the subordinate group cannot escape either the physical or the psychological domain of discrimination.

Female substance abuse can be described as an attempt to control the perceived invasion of physical or psychological boundaries. The control mechanism of drinking or using drugs can provide the illusion of escape through refusal to participate fully in whatever dominant–subordinate relationship is enacted.

Similar to the external invasion-and-control sequence is the loop of internal experience that cycles from pain to numbness to shame and back again to pain. The woman who experiences disqualification, humiliation, inequality, physical or sexual abuse, and/or pervasive low self-esteem might describe herself simply as experiencing pain. She may alleviate the pain by abusing alcohol, drugs, or prescription medicines, thus moving to the numbness or relief part of the cycle. Relief through substance abuse is short-lived, as the loss of control engenders feelings of shame. Shame breeds the potential for disqualification, physical abuse, sexual abuse, inequality, and low self-esteem. Once again, the abuser has cycled back to pain.

The woman's choice to self-medicate through substance abuse may be understood as an attempt to insulate herself against invasion, on both the personal level and the larger societal level. If she is inaccessible because she is intoxicated or drugged, she can still be invaded in the domain of actual physical impact on her personal boundaries, her freedom of choice, decision making, and so on, but her internal experience may be impenetrable because she is anesthetized against the pain and outrage she would feel if the invasions took place in her sober state.

Substance abuse is a distancing mechanism that allows the woman in pain to avoid more direct (and possibly dangerous) responses to an oppressive situation. By choosing substance abuse as an insulating or distancing maneuver, women may attempt to repel feared or actual invasion of personal and physical boundaries. Much of the existing literature concerned with alcohol and drug abuse describes the use of chemicals as a vehicle for distance regulation. This analysis is, unfortunately, genderless. Because the woman has less access to resources (less earning power) and, often, more responsibilities for children and other dependents (aging parents, incompetent siblings or husbands, for example), she may have to find a vehicle for distancing within the relationship. Intoxication provides emotional distance from those with whom she must continue to coexist. She may distance through social withdrawal or through diminishing emotional connectedness. The distance created by the substance abuse allows her to feel less acute pain, fear, and anger.

Secrecy is another significant form of control. Keeping the substance abuse a secret is a form of exercising control against intrusion. Drug, alcohol, or medication abuse often not only is kept secret by the woman herslef, but family members, work colleagues, and professionals may inadvertently collude by avoiding or denying the problem. The secret of female substance abuse may be handed down through several generations, creating a multigenerational pattern of using drugs to manage external intrusion.

In the histories of oppressed groups (any group in a subordinate position whose access to resources, freedom of choice, and opportunity to leave the field are controlled by a dominant group), it is frequently the case that silence and secrecy are forms of control or self-protection. Women, children, prisoners, people of color, homosexuals, and the physically disabled all have traditions of secret codelike language and strategic silences.

The silence or secrecy may be described as a form of controlling access to something belonging to the individual or group. It may also be a way to disguise or control the individual's or the group's impulse to express rage and rebellion against the dominant group. Secrecy controls the potentially dangerous impulse to challenge one's subservient position.

The intoxicated woman may disguise her rage by sounding incoherent or ridiculous and behaving in an out-of-control manner, which allows her an indirect form of rebellion. She may become so impaired that she vomits or loses consciousness—another form of disguised rebellion against the contempt for the control imposed by the dominant group's rules and beliefs about the female role. The inevitable cycling back to shame serves to keep the substance abuser in a subservient position, another way of avoiding the repercussions of challenging traditional gender-determined power imbalance.

Not all women who abuse alcohol and drugs appear to control their anger or maintain a subservient or subordinate position. For some, the state of chemical intoxication provides a release, an opportunity to exercise anger and defiance against oppressive situations or boundary intrusions. Whether or not the intoxicated woman is actually able to exert herself in a more openly defiant and powerful way is doubtful. What is important is that she may experience herself as more powerful and rebellious.

Mary is more likely to be viewed as defying the authority of the system and rebelling against her would-be helpers because she often turns her shame into a defiant, out-of-control relief from pain. Whether or not she is actually chemically impaired, she behaves in a rebellious, unladylike manner, which provokes outrage and rejection or punishment from the helping system.

There is another important concept in the telling of Mary's story. Mary and her husband may have shared a mutually enabling pattern of abusive behavior, including drug and alcohol abuse, but their parental roles were not equal. Mary was responsible for the children, including her accountability for them in the face of their father's physical violence toward them, and toward her also. When she could not, in the eyes of the system, adequately protect them, they were placed in foster care.

Her alternatives were not easy to achieve. She could have left her husband and moved with the children to a safer place. Unfortunately, Mary had little possibility of providing financially for the children, and she was further handicapped by her pattern of abusive drinking. Like many other wives of alcoholics (and children of alcoholics), she may have believed that she would be able to gain control of her own life, her marriage, and her husband's drinking and abusive behavior "some day" in the future.

Once the state had intervened, Mary grew more despairing, and also more enraged. She finally gathered her forces and divorced her husband. The state refused to return her children to her until she was also able to give up her alcoholic life-style.

Mary's dilemma, once she had gained control of her life and her family, was that she was still engaged in a daily series of battles. Her battle with substance abuse continued to rage, as did new battles with her children and with the professional helping network. Beneath the rage was the pain of loss: loss of partner, loss of self-esteem, and the not inconsiderable loss of the self-medicating release from alcohol and drugs.

From a family systems perspective, the story needed earlier "chapters," descriptions of Mary and her family of origin, before the voices of the present and future could be heard. One advantage of exploring Mary's stories of her childhood was that the descriptions belonged to her; she had control of the language to describe that system and she had control of secrets and silences. What is lacking, of course, is the more three-dimensional quality of varying descriptions possible when there is more than one observer telling the story. Mary's description, undoubtedly had many different voices and nuances of meaning, depending on the context of the story telling.

If she had described her family to a substance abuse counselor with a medical model orientation ("the elucidation and treatment of biological abnormalities that predispose the individual to—or create—aberrant behavior," Donovan, 1986, p. 195), she would have been guided to focus on those in the family who were substance abusers, including siblings, parents, aunts, uncles, cousins, and grandparents.

A very different description might emerge if she were talking to an individual psychodynamic therapist or a family therapist. The female client, for example, who tells her story in the chapter on "A Recovering Alcoholic Speaks and Her Family Therapist Introduces Her" (Kaufman & Kaufmann, 1981), focuses almost exclusively on the negative, painful relationship she experienced with her mother. Mary, too, might describe a childhood of neglect and unmet needs. She might choose to explain this by identifying her father as an abusive alcoholic and her mother as overwhelmed and emotionally depleted. Or she might simply say that she was from a large family where obedience and survival of the fittest ruled.

Telling her story in a context that was supportive of her authority-questioning stance and her heroic determination as a single parent, Mary could probably describe her family legacy as having learned to be tough enough to survive and to enjoy life whenever possible.

In a therapy that was particularly focused on shame and shaming events in the family's history (Fossum & Mason, 1986), Mary would be encouraged to describe both the shaming events of childhood and the shaming events in her current family's history. These events, or patterns of shame, might be based on substance abuse, physical or sexual abuse, or compulsive behaviors around money, food, or sex. Mary can be described as someone living in a shame-bound family, a family in which a cycle of control and release, centered in the experience of shame, becomes stereotyped and ritualized, and is passed on from one generation to the next.

"All families explain the events in their history through family myths. Myths in the shame-bound family are born out of distortions and delusions, and through loyalty function as barrier reefs to family shame" (Fossum & Mason, p. 46). To navigate through these reefs to penetrate the secrecy surrounding family shame, Mary and her children need a supportive, inviting context in which family members and all others involved in the problem-determined system construct new meanings together.

TREATMENT

Mary's story of the bicycle in the supermarket nudged one family therapy team[2] to try a new forum for their coevolving meaning system. The team began to notice that their conversations about and with Mary's family seemed to center on themes of playfulness and impatience with convention. Sometimes, the team invited Mary to join them behind the one-way mirror (during a session) to advise them on the therapist's session with the children. Sometimes, 12-year-old Patricia would sit with the team behind the mirror or members of the team would phone from behind the mirror to engage in lengthy, more intimate conversations with one of the children or Mary while the therapist continued his conversation with the other two family members.

Mary's family began to change the team's myths and rules about therapy. The team learned that useful conversations, stimulating changes for the family members and for the team, could occur through more varied forms of therapy than previously had been tried. Simultaneous conversations and shifting membership behind the mirror and in the room freed the team to begin initiating and responding to more varied ideas.

At one session, a series of extremely useful questions about family relationship patterns and beliefs developed through the use of a systemic puppet therapy. Mary's daughter was able to articulate her painful dilemma of realizing that her mother longed for the young child Patricia once was (before the years of

[2]1985–86 Systemic Therapy Training Team supervised by author at the Greater Lawrence Training Institute, Lawrence, Mass.

foster placement). Mary chose to make an opening in her tough guy armor and to reveal through her puppet voice that she was not only overwhelmed by her ongoing battles, but also was acutely lonely. She explained that she behaved like a child much of the time with her children in order to have some kind of peerlike support and companionship.

Another important discovery for the team as part of the observing system was their changing descriptions of Mary and the children. As Mary's family moved out of the shadows of shame and mistrust, the family members became more engaging and complex. When the members of the team were able to exchange a broad spectrum of descriptions and questions, both with each other and with the family, Mary and the children were able to hear themselves described in unexpected ways.

A feminist voice from the team described Mary as a strong, assertive woman, able to be expert in both the domain of her family and the domain of the professional helping network. Another voice of compassion suggested that each family member could choose to separate himself or herself from the causes of shame-bound interactional patterns and could be freed from those patterns through the breaking of family rules about self-hate, self-blame, and toxic secrets. A systemic description offered the family some new ideas about how they interacted in patterns based in family loyalty and mutual concern.

The form of treatment is as important as the issues that are addressed. The use of the reflecting team[3] offers rich opportunities to voice the complexities and ambiguities represented in systems created by the problem of substance abuse.

The reflecting team represents the multiverse of observations and descriptions that may all potentially fit the dilemmas facing those who are implicated in the maintenance or treatment of female substance abuse. While the team offers the family ideas (or asks questions) concerning issues of family history, previous treatments, invasion and control themes, and so on, the therapist is free to pursue a more intensive therapy relationship with the individual client that can be potentially more actively empowering and empathic.

The continuing, reliable presence of the primary therapist is an important part of gaining the substance abuser's trust. Like a naturalist, the therapist must spend time with the client (and with the members of the problem-determined system), simply being there. The therapist spends time in this way not only in observing, but in being observed—something individually oriented therapists may assume as a given, but family therapists often need to learn.

Larger societal issues of gender-based oppression may be raised through the questions and observations of the team, and also in a more in-depth, affectively focused relationship built over time with the primary therapist. Issues of containment and safety, relating both to the client herself and to her children, must, of course, assume primary importance before therapy can take place. The substance abuse must stop. This is most likely to happen in inpatient settings where a strong emphasis of AA or Narcotics Anonymous is an adjunct to the detoxification process. If children are at risk of abuse or neglect, their safety must be assured by social service representatives or other family members.

---

[3]The reflecting team is a new strategy in systemic treatment developed by Norwegian psychiatrist Tom Andersen.

As a more feminist and systemic perspective emerges in the treatment of female substance abusers, the awareness of invasion and control themes may become more visible. This awareness may permit all those involved in helping the client to manage her problem to be more alert to less controlling alternatives for offering safety to both the woman and her children.

CONCLUSION

Women use substance abuse as a powerful form of self-medication. As part of a recursive cycle of invasion and attempted controls, the substance-abusing woman frequently experiences violation of her personal boundaries and searches for relief from pain through intoxication, which, in turn, leads to shame, and finally back to violation and pain. To understand her place in a systemic context, it is crucial to understand the problem-determined system; families do not exist as an entity with one collective set of feelings, behaviors, and thoughts. Rather, the family, like the treatment system, is made up of a number of individuals whose separate (though interconnected) descriptions of self and of the problem compose a cluster of discrete realities, or the meaning system. The description of the female substance abuser may include her own description of pain and shame, as well as descriptions of her by others in the observing system. Her children may offer descriptions entirely different from their mother's. If they are shamebound, they may maintain the constraints of family loyalty, which do not permit them to speak at all about their own shame or their mother's.

Professionals may describe the female substance abuser in a variety of ways, depending on their individual explanations of addiction, their beliefs about the female role in a socioeconomic context, and their own personal histories with regard to both addiction and women.

The descriptions of those involved in the problem, including both family members and members of the treatment system, are reflections of many realities. "The act of observing changes that which is observed" (Anderson, 1986, p. 4). When we see the significant system as including the substance abuser in relation to the substance, as well as the family constellations she is or has been a part of, the helping system, and whoever else is observing the situation, we begin to focus on an evolving meaning system.

Rather than suggesting the paradoxical notion of positively connoting the sacrifice of the woman's health for the good of the whole family, or describing an individual trapped by a medical model-oriented addiction, or a woman oppressed in a patriarchal power system, the second-order cybernetic or feminist therapist should find ways to generate a fluid exchange of descriptions of the situation.

The process by which this building of relationships and coconstruction of a meaning system, including the observing system, will be determined by numerous factors: What are the possibilities for teamwork? Can the team articulate its description of the situation to include the individual experience, as well as all others involved in the problem-determined system? How long is the problem-determined system likely to remain engaged with the same professional membership or the same family membership?

It is possible, even probable, that for genuinely open relationships to be created, change must occur both in the conversational domain of a group (family, professionals, team) and in individual meetings in which the therapist and the woman talk in a more intimate, affectively oriented context. The setting of the larger group may not be the most conducive setting for an individual to expose her experience of pain or shame.

A conversational domain must be created in the client-treatment system in which family loyalties are respected, genuine descriptions of family and individual distress are revealed, distinctions are made between mutually maintained and equally maintained interactions, and new options for change, separation, and growth are imagined.

REFERENCES

Anderson et al. (1986). Problem-determined systems: Towards transformation in family therapy. *Journal of Strategic and Systemic Therapies*, 5, 1–13.

Bepko, C. (1986). Alcoholism as oppression: The dilemma of the women in the alcoholic system. In M. Ault-Riche (Ed.), *Women and family therapy*. Rockville, Md.: Aspen Publications.

Bepko, C., & Krestan, J. (1985). *The responsibility trap: A blueprint for treating the alcoholic family*. New York: Free Press.

Corrigan, E. (1980). *Alcoholic women in treatment*. New York: Oxford University Press.

Donovan, J. (1986). An etiologic model of alcoholism. *American Journal of Psychiatry, 143,* 1–11.

Fossum, M., & Mason, M. (1986). *Facing shame*. New York: W. & W. Norton.

Hoffman, L. (1985). Beyond power and control: Toward a "second order" family systems therapy. *Family Systems Medicine, 3,* 381–396.

Imber-Black, E. (1986). Women, families and larger systems. In M. Ault-Riche (Ed.), *Women and family therapy*. Rockville, Md.: Aspen Publications.

Kaufman, E., & Kaufmann, P. (1981). *Family therapy of drug and alcohol use*. New York: Gardner Press.

MacKinnon, L. & Miller, D. (1987). The new epistemology: Feminist and socio-political considerations. *Journal of Marriage and Family Therapy, 13,* 2.

Miller, D. (1983). Outlaws and invaders: The adaptive function of alcohol in the family-helper supra system." *Journal of Strategic and Systemic Therapies, 2,* 3.

Miller, D. (1988) Family violence and the helping system. In L. Combrinck-Graham (Ed.), *Children in Family Contexts*. New York: Guilford Publications.

Miller, D. (in progress). *Women who hurt Themselves: A systemic view*.

Sandmaier, M. (1980). *The invisible alcoholics*. New York: McGraw Hill.

Part III
Poverty and Family Therapy

10

POVERTY, POLITICS, AND FAMILY THERAPY: A ROLE FOR SYSTEMS THEORY

Jaime Inclan, Ph.D., and Ernesto Ferran Jr., MD

The pervasiveness of poverty and its consequences in a nation as rich as the United States is a critical problem that is now gaining renewed prominence. The failure of liberal programs of the 1960s and early 1970s has been matched by the failure of the conservative approach of the late 1970s and 1980s. The current sociopolitical environment, however, may be one that allows the problem of poverty to be addressed in more effective ways, by permitting the participation of previously discrepant interests. Systems theory can play an important role in the conceptualization of new and meaningful strategies.

In mental health (particularly in family therapy), the interest in understanding psychological problems in their context has opened the door to reconsidering the effects of poverty on the lives of families. This chapter aims to provide an overview of particular issues of poverty, and to suggest a framework for discussion. Social, political, and economic considerations are introduced in order to integrate findings and approaches. Liberal and conservative views on poverty are presented and critiqued from the perspective of systems theory.

Awareness of the problems of poverty at a population level is a must for clinicians in developing respectful attitudes toward their clients and in the formulation of treatment orientations. The authors believe that breaking down the overwhelming problem of poverty into discrete components may help professionals to overcome the sense of awe and impotence that is common in working with poor families. We approach this task having been promoters of the liberal programs of the 1960s and 1970s and observers of the effects of the conservative policies that came afterward.

The discussion is divided as follows: first, we present demographic data bearing on the size and shape of the problem. A sketch of some aspects of the development of poverty over time is provided. Next, the continuum that exists among unemployment, chronic unemployment, and the underclass (those people who live in the margins, with little chance of entering the economic main-stream) is described, as well as some of the original formulations about the culture of poverty concept. We also present treatment considerations and discuss our views on the relevance of systems theory to the understanding of the poverty.

WHO ARE THE POOR?

In 1985, there were 33.1 million poor people living in the United States. They constitute 14 percent of the population. As Table 10-1 indicates, this represents an increase of 8.5 million since 1978 (Gabe, 1986, p. 5).

Table 10-1
Persons in Selected Groups Below the Poverty Level 1959–1985
(in thousands)

Census Year	Total	White	Black	Spanish Origin
1985	33,064	22,860	8,926	5,236
1984	33,700	22,955	9,490	4,806
1983	35,515	24,189	9,888	4,641
1982	34,398	23,517	9,697	4,301
1981	31,822	21,533	9,173	3,713
1980	29,272	19,699	8,579	3,491
1979	26,072	17,214	8,050	2,921
1978	24,497	16,259	7,625	2,607

Although the figures represent an improvement from the 1983 high of 35.5 million, several points deserve mention.

McQueen (1987, p. 10) reports that the Census Bureau "noted that the income gap appears to be widening between Whites and Blacks and between the upper and lower fifths of the range of household income." The number of Hispanic poor continued to rise, and in 1985 numbered 5.2 million. Gabe also notes that in the same year, 12.5 million children were considered poor, a total of 20 percent of all children under the age of 18, and more than half of them were living in female-headed households. In 1980, the total population of the 50 largest U.S. cities was 37.8 million, a decline of 5 percent over ten years. But the overall population for these cities with income below poverty levels rose 11.7 percent to 6.7 million. Economic upturns in some of these cities have not been strong enough to stem either the decline in their number of White residents, or the increase in their number of poor residents (Herbers, 1987).

The recent coexistence of increasing economic strength in large northern cities and a growing core of poverty in their urban centers makes incomplete any single explanation for unacceptably high poverty rates. For example, for the first half of 1987, national unemployment levels, frequently cited as a barometer of the economy's well-being, ranged from 6 to 6.5 percent, the lowest levels since 1979 (Hershey, 1986). Yet these figures are acknowledged to reflect a decline in manufacturing jobs, and with them entry-level positions, while service and high-technology jobs provide the new opportunities. New York City gained 239,000 jobs from 1980 to 1986, an increase of 7 percent. But manufacturing jobs declined 108,000, or 22 percent, to 390,000, and service jobs increased 183,000, or 21 percent, to 1.1 million (Herbers, 1986).

The economic effects of these shifts do contribute to the existing levels of poverty, but responses and explanations have as yet not provided for any comprehensive improvement.

HOW DID WE GET HERE?

In the developmental views on the deterioration of minority communities and the resulting social threat that poverty represents today, attention is focused on the post-World War II period to the early 1970s. Emphasis is placed on (1) migration patterns and consequences, (2) differences between first- and second-generation migrants, and (3) the change in values and culture that obtain for a significant segment of the poor, the underclass. Lemann's (1986) views on these issues have guided this discussion.

The major Black and Puerto Rican migrations to the urban centers of the North followed the economic boom of the post-World War II period. As was true of the depression of the 1930s, the trend of migration ended in the 1970s because of economic crises in the host urban centers.

The experiences of these first Black and Puerto Rican migrants had much in common. Their primary motive for migration was to escape poverty. They withstood the abuses of second-class citizenship in a new environment in exchange for a chance to make a decent living. Displaced by the process of industrialization taking place in their mostly agrarian communities, they were more motivated and better educated than their peers who did not migrate. They traveled along prescribed routes, whether Highway 51 (which gave to Chicago migrants from Alabama, Louisiana, and Mississippi) or the *Marine Tiger* (the name of a popular merchant ship traveling between Puerto Rico and the northeastern United States). They settled in communities already established by other Blacks and Puerto Ricans.

Also typical of the first generation of migrants was the fact that they tended to improve their standards of living initially. They valued the two-parent family, endurance, strength, the work ethic, pride, and discipline. As in their communities of origin, honor and respect for authorities and elders were expected and enforced, through a network of close family and social ties.

Although this was soon to change, the communities in which Blacks and Puerto Ricans arrived and developed were ethnically segregated but moderately integrated by social class. This had positive implications for role models, value incorporation, socialization, schooling, and the like. As teachers remind us, "difficult" children could be handled when they were the minority. Parents and neighbors could more readily deal with problem children when they were the exception.

Beginning in the 1960s, however, a second wave of migration took place. The middle class and emerging middle class moved away from the poor communities and ghettos. By 1970, the ghettos were transformed from having differentiated Black or poor Hispanic social classes to being exclusively poor Black or Hispanic.

In urban ghettos, the demographic phenomenon of the 1960s and 1970s was depopulation. The South Bronx lost 37 percent of its population between 1970 and 1980. Those who could leave did so in search of better schools, safer neighborhoods, and better-paying jobs. What Lemann (1986) called "the victory of disorganization" ensued (p. 36). Communities were "red-lined," and legitimate commerce disappeared. The structural controls provided by family, neighborhood, and religion began to loosen as the more stable and entrenched elements—for example, community leaders and working residents—moved out. These communities also faced handicaps different from those experienced by Eurpopean immigrants earlier in the century. Existing housing stock had, by the 1960s, deteriorated to the point of abandonment, demand for unskilled labor had greatly diminished, and the language and color difficulties experienced were more destructive and powerful than those experienced by Europeans. Many Blacks and Puerto Ricans who left their neighborhoods now live upwardly mobile lives in integrated communities. Those who remain live amid greater relative poverty than previously experienced and in isolated and segregated ghettos.

Diverse explanations for the decomposition of the social fabric of poor communities are being advanced. First, the process is inescapably linked to the general economic crisis that has affected the national economy, and inevitably is harsher in poor communities. Support services, including housing development and rehabilitation, police and fire protection, health and preventive services, and the educational system, head a broad list of ecological supports necessary for community development that were scaled down or dismantled during this period. Second, the changing nature of economic opportunities from manufacturing to service and technological fields made access to means of self-support for many in poor communities more difficult. Third, the drug epidemic intensified the flight away from the ghettos. Fourth, community-based advocacy and political groups, before able to provide leadership for neighborhood empowerment, lost the momentum that provided a sense of hope and direction for youth and other elements within the poor communities.

The final and least discussed explanation for the decomposition of poor communities is the ideology of defense of the ghetto that limited the potentials for incremental positive change that might have occurred. Let us explain. A strategy of defending the ways of the ghetto was developed by activist residents and outside liberal sympathizers during the 1960s. As a response to racist perspectives that viewed minorities living in urban ghettos as inferior, it framed the strategy in a relativism that upheld poor neighborhoods as different and not inferior. These people did not passively accept "deficit findings" such as low-birth-weight new borns and Black English as just unfortunate "givens" in explaining the plight of the poor. Such findings were often feared to be racist value judgments inflicted by a majority culture that did not understand ethnic differences. The fear was that all deficit findings would be clustered together and that any one valid finding would be used to defend the others. Low birth weight is clearly a risk factor for infant mortality that can be caused by suboptimal prenatal care. The causes of suboptimal care are debated to this day. The needed health-care settings are not always readily available, but when they are, explanations for their ineffective utilization are conflicting.

Use of "Black" or nonstandard English has been associated with a speaker who is inferior or incapable of adhering to majority norms. This view can preclude the recognition of potential in many young people, and contributed to controversial decisions on the use of psychological testing in Black children.

The net effect of the aforementioned strategy was to provice meaningful defenses against wholesale racial stereotypes of ghetto residents, but it also prevented an introspective examination of the community's own responsibilities for improvement.

The debate on what went on in the ghettos reached national proportions. Oscar Lewis' (1965) portrayal of slum dwellers in Puerto Rico as living in a "culture of poverty" and Moynihan's (1965) report on the Black family were viewed as racist. The fear was that implicit in these descriptions was the notion that the poor were inherently inferior. The predominant counterargument was perhaps best portrayed by William Ryan (1971) in his book *Blaming the Victim.* which he explains as an attempt by the well-to-do to redefine the problems of the distressed and disinherited as their own fault.

Ryan's observations, although correct in rejecting causation as induced by the victim, is incomplete. It was framed in linear logic, which, when extended to account for causality, resulted in "defeatism clothed in hope" (Lemann, p. 58). Namely, if there is not a self-defeating culture of poverty in the ghettos, and yet the ghettos have problems, the problem must lie in racist White society. Therefore, changes in basic "power relations" would have to take place for the problems of the ghettos to be solved. Defeatism is inevitably engendered, since to have poor Blacks and Hispanics await structural changes in order to better their collective condition was, in effect, a dismissal of them. Given the historical reluctance of this nation readily to undergo such structural changes, the ghetto population is doomed to an existence that cannot improve in the near future.

Ryan's blame-the-victim argument is linear and not systemic. First, not recognizing differentiated subgroups among the poor led to sweeping generalizations, which, in turn, contributed to a polarization of the arguments: either poor minority people are inferior or society is racist. Second, the need to combat racist views was more urgent at the time. It resulted in less attention being paid to the indentification and resolution of specific problems such as the drug epidemic. Third, liberal and activist ethnic and cultural defense strategies, framed in linear thinking, were not able to accept the fact that if poor minorities are oppressed, it follows that they will have more problems. If not, why is it necessary to change the system? Fourth, the argument ignores the systemic principle of homeostasis, which posit that, in closed systems, a set of behaviors, regardless of the etiology, will tend to perpetuate themselves. Fifth, the argument did not take into account the sociological changes in progress, namely the exit of an emerging middle class from the ghetto communities. These five factors eroded the possibility of the community existing as an open system capable of transformation through input of differences.

Linear thinking did not allow for the possibility of two realities: (1) that structural problems exist and (2) that microsystemic problems at family and community levels also exist. Black and Puerto Rican cultures are different from mainstream American norms. The culture of nonintegrated, poor ghettos is radically different. The values, hopes, and energies of the first generation of migrants have been seriously weakened in the second generation. The educational system, language, economy, and social and human values that prevail in class-segregated communities do not prepare those who live in these communities to interact in the mainstream society. This is the reality of the social system that many poor Blacks and second-generation Puerto Ricans grow up and live in.

The institutions in all poor Puerto Rican and Black neighborhoods do not, and perhaps cannot, by themselves, promote the integration of second-generation migrants into the mainstream. Their goals have subtly but dramatically changed from transformation to containment of the problem. The schools do not worry about learning achievement, but instead are concerned about whether there will be enough students to avoid layoffs and keep the schools open. The police do not worry about local drug consumption. Their interest lies in preventing the person driving the car with out-of-state license plates from coming into the ghetto to buy drugs. The housing authorities do not screen for social class and ethnic integration but for social class and ethnic segregation. The health and mental health clinics worry not about solving problems and promoting health, but about how to avoid a potential lawsuit or media scandal, or how to keep the statistics high so that the funding stream does not dry up.

But the strategy of containment, built on top of higher unemployment rates and reduced entitlement benefits, is not working. There are a growing number of poor people who are unemployed or chronically unemployed, and an increasing underclass in poor minority communities. Negative leadership, fostered by the parallel economy of drugs and crime, has provided poor and inappropriate role models for many young people. The subculture of poverty has become the dominant culture in many pockets within minority comminities.

RELATIONSHIP TO THE MAINSTREAM WORK WORLD

To avoid the errors of the past, we must understand particular circumstances and subgroups within the poor. There is much confusion (and varying terminology) in current attempts to define and understand poor people. One useful way to break down the number of poor people is by considering their relationship to mainstream work life. Three terms are used here to help clarify the diversity of the people in question: unemployed, chronically unemployed, and underclass. Although further refinement of these categories into subsets, such as working poor or underemployed, is possible, we see this basic categorization as useful for clinical purposes.

The underlying premise for choosing this method of classification is that the relationship of individual(s) to the work world is an essential determinant of organization, both psychological and structural. Specifically, the way one views society, the view of society passed on to children, and the manner in which families are organized (affectively, cognitively, and structurally) are directly affected by the relationship of family members to the work world.

We will consider the unemployed as consisting of those people who, although currently out of work, have a work history of having been employed for at least five of the past seven years. The chronically unemployed are those persons who have been unemployed for at least five of the past seven years and who have ceased to look for employment but may still continue to value work as a measure of self-esteem and survival. The underclass is that group of individuals who have been unemployed for at least five of the past seven years and who exhibit a value system that makes their effective reincorporation into the world of work unlikely.

One employment status category can turn into another—unemployed to chronically unemployed to underclass. Unemployment can be an acute condition that lasts a short time or it can become a chronic condition. The progression is not purely a quantitative one. In addition to length of stay in the unemployed condition, the person must cease to look for employment in order to be con-didered chronically unemployed. (Economists use the term "labor force partic-ipation rate" to describe those who are employed or looking for employment.) Clinical data suggest that a psychological transformation occurs at some point during this passage. In systemic terms, the family, initially in crisis because of the unemployment of a spouse, reorganizes itself into a new homeostatic balance and structure—that of a family with a spouse (or spouses) who do not expect to work.

When a passage from chronically unemployed to underclass takes place, it is a qualitative change, a move that can be defined as internalization of the "culture of poverty" mentality. Structural changes leading to chronic unem-ployment usually precede consciousness or value transformation. Conversely, the development and incorporation of the values of the culture of poverty charc-terize the underclass. The underclass and the culture of poverty concept will be discussed later.

What has been presented thus far should not be construed to imply a negation of microsystemic personal and subjective influences in favor of macrosystemic structural and economic forces affecting poverty. On the contrary, changes and progressions outlined here take place in interaction with, and mediated through, the personal, idiosyncratic resources of individuals and families. The model suggested by Allen and Britt (1983) to understand psychological disorder is here adjusted to permit an understanding of poverty and its consequences (see Figure 10-1).

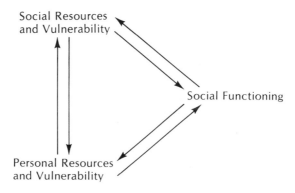

Figure 10-1

The model suggests dynamic interaction between social factors such as employment status and personal factors such as family organization and social functioning (defined as the ability to perform and derive satisfaction in the mainstream society). It is the relative weight of these factors that can provide a dynamic understanding of the process and focus of intervention.

The Unemployed

The 80 percent of the unemployed population looking for work at a given moment make up the unemployed. At a population level, economists are concerned about the decreasing rates of participation (those working or looking for work). Lemann (1986a) describes the labor-force participation for Black teenage boys as falling from 60 percent in 1940 to 36 percent in 1970, a drop he calls "too great to be accounted for by just unemployment or by the increasing proportion of Black teenagers in school." Even more extreme indications of difficulty are provided by figures coming from Puerto Rico, where unemployment has been calculated at 20 percent during the past five years, and where the labor-force participation rate for the whole work-age population is 42 percent (Delgado, 1986).

As cited in Auletta (1982), Homer Kincaid, director of West Virginia's supported work project, presented his view on the plight of a group of the unemployed:

> These people are victims of society. Let me give you an illustration. Technology hit the coal mines. Before that, you had families that saw no reason to get an education. They just went into the coal mines. Yet what happened in the fifties? These people were put out of work. No training programs, no jobs. They lost their self-image. They went on welfare. Pretty soon the father was an alcoholic because government didn't do something about it. If we had had training programs we would have *done something before their spirit was broken*.

The Chronically Unemployed

It is estimated that about 5 percent of the unemployed are chronically unemployed (Duncan, 1984), a group that has received much attention in the national and local debates on welfare policy. Conservatives insist that the growth of social welfare programs, combined with other factors such as decline in discipline in the schools and the family, are responsible for the chronically unemployed person's decline in willingness to take responsibility for himself or herself through such means as work. The liberals view this population group as victims of society and its institutions, which have failed to provide the necessary employment and educational opportunities. This debate has been carried out within a linear framework that encourages blame and polarization.

There is a diagnostic distinction to be made between the chronically unemployed and the underclass. Although the chronically unemployed share with the underclass a lack of participation in the mainstream work world, they typically do not exhibit the culture-of-poverty syndrome. The chronically unemployed tends not to reject the values of mainstream society, and many of these mothers and fathers do come to clinics for help. They believe their children should be in school, and that street life and drugs constitute intolerable dangers. They often have religious convictions, even if they do not practice them; they believe that children ought to show respect and be disciplined, that academic achievement is the road to success, that two-parent families should be preserved, and so on. Parents who are chronically unemployed, however, tend to view themselves as victimized, unable to implement their beliefs, incapable of being full participants in the mainstream social process. The underclass has generally given up on mainstream society and takes part instead in its own culture, economy, sets of values, and so on. More typically, they will express such sentiments as, "What good is school anyway?" "You've got to get over," and "Look out for yourself."

Two specific subgroups within the chronically unemployed tend to utilize the mental health system: the passive poor and the traumatized, a growing group in the past decade (Auletta, 1982, p. 44). The passive poor make up the largest group of patients from poor communities who seek services in public clinics. Usually, they are long-term welfare recipients, with multiple agency involvements over many years, often with very intensive use of medical services. They are the ones with the thick charts.

Those who work with the passive poor have learned that ecological models and treatment approaches that include the family, extended family, providers from other agencies, friends, and acquaintances are usually necessary for effective intervention. Therapy with the passive poor needs to address two critical issues: resolving the passive-dependent attitude toward the world and creating a realignment in the ecological network that supports the passive-dependent attitude. Group therapies, self-help groups, and community advocacy groups have been successfully employed to change attitudes of dependency. Similarly, cognitive therapies, specifically learned-helplessness theory, show promise in this area. Aponte (1985), Imber-Black (1986), and others have described ecological and larger-systems treatment models that are effective in focusing efforts of support networks on directions that promote competency.

Auletta (1982) described the traumatized as the "drunks, drifters, homeless shopping bag ladies and released mental patients who frequently roam or collapse on city streets" (p. 44). In the past decade, this group has received more attention as a result of the middle-class social protest against the conditions of the homeless and ex-mental patients. Unlike the passive poor, the traumatized tend to violate unspoken, unseen boundaries of turf, decor, and the like, which brings them to the attention of those outside of their ghetto communities. Much of the national attention paid to all groups of the poor has been inspired by this interaction.

The Underclass

Estimates differ concerning the number of people who are more than periodically or chronically unemployed. Conservative Edward Bansfield (1968) agrees with the anthropologist Oscar Lewis, "rough guessing" that about 80 percent of the poor in the United States suffer only from poverty defined as having insufficient income as a result of temporary unemployment. They suggest that the passage of time, and the greater availability of job opportunities, would resolve the problems of this group. In their estimate, this would leave 20 percent of the population with more severe difficulties resulting from their poverty status.

Duncan (1984) estimates a lower percentage of persons in chronic poverty conditions—5 percent of those unemployed having been so for five of the past seven years. A subgroup of the 5 percent chronically unemployed has also developed values consistent with Lewis' description of the culture of poverty. They constitute the underclass.

The underclass has also been called the long-term poor, the dependent poor, the lumpenproletariat, the acute poor, the chronically poor, the disenfranchised, and the disadvantaged, among others. As these labels suggest, this group has been described and treated with derision by most observers. DeTocqueville described how "the lower ranks which inhabit these cities constitute a rabble" and Marx refered to them as "the social scum, that passively rotting mass thrown off the the layers of old society" (Auletta, 1982, p. 26). Moynihan borrowing from Kenneth Clark called them a "tangle of pathology" (Lemann, 1986b, p. 58).

What distinguishes this subgroup of the 5 percent chronically poor population is not its members' status of poverty, but their world view, values, attitudes, and behaviors that are a consequence of their prolonged stay in this disadvantaged state. It is this underclass status, Lewis' culture of poverty, that distinguishes the underclass from the chronically unemployed. There is an interaction of social and personal resource vulnerabilities that promotes the development of an underclass. However, in line with their political ideology, liberals put the weight of responsibility and blame on such structural factors as unemployment and racism, whereas conservatives blame family and individuals for the social failure of the subgroup.

The underclass does not use the array of mental health services that are available to the general population. They live by the norms of their subculture, its values and institutions. They have, to a great extent, given up on, and been given up by, the family and the social institutions that embody the mainstream culture. Systemically, their subculture is organized along closed-system principles that make access and intervention more difficult.

Auletta further distinguishes between two subgroups within the underclass:—the hustlers and the hostile. The hustlers are those individuals who earn their livelihood in an underground economy but who do not typically commit violent crimes. The hostile are those who live a life of crime. They are frequently connected to the drug world as users and traffickers. Since they do not use mental health services, these two groups are best known by the police and find themselves more frequently in jails and prisons. Their being poor is not necessarily defended by their lack of money. They are not necessarily dependent on the system or on public assistance. Their street activities are understood by them as work, and indeed they spend long hours at them. They wish for, and often have, many of the material commodities accorded to the middle class of mainstream society. These are obtained, however, through the means available to the subculture of poverty.

Members of the underclass tend to be cut off from their own families, who give them up as lost to another world. They tend not to form stable marital relationships. Instead, relationships usually are temporary and do not include a commitment to spouse or children. As a result, the underclass are fathers or, more typically, mothers in single-parent families.

The underclass culture stands against mainstream society as a competing pathway to success in poor ghetto communities. Drugs, in particular, have produced an alternative economy that provides high wages and a source of self-esteem to people in ghetto communities who have not gained either in mainstream society.

THE CULTURE OF POVERTY

The culture-of-poverty concept, controversial when first introduced by Oscar Lewis (1965), has been globally invoked to mean so many different things. Yet it remains crucial to understanding the underclass phenomenon. Some of its salient features, as presented by Lewis, are described in the following.

Lewis estimates that 10 to 20 percent of the poor experience the culture of poverty as a self-perpetuating or difficult-to-escape condition. Social and personal resource vulnerabilities place at risk unemployed, poor, single- or teenage-parent, Black, and Hispanic families.

The description of the psychological state, and behaviors observed at the level of the individual, includes a primary orientation to the present time mode; a failure to postpone gratification and a tendency to action and impulsivity; a sense of human nature as fixed and, therefore, of one's fate being both predetermined and unchangeable; a resentment of authority and a sense of being blamed and victimized; a sense of aloneness and inability to trust others or form lasting attachments; an inadequate sense of rigor, discipline, or perseverance; a tendency to dependency rather than self-reliance; and a disinclination to adhere to salaried jobs.

Other features include a lack of participation and contribution to the major institutions of the larger society (school boards, local governing units, etc.), poor housing conditions and crowding leading to a minimum of organizations beyond that of the nuclear or extended family, familial disorganizers such as the absence of childhood as a distinct protected stage, early introduction to sex, lack of privacy, low self-esteem, helplessness, and anomie.

Lewis also proposes a macrosystemic understanding of the culture of poverty. Societies that expose a set of values for the dominant class that stress the accumulation of wealth and property and explain low economic status as the sole responsibility of the individual tend to foster a culture of poverty. Those who live in the lower strata of a changing society and feel alienation from it are the most prone to developing this condition.

The culture can be broken, if not poverty itself, by creating basic structural changes in society—by redistributing wealth, organizing the poor, and providing a sense of belonging and leadership. People who begin to see themselves as attempting to work within mainstream society also represent change and escape from this cultural stranglehold.

It appears, then, that Lewis' original observations on the culture of poverty are accurate portrayals of a reality lived by many today. His ecological understanding of the phenomenon is particularly relevant to systems theory.

TREATMENT CONSIDERATIONS

The need for better integration of the treatment of the poor has been described as ecologically oriented therapy. Others may prefer the term "holistic." These are two essential features of ecologically oriented therapy: the understanding of families within their cultural, historical, and class background, and the orientation of the treatment of families to the matrix of their social-ecology, where the dynamics of the individual, the family, and society meet (Aponte, 1985).

The concern of economists about levels of labor participation should be shared by therapists working with the poor. Specifically, it is suggested that a social diagnosis include, along with evaluations of support networks, drug abuse, and criminal histories, the following.

1. Quantitative criteria—work history: a. How long has the person been employed during the past ten-year period? b. What is the family of origin's work history?
2. Qualitative criteria (differentiating subgroups: a. Unemployed and looking for work. b. Unemployed and not looking for work.

Assisted by this information, therapists can proceed to a clinical evaluation of the personal resources and vulnerabilities of their patients and families in view of their social functioning status.

The treatment that follows from the evaluation is guided, in general terms, by defense and offense strategies. The defense strategy can be viewed as preventing the unemployed condition from becoming a chronically unemployed condition. The offense strategy is the step-wise reincorporation of the individual into the work world.

Therapy that aims to prevent an unemployed condition from turning into a more severe one is often supportive and educational. The educational component often consists of relabeling the interpersonal and family conflicts and tensions that may be exacerbated at this time as derivative from and precipitated by a change in employment status. A reframing of difficulties experienced at this time as transitional and caused by outside forces can enable families to make accessible personal resources that are necessary at this time of crisis.

It is also important to be supportive to the individual and the family that experienced the job loss. Support can be provided concerning issues of self-esteem, and the feelings of anger and depression that are frequently present. This is especially true for the many people who lose their jobs as a result of the economy over which they have no control but which force them to seek new employment, often at a lower salary. People work long and hard hours to try to fulfill their dreams. When these are shattered, therapists must be available at a human level as they also entertain systemic interventions for the promotion of change.

Unemployed patients who have strong work histories and personal resources can be helped through advocacy efforts on the part of their therapists. It may include referrals to retraining and educational programs that can further prepare them to perform in today's technological and service-oriented work world.

The treatment of patients with strong work histories but more limited personal and family resources requires different advocacy efforts. Industrial, manual, and mechanical jobs constitute the choice job-placement settings for this group of the unemployed. Implicit in the above are linkages between mental health agencies and training and employment agencies, currently an underdeveloped partnership. Therapists must better appreciate and utilize the available case-management strategies or advocate for such strategies.

Clinical determinations to be made in the treatment of the unemployed include: (1) an assessment of their general view of the world, value orientation, and orientation to work, and (2) an assessment as to whether the personal and family difficulties that are being experienced are temporary adjustment disorders basically ascribable to the person's change in employment status. Prompt interventions for such people can enhance their effectiveness. Interventions should take place before the new structural condition, unemployment, erodes the sense of self and/or results in a reorganization of family and ecology into chronic unemployment status. Once the dynamics of self and system consolidate into qualitatively different structures, with concomitant sets of values and mutually reinforcing feedback mechanisms, it becomes necessary to intervene in more comprehensive ways.

Currently, there is great interest in developing effective intervention strategies for the chronically unemployed when mentally ill. Mobile crisis teams (Cohen, in press) reach out to these individuals as they tend not to come to clinics. Treatment for this group has emphasized also casework and case finding, but obtaining reliable personal and treatment histories is difficult. Mobile crisis teams are beginning to identify the population, quantify it, and establish trust relationships that may lead to treatment. Workers in this field are defining—legally and clinically—the treatment options available given the complex civil rights issues involved. Mobile crisis teams typically network with existing services in the community for the provision of care for the traumatized. Although the focus at this time is on containment of the problem, the future task in this area is one of developing and implementing treatment models. Family and systems therapists could play a creative role in developing approaches not meant to negate the roles that can be played by individual and group therapists, and the intergenerational perspective afforded the family therapist provides for unique observations.

The culture-of-poverty mentality has made traditional mental health programs unavailable to the underclass. Their needs seem so far to have been best met by groups able to provide a different outlook vis-à-vis problems in their lives. Religious groups such as the Muslims in the Black community and Jehovah's Witnesses in the Hispanic community have been observed to intervene effectively in the lives of the underclass. Social action and political groups have similarly been able to effect changes in the underclass group. In our recent past, we observed how the Black Panther party and the Young Lords were able to recruit members of the underclass (among others) to their ranks and, through involvement in their organizations, transform the culture-of-poverty mentality of Black and Hispanic youth from social alienation to social participation.

Participation in organized groups, religious or political, can afford an opportunity for "a new life" for members of the underclass. First, these groups provide a philosophy of life, a way of understanding the world and acting upon it, that confronts the narrow vision of the culture of poverty. The commitment required is full-time, and the changes required total. Second, and more important, the groups themselves provide a new interpersonal context capable of bringing meaning to their lives. Feedback is always available, hope is entertained at all times. Failure to adhere to an agreement is readily followed up on, short-term and long-term plans are demanded, and so forth.

Two direct implications for treatment are derived from the above. First, mental health centers and providers working in poor communities mght support, help develop, and coordinate care with social, religious, and grass-roots political groups in the community. It would seem an important partnership that could facilitate meeting the needs of a significant and growing underclass. Second, a rethinking of and a commitment to addressing the mental health needs of prison inmates, overrepresented by Black and Hispanic members of the underclass, need to become a national and local priority. Access could be facilitated for providers who have an interest in and the ability to intervene with this segment of the underclass. Systems-oriented therapists need critically to review their historical failure to work with and write about this group.

THE ROLE OF SYSTEMS THEORY

Conservative and liberals have tended to operate with a linear model. Ryan (1971) typifies the liberal argument that society (social resource vulnerability) is responsible for individual behavior and, therefore, for the development of the underclass and the psychological disorders that ensue from being a part of it. Bansfield, (1968) and Sowell (1981) present the conservative argument that individual factors (personal resource vulnerability) are responsible for poverty and the underclass.

An integrative model, as proposed in Figure 10-1, allows us to understand the phenomenon better and to avoid the polemics that have governed this field of study. Most important, it allows for the design of strategies that are specific to defined groups, and that can include different segments of society in the resolution of the problem.

The proposed integrative model is systemic. Concepts of systems theory that are useful in this integration are hierarchical organization, isomorphism, and self-responsibility versus blame.

Hierarchical Organization

Systems theory views the world as organized at levels that range from the microsystemic (the individual) to the macrosystemic (society and its values). Systems thinking further suggests that to describe a phenomenon properly, one must be cognizant of the hierarchical level of organization that constitutes its context. In other words, a progression from individual rules to societal rules and mores presents different levels of organization. The validity or "truthfulness" of observations is thus contingent on and limited to its context, that is, its hierarchical level. Thus, to state that when society and its institutions fail to offer meaningful social programs demonstrates social resource vulnerability. That it then fails poverty-level families is an observation at a macrosystemic level. Its truthfulness or validity must be ascertained by observation and the study of macrosystemic processes.

The position that personal resource vulnerabilities—family structure disorganization and limited values orientation—of poverty-level families impede or limit the ability to function in mainstream society is a proposition at the microsystemic level. Its validity is to be determined by observation of microsystemic processes.

A common error, according to systems theory, derives from the comparison of data out of context. This error can be grave when the contexts that are ignored concern differing hierarchical levels. One cannot directly challenge the proposition that society must change for poverty to diminish with the proposition that individuals and families must change for poverty to diminish. One view does not negate the other.

Instead, systems theory proposes that there are different "truths" that can aptly describe a given phenomenon. This follows from the proposition that there are different levels of hierarchical organization. Thus, the proposition that social resources vulnerability is a determinant of poverty and poverty's consequences is as accurate a statement as the one that personal resource vulnerability is a determinant of poverty. Individual determinants and vulnerabilities are not ignored in a therapeutic context in defense of a view that blames society, and conversely.

Isomorphism

If there are different contextual realities, are there connections between these? Are there inferior and superior levels of organization? Where does the causal question become relevant?

Prior to systems thinking, observations across levels of organization were guided by the linear quest of causality. In terms of the poverty debate, the question has been: Is societal neglect causative of poverty and its manifestations or is family disorganization the cause of the failure to participate in the mainstream society? This debate reached a heightened intensity in the 1960s with Glazer and Moynihan's report (1963) that defined the political terms of the debate: What do poverty families need, jobs or family reorganization? Liberals have tended to argue for jobs through governmental initiatives. The conservatives' emphasis has been on letting poor families rely on their own initiatives, so they may reorganize themselves to participate in the productive activity of mainstream society.

Isomorphism is a systems concept that makes possible descriptive comparisons across levels of organization. It refers to the degree of congruence between phenomena at two different levels of organization. It avoids the tendency toward causality inherent in linear thinking and favors relationship description. Isomorphic descriptions can have content and process dimensions. One advantage of a comparison made on the basis of isomorphic relationships is that it readily suggests the possibility and need to attack the problem at different levels while avoiding the polemic of which level is more important or causative. Isomorphic descriptions comprehend the dialectical relationship of phenomena at various hierarchical levels. At the level of intervention, isomorphism implies the need for differentiated responsibilities and actions. As such, it makes possible the integration of apparently dissimilar approaches—and thus its relevance as a framework for understanding a problem so complex and insidious as poverty.

It is possible to think of isomorphic relationships between, for example, the organizations of government, public service agencies, and families. We can describe a system of governmental agencies that exist without a clear philosophy or mandate (absence of a national or local family policy) operating a wide variety of public services, which, in an uncoordinated fashion, are trying to meet the needs of poor families, who are themselves disorganized as to structure and purpose. Similarly, it is possible to focus on the multiple levels of the problems faced by many young Black and Hispanic males. They tend not to be adequately engaged and treated in mental health centers, not to participate significantly in the mainstream economy, and not to be addressed in national welfare policy (most states limit public assistance to single-parent families). These examples suggest responsibilities for a very large number of people—clinicians, administrators, policy makers, and the like—who interface in the delivery of care to the poor.

Self-Responsibility versus Blame

An analysis based on linear reasoning tends to lead to cause-and-effect relationships, which, in turn, tend to result in blame allocation. Who or what is to blame is decided in relation to one's view of cause and effect. Liberals blame the system for causing poverty, as they view structural unemployment and racism as the cause of family disorganization. Conservatives', however, are quick to point out that in the 1960s, when unemployment decreased, crimes and welfare still expanded. Conservatives, therefore, argue that the family, with its culture and organization, is to blame for poverty and its consequences. This position, when held nonsystemically, is considered offensive, in that it implies that the poor are inferior. As stated previously, Ryan (1971) called this point of view "blaming the victim," which suggests that the system is to blame. And so on and so forth—this debate can go on ad infinitum. Linear thinking on the question of poverty has stymied the development of an approach to the problem that is integrative conceptually and operationally. Systems thinking can help to deliver us from the drive to allocate blame and support instead of the need to assume responsibility.

Without the notion of responsibility, systems thereby would be incomplete and inadequate. The idea of hierarchical levels suggests multiple realities and, therefore, multiple responsibilities. Within this framework, we can simultaneously stress that the system is 100 percent responsible for the problem of poverty and its consequences and that the family is 100 percent responsible for the problem. Each will have to do something different if there is to be an overall change. Each will have to mobilize resources within its level of organization to achieve this change. And the responsibility of both, each at its contextual level, is to operate to achieve change within its field of operations.

Internalization of the dialectical nature of the realities involved, and of the need to assume responsibility relative to these realities, could provide a more effective focus for the energies of the many people, within and outside of the mental health fields, who are concerned with alleviating the problems of poverty. For example, cognizant that families and their community organizations must change, agency bureaucrats and politicians can best serve the poor by operating on the premise that they, society and its organization, must change and are the source of the problem. And cognizant that society and its institutions must change, community organizers and therapists can best serve their poor families by operating on the premise that poor families must change and are, as currently organized, the source of the problem. Providers can cross levels by helping to mobilize families to change society.

An important assumption in the integrative approach suggested is that it is in the interests of all involved to solve the problem of poverty. The Roman Catholic Church of the United States shares this assumption and expands upon it. In the Bishops' pastoral letter on the economy (cited in Excerpts, 1986), they understand the problem of poverty as a "social and moral scandal" and its resolution as a moral question. "The fundamental moral criterion for all economic decisions, policies and institutions is this: they must be at the service of all people, especially the poor" (p/ A14). The Bishops' letter further states: "Decisions must be judged in light of what they do for the poor, what they do to the poor, and what they enable the poor to do for themselves." The Bishops make broad recommendations on the responsibility of government for the welfare of the poor. They range from policies to promote full employment to policies that focus on the individual. The cornerstone concern of the Bishops' letter is the system of distribution of wealth in the United States and its prejudice against the poor.

THE ECONOMICS OF POVERTY

The increasing economic gap between the poor and the rich in the United States threatens the middle class and portends further social discontent (Koepp, 1986). The growth of more "haves" and "have nots" has resulted in a thinning out of the middle class.

An exhaustive review of research on economics and psychosocial dysfunction (Seidman & Rapkin, 1983) singles out the perniciousness of relative poverty, that is, the experience of poverty relative to one's reference group. By implication it suggests that the growth of riches can be stressful to all and lead to greater psychosocial dysfunction among the poor.

In a study commissioned by the Federal Reserve Board in 1983 (cited in Carter, 1986), it was found that the wealthiest 10 percent of U.S. families—7.5 million households—own 84 percent of the nation's assets. An even more staggering statistic is that the richest 1 percent—840,000 households—own half of the country's wealth.

The heyday of the middle class is clearly over. The U.S. family income, adjusted to today's price levels, leaped from $14,832 in 1950 to $27,338 in 1970. For 1985, however, it was $27,735, barely an improvement for the past 15-year period (Koepp, p. 55). The middle class is not improving its economic position. Instead, the rich are getting richer and the poor are getting poorer. Clinical and research data suggest that greater relative poverty is likely to result in greater psychosocial dysfunction. What can be done? Is it or is it not in the interest of all to obtain a fairer redistribution of wealth?

Although most economists and political observers see the problem of poverty as an aberration of the system and solvable through the system, radical critics of capitalism understand the problems of poverty to be the natural consequences of growth and development within a capitalist system. Marxists claim that economic growth in a capitalist system will inevitably bring with it greater unemployment. The argument is that the growth of social wealth in bourgeois society inevitably leads to increased social inequality or the expanded bifurcation of society (Marx, 1958).

In the United States, however, there is a renewed interest in finding solutions to the growing problem of poverty. There is talk about potential new political coalitions emerging that can reach further than the previous stalemated liberal and conservative camps. Professional mental health organizations are putting issues of poverty back on their agendas. It appears that an opening exists for systems-oriented therapists to play a role in the search for new conceptualizations and in the implementation of innovative programs that address the gamut of needs of poverty-level families.

CONCLUSION

A comprehensive understanding of poverty and its consequences requires its contextualization. Insights from a broad range of disciplines can help to broaden this understanding. New conceptual schemes, political alliances, and program initiatives are needed to reverse the alarming and growing trend toward an increasingly bifurcated society. History warns us about the social dangers that a bifurcated society represent. The words of Sen. Patrick Moynihan (D. N.Y) afford optimism: "We may just have one of those rare alignments that bring about genuine social change" (cited in Morganthau, 1987, p. 24). To act responsibly at this juncture requires boldness and the courage to break with old intellectual schemes and political allegiances. There is a growing awareness, at all levels of society, of the need for broader participation in antipoverty campaigns. The U.S. Catholic Bishops' positions should be emulated. Twenty national organizations, including the American Public Health Association, have taken the position, endorsed by 70 others, that "the fact that one out of every seven Americans lives below the official poverty threshold is unacceptable, especially when 40% of these persons are children" (Groups, 1986). Governor Michael Dukakis of Massachusetts thinks that the employment program "should be part of a national deficit-reduction strategy" (Morganthau et al., 1987, p. 25).

Also hopeful is that although there is a wider participation and broader focus on poverty concerns, there is also a growing sophistication in understanding the complexity of the problem. All the "poor" are not lumped into one group. There is instead greater emphasis in delineating subgroups within the poor that can be assisted through specific initiatives. Adequate progrm planning and implementation can, in turn, avoid demoralization and burnout in the staff providing the services. Specifically, one needs to be aware of the differences within the poor and of differing etiologies of poverty, in particular, of nonlinear relationships that derive from the transformation of phenomena into qualitatively different ones.

The interface of poverty with education, child care, health, housing, and, of course, training and employment, is now being emphasized. This should be very appealing to systems thinkers. Furthermore, there is an emerging sophistication about the psychological issues of poverty and of its extremes—the culture of poverty. The Massachusetts Commissioner of Public Welfare, Charles Atkins, puts it in this way: "It takes time and money to get at the people who have been stuck on welfare for years. You have to break through their psychology of despair. They need intensive hand holding" (Morganthau et al., 1987, p. 25). Although systems-oriented therapists may have contributions to make that go beyond hand holding, they may have plenty to learn about humanism being at the core of mental health delivery.

Systems thinkers could add sophistication to the debate on poverty by underscoring processes where quantitative and descriptive data have prevailed, most notably by being able to distinguish between subsets of the unemployed.

The process by which a phenomenon (such as unemployment status) leads to a qualitative change in how a person interacts with his or her world has generally been neglected in studies of unemployment and poverty. Consequently, the implications for policy and therapy with regard to transformations within the employment status continuum have been misunderstood. A change in status that does not imply qualitative change—such as from employed to unemployed—can be reversed linearly, that is, by providing employment to the unemployed. However, the provision of employment to the chronically unemployed and the underclass will not so readily obtain the same positive results. For one extreme group, poor families of the underclass, interventions that address the culture of poverty mentality and its supportive ecology need to be considered.

Family therapists have a significant role to play, but where are they and their professional organizations and journals, in this current debate on poverty and its consequences? Where and with whom do systems-oriented therapists work? The trend to have one task force or one plenary session on the poverty issue every so often may need revision. The pathway of frustrations in attempts at dealing with bureaucratic and public systems often leads to a retreat into private practice; this needs to be challenged. For example, a leading family therapist travels the lecture circuit accumulating sympathy for himself and inadvertently justifying others' lack of involvement in the public system by telling stories of how the doors of public institutions in New York stayed closed even when he uttered the open sesame, "I'm available." Constructive criticisms by therapists on the question of poverty can achieve the reaffirmation that the field had a concern with the issue at its foundation. Joining in the evolving national priority and debate on poverty may provide systems-oriented therapists the opportunity to contribute to the development of socially relevant programs and therapies.

Programs that assist the poor need to be better contextualized. At the program level, cooperative agreements, agency consortia, and integration of services to offer multiservices are called for. In particular, mental health centers need to develop a more integral partnership with training, retraining, and employment centers. To achieve this, we must consider how individual's and family's relationships with the work world influence all its processes in a direct and vital way. We must have the integrity to uphold this relationship and advocate for programs that address it. Our personal experience and our research support it. We must be prepared to debate and defend this position, not shy away from it for fear of red baiting.

The need to integrate political efforts, programs, and treatment orientations when working with the poor requires a review of 1960s and 1970s sociopolitical concepts that had been used to define and categorize poverty populations. The analysis presented here, in revising controversial subjects such as the culture of poverty and the underclass, is an attempt to remind us that the drive to understand and treat "the system" has, to a great extent, replaced the need to care for poor people. Systems theory and ecologically oriented treatment modalities present an opportunity to correct this "deviation" and provide a better framework for effective interventions.

REFERENCES

Allen, L., & Britt, D. W. (1983). Social class, mental health and mental illness: The impact of resources and feedback. In R.D. Felner, L.A. Jason, J.N. Moritsugu, & S.S. Farber (Eds.) *Preventive psychology: Theory, research and practice* (pp. 149–161). New York: Pergamon Press.

Aponte, H. J. (1985). The negotiation of values in therapy. *Family Process, 24*(3), 323–338.

Auletta, K. (1982). *The underclass.* New York: Vintage Books.

Bansfield, E. C. (1968). *The unheavenly city: The nature and future of our urban crisis.* Boston: Little, Brown.

Carter, A. L. (1986, Sept. 23). How about a capital accumulation tax? *The New York Times,* A35.

Cohen, N., & Sullivan, A. (in press). Developing mobile crisis intervention services for the chronic mentally ill in New York City. In N. Cohen (Ed.), *Psychiatry takes to the streets*. New York: Guilford Press.

Delgado, A. (1986, Aug. 30). Todos consumen y pocos producen [All consume and few produce]. *Claridad*, 25.

Duncan, G. L. (1984). *Years of poverty, years of plenty*. Ann Arbor, Mich. Institute for Social Research, University of Michigan.

Excerpts from final draft of Bishops' letter on the economy (1986, Nov. 14). *The New York Times*, A14.

Gabe, T. (1986, Sept. 15). *Progress against poverty (1959 to 1985 and the poverty debate* (Order Code No. 1B84013). Washington, DC: Congressional Research Service.

Glazer, N., & Moynihan, D. (1963). *Beyond the melting pot*. Cambridge, Mass.: MIT Press.

Groups urge U.S. to end poverty (1986, Dec. 23). *The New York Times*, B5.

Herbers, J. (1986, Oct. 22). Mismatch in jobs and skills is found in survery of cities. *The New York Times*, A24.

Herbers, J. (1987, Jan. 26). Black poverty spreads in 50 biggest U.S. cities. *The New York Times*, A27.

Hersey, R. D., Jr. (1987, July 3). Jobless rate at lowest point since '79. *The New York Times*, A14.

Imber-Black, E. (1986). Systems consultation. In L. Wynne (Ed.), *The systemic consultant and human service providers* (pp. 357–374). New York: Guilford Press.

Koepp, S. (1986, Nov. 3). Is the middle class shrinking? *Time*, 54–56.

Lemann, N. (1986, June). The origins of the underclass (pt.1). *The Atlantic Monthly*, 31–55.

Lemann, N. (1986, July). The origins of the under class (pt.2). *The Atlantic Monthly*, 54–68.

Lewis, O. (1965). *La Vida*. New York: Random House.

Marx, K. E. (1958). *Capital Vol. 1*. Moscow: Forezulg Publishing.

McQueen, M. (1987, July 31). Poverty rate falls to 13.6%: Decline is third straight. *The Wall Street Journal*, 10.

Morganthau, T., McDaniel, M., Doherty, S., & Anderson, M. (1987, Feb. 2). Welfare: A new drive to clean up the mess. *Newsweek*, 24–25.

Moynihan, D. (1965). *The Negro family: The case for national action*. Washington, DC: U.S. Government Printing Office.

Ryan, W. (1971). *Blaming the victim*. New York: Random House.

Seidman, E., & Rapkin, B. (1983). Economics and psychosocial dysfunction: Toward a conceptual framework and prevention strategies. In R. D. Felner, L. A. Jason, J. N. Moritsugu, & S. S. Farber (Eds.), *Preventive psychology: Theory, research and practice*. (pp. 175–198). New York: Pergamon Press.

Sowell, T. (1981). *Ethnic America*. New York: Basic Books.

11

MENTAL HEALTH SERVICES FOR THE URBAN POOR: A SYSTEMS APPROACH

Donald B. Brown, M.D.,
and Myrtle Parnell, M.S.W.

In 1976, the authors became the first program director and chief social worker of a newly created community mental health program in the South Bronx in the city of New York. As part of the Morrisania Neighborhood Family Care Center (NFCC), the program was designed to serve the particular needs of a largely minority population in an area that had been devastated by the effects of poverty and racism. The program was based on a family and social systems clinical model.

Family therapy taught us to be aware of the particular family and kinship network within which our patients function, and to make use of this in our interventions. Further experience has shown the importance of understanding and developing the ability to bridge the dramatic, and often critical, differences between the family experience of most of the clinicians and those of clients of different class, racial, and ethnic groups (Parnell & Vanderkloot, 1989).

Systems theory has taught us to be aware of the influences of the patient's total social network, including health and social services, the educational system, the police and court system, the job market, and the welfare system. Although the clinician cannot expect to change these systems the better to meet the needs of patients, he or she can be instrumental in helping the patient understand these systems and negotiate them successfully.

The unique circumstances of poverty present many seemingly intractable problems that are generally considered well beyond the scope of the mental health practitioner. To live in poverty means facing limited access to such basic needs as food, psychological nurturance, adequate housing, education, and opportunity. The resultant psychological damage to a poor person can be greatest when he or she perceives that the society blames the person and family for their lack of resources, and also that most legal avenues out of his or her situation are closed to him or her. If the person perceives that the school and job training programs do not prepare him or her for jobs in the mainstream, there would seem to be no hope and no way out. To many children these issues are clear by age ten and inform them that their options consist of a life of crime for boys and motherhood at an early age for girls.

The poor person is acutely aware of the affluence in the world beyond the immediate neighborhood, and this experience of poverty in a world of plenty is especially frustrating and damaging to self-image and sense of self-confidence. The person must learn to deal with the very systems that have held out false hopes of meeting his or her basic needs. It is only after he or she has been able to achieve some reasonable stability in income, housing, and personal safety, that other issues of personal development and fulfillment can be addressed in a mental health clinical treatment setting. For a significant number of our patients, the resolution of the basic survival issues in itself provides the freedom and motivation to enroll in school or obtain a job. Further help from a mental health professional is then not needed.

Decisions regarding programs and services for the poor, especially concerning the delivery of medical and mental health services, are often made by decidedly nonpoor professionals who have invested in years of training and professional development that do not adequately prepare them to address the problems of the poor. Most clinicians do not deal with the public policy decisions that affect their patients. They, like the poor they serve, can become overwhelmed by day-to-day survival issues. They have to struggle with efforts at multilevel systems interventions vital to the survival of their patients, and do not have the energy or opportunity to gain sufficient knowledge to become involved in the political processes that so critically affect the lives of both their patients and their programs.

Many of the "intractable" problems of poverty and the seriously mentally ill in the community are actually created, or greatly exacerbated, by the implementation of governmental policies that, on faith, seem to be constructive. Many policies may actually be quite effective in one area, but can have catastrophic effects in other areas. Policy planners and politicians are, too often, overly concerned with their own immediate constituency and short-range goals to be aware of the devastating effects that the implementation of a program may have on people and neighborhoods other than their own.

An example is included in our description of the community we served, which shows how the establishment of middle-income housing rapidly depleted the Morrisania area of its middle class, leaving a poor, underorganized population unable to build necessary supports for community living. On a national level, the serious failure of our policies of deinstitutionalization to foresee the need for more adequate services for the chronically mentally ill in the community only recently has been acknowledged.

In our concept of the organization and structure of a mental health clinic to serve the innercity poor, we have found that a general systems approach to the social context of race and poverty is absolutely essential (Feiner & Brown, 1984). This approach is vital in properly understanding the population to be served, the problems to be addressed, and the clinical methods and techniques to be utilized.

In this chapter, we will describe our experience with the way in which contextual factors have influenced the development and functioning of our clinical service program for the urban poor. We will look at the influences of the social and economic organization of the larger community and aspects of the public mental health service system context, and address those factors from our professional practice systems that we believe affect our ability to do systems-oriented clinical work.

THE EXTERNAL ENVIRONMENT OF THE CLINIC

The Community Served

In the ten years preceding the establishment of the Morrisania NFCC, the southwest Bronx community had undergone drastic changes. It had been a well-established homogeneous middle-class Jewish family neighborhood centered on the broad and elegant boulevard known as the Grand Concourse. This community, however, was experiencing tensions on its fringes as a result of the in-migration of poor, transient Puerto Ricans and Blacks. The more affluent families began to move to less stressed neighborhoods in nearby suburbs, thus beginning a process of "White flight".

Greatly accelerating this flight was the opening of Co-op City, a housing complex with its own schools and services. It was a new middle-class enclave for 60,000 people in a well-protectd section of the Bronx that was well insulated from the encroachment of urban blight by its remoteness and inaccessibility by public transportation. Having been subsidized by the state to be affordable to middle-class families, the complex allowed the remaining middle-income families of the Morrisania area to move out en masse, leaving behind a neighborhood bereft of effective leadership, social cohesion, and political clout.

Unfortunately, the city did not take a "systems view" of the citywide housing problem. It did not stop to wonder what the effect of the creation of an opportunity for many thousands of middle-class people suddenly to leave their old neighborhoods for "the better life" would be on threatened neighborhoods.

Without Co-op City, the Morrisania neighborhood would probably have deteriorated slowly, as have many urban neighborhoods under the pressure of increasing costs of housing maintenance, but it would have survived and changed slowly enough to allow new leadership to develop among its new residents to deal with its problems.

Moving into the area were large numbers of poor Blacks and Puerto Ricans, attracted by good housing stock that was vastly superior to what they had left behind. Many of these new people were working poor and many were on welfare. They could not afford the kind of rents the buildings had previously maintained. The housing stock rapidly deteriorated. An epidemic of arson was partially fueled by landlords who turned to insurance companies for their profits. Vacant lots containing piles of the unsightly rubble of burned-out buildings became this area's most striking feature. The family-oriented shopping and services that the area had previously known left. Drugs, violence, and crime became omnipresent. Community cohesion and political power had not developed, at least in part, because of the transient nature of the population.

A proposal to close the antiquated Morrisania City Hospital because it was "underutilized" and move it to new facilities some five miles away brought the situation to a head, as it would have left the overwhelmingly poor population of this area without essential medical services. The city agreed to establish an ambulatory health care clinic, the Morrisania NFCC, across the street from the soon-to-be-closed hospital.

THE MORRISANIA MENTAL HEALTH PROGRAM

At the time Morrisania City Hospital closed, construction of a new wing to the NFCC, the Mental Health Annex, was completed. It was funded by some of the very last federal monies appropriated for the construction of buildings as part of the original Federal Community Mental Health Centers Act. The new psychiatry program, which we were to lead, was funded by the New York City Department of Mental Health to replace and expand the previous hospital's Mental Hygiene Clinic. Our mandate was to offer a comprehensive range of outpatient and acute day hospital services for a catchment area of some 130,000 people.

As is common in the public hospital system in New York City, our program had an affiliation contract with a voluntary hospital, Montefiore Medical Center, which is part of the Albert Einstein College of Medicine. This allowed our program to be a training site for medical students and residents, and allowed the Morrisania doctors to hold faculty appointments in the medical school.

Goals

As has been described in detail elsewhere (Brown, in press), in creating a totally new work system, we initially had many opportunities for innovative and radical departures from the way of working in other mental health programs. Making our clinical services relevant and useful to the community we were to serve was our primary goal in developing and running this new program. We knew that poor people need mental health services that would respect them, their belief systems, and their way of life.

We set out to provide clinical services that were specific to the needs of our patient population. For the chronic mentally ill patient, we provided traditional psychiatric and support services. For the majority of our patients, we planned clinical services, based on the ecosystemic and family therapy concepts. This led to a nonblame treatment model that emphasized competence and identified and utilized the strengths in the patient/family system, social network, and community to resolve the presenting problem. The interventions were made with careful attention to the patient's culture and value system.

The therapy was to begin at intake and was to be brief, as the presenting problem was viewed as a temporary setback in the functioning of the patient/family.

In order that there be continuity of care, which was a very high priority, patients were assigned a therapist in the first visit, who would continue to treat the patient/family through all subsequent case reopenings.

Our Patient Population

A typical case in our clinic is a single parent, mother of several children, living in a deteriorated building that has no locks on the entrance door and where the mailboxes are regularly violated. The apartment door may have several locks, attesting to the degree of concern about intruders. There may be one or more abandoned buildings on the block.

The presenting problem may be the mother's "nervousness," depression, or disorganized behavior, or one of the children misbehaving in school. The mother regrets that she dropped out of school and wants her children to do better.

The family subsists on welfare assistance, food stamps, and Medicaid, and has a two-party rent check (requiring the signatures of both the tenant and the landlord) because of previous nonpayment. For a family of three, the New York City Dept. of Social Services, Income Maintenance office provides a cash allowance of $100 semimonthly and a rent allowance of $244 a month. As apartments for the amount of rent allowed are extremely rare in New York City, part of the cash allowance would be added to the rent. The cash allowance also covers utility bills, clothing, and all other family needs.

The children are likely to be kept indoors after school because drugs and violence are so prevalent in the neighborhood. Many of our families have been the victims of burglaries, muggings, physical and sexual abuse, and murder, or have been touched by crime through family or social network connections.

There is usually a strong kinship network that includes friends and fathers of the children, which is essential to the family's survival. Resources, social and financial, are not the exclusive possessions of an individual or family. It is understood that in times of crisis "what's mine is yours." This system of reciprocal obligation is a major survival mechanism among the poor (Stacks, 1974).

The religions may be different from those of the middle class. The poor prefer the Pentecostal Church, Espiritismo, or Santaria. Ministers, sisters of the church, and faith healers are the natural helpers in time of emotional or spiritual crisis.

Our patients know that, at best, they are not valued, and, at worst, they are seen by the larger society as burdens, lazy, dumb, and worthless. Their existence is one of vulnerability to the exigencies of welfare case closings, poor job market, and violence in the streets. Life is a series of crises held together by their relationships with, and the resourcefulness of, their family, friends, and religion.

Our patients come to us as "self" referrals, or from other parts of the psychiatric care system, the NFCC medical services, schools, and other human service organizations in the community. We service a wide spectrum of patients with mental health problems, which can be roughly divided into three categories.

Approximately one-third of the patients under our care have a history of chronic or episodic mental illness with psychotic symptoms, and most of this group have had one or more hospitalizations. Another third present with a history of one or more periods of significant difficulty in managing their lives. They may typically have disabling anxiety or depression, either in response to important stressors or as a feature of a long-standing disability. Approximately one-third seek help for anxiety or demoralization stemming from situational or long-standing relationship or family problems, or the stresses of struggling to survive in poverty. Children with behavioral problems are included in this group, as well.

In all three categories, anywhere from 20 to 30 percent of our patients use alcohol or drugs in a way that we view as a secondary problem. We do not treat those patients whose substance abuse is considered a primary problem unless they are successfully engaged elsewhere in a specialized substance-abuse treatment program.

Value of the Systems Theory Approach

We believe that upon making a shift from the traditional individual clinical approach to one that encompasses the organization of the social world around the distressed individual or family, our therapeutic effectiveness can be enhanced in a number of ways.

First, we become more attentive to cultural values and the norms of our patients and the communities in which they live. For example, in the Black and Hispanic cultures, the darker color of a family member might be viewed as a negative feature, resulting in scapegoating of that child. Also, in both the Black and Hispanic cultures, cooperation, rather than competition, is a dearly held value. It is the core of family and community life. For a therapist to encourage competition among family members and friends would violate this norm. Such misunderstandings may lead to an assessment that the patient is unmotivated and resistant when, in fact, he or she may simply be rejecting the different value inherent in the intervention or treatment goal.

Second, many options for intervention are open beyond solely offering help to the individual. They include working with natural support systems as well as other institutions important in the patient's life. Clinicians can work as systems brokers, helping patients in their dealings with, for example, the Bureau of Child Welfare, other health and mental health providers, income maintenance, the courts, schools, or housing.

The third reason for using a systems clinical approach is that it easily allows us to be problem oriented and pragmatic—emphasizing the present rather than the past. Systems clinical theory provides an excellent basis for understanding and treating the crises of the poor and vulnerable mentally ill in terms of relevant changes in the immediate context of the life of individuals and families. Additionally, systems theory removes, or shifts, the stigmatizing label of the problem as belonging solely to the identified patient. Blame is decreased. Our focus is shifted toward the view of maximizing strengths and coping abilities in a particular context.

The following example illustrates these points. A boy is presented as having behavior problems in school. A genogram done in the first or second session reveals that this family has had a number of losses in the previous two years and the mother's favorite brother has recently been murdered. The family's emotional resources and functioning have been impaired by these events. As both the school record and the mother indicate that the functioning of the family was adequate before the initial losses, the treatment focus is on the mourning, and interventions to help the family deal with the violence and general vulnerability they experience in their environment.

The child is encouraged to participate in some physical activity, karate or a sport, that will help him develop confidence in his ability to take care of himself. The parent is encouraged to survey the living quarters and building to determine whether and how security could be improved. When this is done, she has the option of contacting and working with her landlord and/or other tenants to have them join in bringing about the necessary changes to improve the safety of the building. The result of this approach is that the parent regains a sense of competence and she takes charge of providing a safe environment for her family.

Multiethnic Staff

The clinic opened with a multiracial/multiethnic staff, some from the community we were to serve. All were newly hired on the basis of their commitment to working with the poor and a willingness to learn this new ecosystemic family therapy modality. The professional staff was made up of six psychiatrists, three psychologists, seven social workers, five nurses, and three occupational and recreation therapists. Because of the inadequate numbers and unavailability of minority professionals, of the 13 highest trained professionals (the psychiatrists, psychologists, and supervising nurses and social workers), ten were from the majority White, Anglo-American culture, with only two Blacks and one Hispanic. The importance of this early racial and cultural imbalance of the staff was to become clear within the first few years of the program's development.

The clinic's initial staffing pattern included nine paraprofessionals called mental health assistants—all minorities, and all of whom lived in, or very close to, the area we served. They had various degrees of education and experience, ranging from grade school to several years of college combined with many years of volunteer community service. The mental health assistant worked in the crisis team doing assessments of walk-in patients and carried a caseload. This was done under the supervision of the team psychiatrist and/or social work supervisor.

The most significant contributions of the mental health assistant took place in team meetings where professionals and paraprofessionals shared their thinking about cases. They taught the middle-class professional about the family life, cultural values, belief systems, strengths, support networks, and strategies for economic survival—in short, how the poor really survive.

During our early years, the paraprofessionals' knowledge and experience of the community were so vital to the success of our work that they were almost equal in status to the professional. Many cases would not have had satisfactory outcomes without the help of the mental health assistant. They could explain the functioning of the family in a way that highlighted the strengths, providing a helpful way to intervene in the system. The mental health assistants' connections with the community agencies and institutions made it possible to resolve extremely complex problems regarding patient finances or other needs. In this way, they became the primary patient advocates for the clinical program.

On the part of minority staff, there was a strong feeling that these patients were "our people," and in this setting, the minority patient would be given quality care. The minority staff was in a position to teach the White male supervisors about cultural and religious issues concerning this population. Sharing and cooperation, which are values intrinsic to the survival of minorities, set the tone of the clinic. With this constant free exchange of information, customs, holidays, and ethnic foods, and an egalitarian approach in which decisions seemed to be made by consensus, the clinic developed the ambience of a multiracial/multiethnic family. The promises of this family operation could not be kept owing to pressures from within the program and from the larger systems (Brown, in press).

Staff Training and Support

From the outset, we specifically recruited staff members who were already well trained in systems clinical theory and its application and/or committed to wanting to work in that way. This priority in hiring eventually was modified.

Systems theory helps us to understand that the characteristics of the interpersonal context in which psychiatric service delivery takes place will affect the nature of the service that is delivered. Thus, to the extent that we could succeed in providing the staff members with an effective support system, and opportunities for their own personal skills development, we expected that they would have a much better chance of achieving similar goals with their patients.

Upon starting our program in its new building, we set up several one-way-mirror rooms with intercoms and videotaping equipment. These basic tools for learning and doing systems work were easily accessible to everyone. From the beginning, in addition to the basic training in family therapy required of every staff member, each clinician participated in at least one weekly small-group supervision that emphasized work with live families using video as a secondary backup.

Our grand rounds program during the first few years consisted almost exclusively of presentations by visiting family therapists, including many "big names" in our field at that time. In later years, many visitors have presented on topics relating to culture, ethnicity, and other clinical issues in community mental health practice.

Clinical supervision of the staff was set up according to the model of the supervisor as a consultant helping to increase competency and promote growth in the treatment social system, just as the therapist intervenes with similar goals in the social system of the identified patient and family. Thus, wherever possible, supervision is live. It is conducted as a practical, live consultation built into the actual service delivery. Supervisors work using the one-way mirror or sit in with the primary therapist to help untangle some complications in a case or to help evaluate the patient or family and develop a treatment plan.

To maximize mutual support and sharing of skills, services are delivered by interdisciplinary teams consisting of approximately six to ten members (including trainees from various disciplines). Team leaders run weekly team meetings in which an open interchange among staff members is encouraged regarding work-related problems, as well as collaboration and mutual learning about cases by members from different disciplines and of different cultural backgrounds.

Case conferences are held regularly. Everyone on a treatment team typically has a chance to observe and comment upon a live case as it is being supervised. In being observed, all clinicians (including the supervisors) are forced to confront issues of trust and fears of exposure in ways that are similar to what patients experience in any therapy situation Once that trust has been established, a sense of support develops that increases the possibilities for both staff and patients to take risks and try new behaviors.

The Therapist's Own Family

Another way in which we made our training structures into a way of building a staff support system was through a Family-of-Origin seminar. This seminar was a biweekly luncheon meeting that was held off and on over many years on a voluntary participation basis. A staff member presented his or her own family of origin to colleagues for analysis and discussion. The focus was on the commonality of life problems and patterns, and noted how racial, ethnic, and socioeconomic factors shaped or reinforced the pattern. We learned about the various cultures in a very intimate way as each person shared his or her life experience. The agenda included personal growth issues for the presenter. The experience led to staff and group mutuality and support, as well as giving us a unique opportunity to learn about cultural differences withi our work group.

Other supports were provided when our psychiatrists made an arrangement to share part of the full reimbursement monies they received for conferences (which the personnel system provided only for M.D.s) with line staff so that they, too, could attend family therapy conferences. In addition, paraprofessionals were encouraged to complete their education and flexible work schedules were arranged. For those who were eligible for graduate school, we created work-study arrangements.

Our ongoing staff training program, now broadened beyond its earlier focus on family therapy, continues to provide an important basis for maintaining a work environment that supports the growth and development of staff and patients.

Our affiliation with the Einstein medical school offers the benefit of having students and trainees work with us, and our distance from larger institutions, both administratively and geographically, has afforded our program independence and autonomy. Our independence has meant that systems thinking has not had to compete with the individual psychodynamic models that characterize the working culture of these other settings.

The Clinical Services

In keeping with the social realities of the patient population, our outpatient services were structured to offer immediate crisis-oriented interventions that were well integrated with longer-term psychiatric treatments. We wanted to be sure that we never had a waiting list.

The outpatient service structure was designed to fit our systems theory concept that requests for help arise at a time of failed adaptation and crisis. The first goal of clinical interventions was to help individuals and families attain a new level of adaptation. Some patients would not be expected to return for months or years until another crisis exceeded their problem-solving capacity. Others would continue for supportive or growth-oriented psychotherapies, and still others, benefited sufficiently from the brief intervention to go on with their lives without further help.

Continuity of patient care was achieved by organizing staff schedules for the outpatient department (OPD) so as to allow each clinician time to see his or her crisis or walk-in patients for follow-up appointments. Interventions were made at the first meeting. More thorough evaluations were made over subsequent visits. The possibilities of change were assessed by seeing how the patient (and family) responded to immediate efforts at change rather than through prolonged assessment interviews.

The crisis/walk-in services, staffed by a psychiatrist and several clinicians, including students and paraprofessionals, has become the hub of the OPD. The service is the focal point for much of the learning. There are an openness and sharing and sense of real satisfaction about the work.

Patients come in without appointments, and frequently in crisis. The presenting problems range from survival issues (no money for food, family undomiciled) to "ataques", depressions, psychotic episodes, addictions, incest, and family violence. There is a high level of both excitement and tension as the nature of the problems presented might be very unusual, challenging, or complicated.

During the first interview, not only are the mental and medical (when indicated) state of the individual patient assessed and individual crisis treatment initiated, but information is gathered about family members and significant others in the patient's social field. The problems presented by our patients are varied, requiring, at times, medical/psychiatric assessment and intervention; social system, family/individual assessment; and interventions by a therapist or advocacy and support by the paraprofessional.

In establishing our program with a systems clinical theory working culture, we were putting into operation new ideas about minorities and the poor. We were clear among ourselves that poverty itself is not a mental illness. We, therefore, assumed that our patients have strengths and organized our assessments to elicit the positives and coping abilities in individuals, families, and social systems, rather than the pathology.

We assumed, also, that patients know what they need and our job is to help them with the problems presented. Our goal is to resolve the crisis and help restore the person or family to their previous level of functioning as quickly as possible. It is often possible to achieve this goal by intervening in the social system and advocating for the patient.

For example, the clinician might contact the Legal Aid Society to explain the details of the patient's ongoing complaints against his or her landlord, so that the patient will be properly represnted in court. We also intervene with the patient when he or she is required to appear in court, attend a school conference, or attend an income maintenance fair hearing.

Our purpose is to teach the patient about the particular system and how it works, so that he or she can eventually manage independently. Instead of escorting the patient ourselves, we may identify some person in the client's network who has the skills and is available to help the patient. For the clinician, resolving these issues is a very tedious and protracted task, requiring numerous calls and resulting in extreme frustration as the policies and procedures in other agencies, as well as the assigned worker, change so frequently.

Patients who first come alone are told that the possibilities for help would be increased if all relevant people involved came in for an assessment as part of a group meeting. Patients too frightened or ashamed to discuss their problems with anyone else are given the private help they request, and the involvement of others is later encouraged.

Our charts are organized to include a time line, a genogram modified to include nonfamily members (important caretakers, godparents, and friends), as well as other agencies involved. The genogram structures information so that existing supports can be assessed for the patient and family, along with the potential for therapeutic interventions.

We recognized at the outset of our program that our ideal of systematically making home visits as part of crisis treatment—and even offering ongoing family therapy in the home—would not be feasible.

This represented too drastic a departure from the usually expected services for which we were funded. NFCC administrators viewed it as an extravagant use of clinicians' time, as not cost effective, and as pampering the patients. We continue to make home visits when there is a concern about a patient who is not keeping appointments and may be in need of hospitalization or where the home situation needs to be assessed for safety or habitability.

Changes have been made in the staffing and hours of the crisis team, but it has continued to be the unit where innovation is encouraged and team work is an essential component of the treatment. We learned that it was not realistic to expect all staff to be sufficiently skilled in crisis work, and some differentiation and specialization of jobs became necessary. A group of clinicians in the OPD has specialized in crisis work, whereas others carry a caseload of longer-term cases.

For every patient admitted to our day hospital, an agreement is made that at least one family member or friend will participate in regular program meetings. Treatment plans have varied to include family therapy sessions, multiple family groups (McFarlane, 1981), and, later in our development, family psychoeducational groups (Anderson, 1980). In a chapter on "Family Therapy of the Schizophrenic Poor," the clinical leaders of the day hospital describe some of the innovations developed in that program to address the needs of their patients (Goldstein & Dyche, 1983).

FACING REALITY: EMERGING PROBLEMS

Our initial enthusiasm for and idealism about the innovative application of systems theory to community mental health care for the urban poor began to fade after several years. We were soon involved in facing the realities of issues of ethnicity and power, working out professional differences, dealing with diverse patient needs, the limitations of time and financial resources, and dealing with the demands of the bureaucratic system.

Our program opened at a time when the city was undergoing a fiscal crisis and a decidedly more conservative political climate was developing locally and nationally. This did not affect the clinic's funding, but nonblame attitudes were not in vogue in the larger community. The Puritan ethic, which asserts that one is responsible for one's own plight, was beginning to resurface in the larger society.

Within the clinic, the liberal social reformist issues of the 1960s and early 1970s were alive and percolating. The staff, not recognizing the changes that were occurring, were attempting to hold to the political and civil rights agenda of the 1960s. Despite the egalitarian philosophy, the power was clearly held by five White males, who were administrators and family therapy supervisors (family therapy supervisors had the highest status in the clinic). Many within this group had very close collegial ties and personal friendships both within and outside of the clinic.

The line staff members, both White and minority, felt their concerns were ignored and that they had no input into the decision-making process. As workloads increased, it was the Hispanic paraprofessional who carried the greatest burden because of the large number of Spanish-speaking patients. Many of these patients also had great difficulties with negotiating the various systems because of their inability to speak English. They, therefore, required a great deal of help with survival issues. The large caseloads of the Hispanic staff made it difficult for them to find time for the extra supervision that was more readily available to the less-burdened, White English-speaking staff.

It appeared that the White staff members were positioning themselves for promotions, whereas the paraprofessionals would be unable to do so. The city personnel system offers no promotional opportuniites for paraprofessionals without formal education, despite the competence gained from their on-the-job learning.

As will be desribed below, pressures from the administration of NFCC began to build for more structure and accountability in the program. Formal systems for evaluating staff had to be used, creating additional tensions as it became evident that the paraprofessionals were not faring well under this scrutiny. Charting was a particular problem because, without formal training, clinical concepts were difficult to put into written form. The training in the clinic was "hands-on." Thus, a paraprofessional could be quite good as a cotherapist, or even, in some cases, as a primary therapist with live supervision, but could not translate the session into chart notes in a way that would pass an audit. The paraprofessional's position in the clinic were diminished. They were no longer the asset that they had been in the first few years of the clinic's existence. Also, the paraprofessional's experiential and intuitive ways of knowing the patients and families were unfamiliar to the newer supervisors. There was no format to discuss these issues and a high level of tension developed.

The Minority Coalition

Out of the strong feelings aroused by these issues, the minority staff members, and paraprofessionals in particular, were disappointed and embittered when it appeared to them that the issues and problems of the larger society with regard to race and ethnicity were being repeated in the clinic. What began as an egalitarian multiracial/multiethnic family gradually evolved into a system where the minority staff members, especially bilingual members, carried huge caseloads of multiproblem families whereas the White professional staff had fewer cases and fewer of the really difficult families. People who do not speak the language of the dominant society are isolated, and, therefore, have less access to the resources and options of the mainstream. The White professional did not treat these patients because he or she did not speak Spanish. The minority staff was especially angered by the inability of the supervisory staff to help with difficult interviews, or really to understand the needs of the patients. The staff members felt they were working extremely hard and getting little help from the higher-paid White professional. The paraprofessionals and other minority staff members resented the freedom and promotional opportunities available to those who were less burdened. With the increased accountability also came evaluations of staff, which increased the tensions between the mostly White staff giving the evaluations and the paraprofessionals receiving them.

These issues were brought to the program director with the request that a minority coalition be established to work with the administration to address these issues. Agreement was given, and a interdisciplinary group was formed that included all levels of staff, from psychiatrists to paraprofessionals. The minority coalition dealt with three issues:

1. Hiring of minority professional staff, especially psychiatrists. Members joined administration in recruiting staff.

2. Increasing the number of Spanish-speaking staff as vacancies occurred through the creation of staff lines designated as bilingual.

3. Improving the performance of the paraprofessionals by giving each one a minority supervisor. In some instances, this approach was helpful; in others, there was either no change or the paraprofessional left the clinic before an assessment could be made.

Before the formation of the coalition, a challenge was made to the White male dominance of the training program—first, by a White female psychiatrist who succeeded in opening up the supervisory group for herself, and the chief social worker, who was Black. Soon after, a Hispanic psychologist, who later organized and led the minority coalition, joined the group.

This was an example of staff empowerment working at its best. Staff complaints were heard by administration, and members' requests for input and a role in resolving the issues were welcomed. Coalition members became very involved in recruiting new staff, began to understand some of the difficult realities of the hiring system, and were successful in finding appropriate applicants. It was a positive experience for the clinic.

Professional Difference

Perhaps the most powerful reality determining the limitations of our ability to apply our systems clinical working model as completely as we set out to do is our embeddedness in the culture and traditions of our professional/disciplinary identities.

in 1968, Edgar Auerswald optimistically reported that "a relatively small but growing group of behavioral scientists, most of whom have spent time in arenas in which the 'interdisciplinary approach' is being used, have taken the seemingly radical position that the knowledge of the traditional disciplines as they now exist is relatively useless in the effort to find answers [for the complex problems of crime, delinquecy, drug addiction, violence, prejudice and psychosis]. A re-alignment of current knowledge and re-examination of human behavior within a unifying holistic model, that of ecological phenomenology [is called for]" (pp. 309–310).

Auerswald went on to point out that the bridges formed between the conceptual systems of single disciplines by using an ecosystems model can threaten the sense of professional identity and the meaning we derive from belonging to a discipline's traditions. Jay Haley (1975) pointed out that the special status and expertise of each mental health professional will be undermined when compentency in family therapy is what is valued most.

Our application of systems theory led to critical conflicts and tensions around the central professional role of the psychiatrist. Our state regulatory system requires that psychiatrists make a diagnosis and approve treatment plans for every patient. A medical/psychiatric diagnosis is required in order for reimbursement to occur. Empowered with the final authority for a patient's treatment plan, our psychiatrists have overall responsibility for the clinical work done by any non-M.D.

Thus, the program required psychiatrists with good skills in the individual biological basis of patient diagnosis and treatment and, who, at minimum, had a good working knowledge of and respect for a systems approach. When a psychiatrist lacked an appropriate ability to balance or integrate these skills, problems arose.

For example, one psychiatrist, a brilliant and innovative family therapist and teacher, had little interest in evaluating patients for diagnosis and reviewing treatment plans. She consistently neglected to adequately record her findings in the medical record and was not interested in working with other physicians on coordinating treatment of the medical problems of patients.

In contrast, another psychiatrist was unable to broaden his view beyond one limited to an individual model of diagnosis and treatment. Typical of conflicts that arose with his patients was the case of a patient with disabling episodes of anxiety who was assigned to a social worker. The psychiatrist believed that this patient should be treated with medication and individual therapy sessions only. The primary therapist and his family therapy supervisor felt strongly that a family treatment approach would be most effective, and that medicating the patient would inappropriately locate the problem within the identified patient.

Not only did conflicts arise between the differing clinical models held by different supervisors, but the context of our program within an ambulatory health center also powerfully influenced the adherence to a disciplinary model of organization of services. Within the facility, there were a medical board and medical director, and directors of social work and nursing. Each discipline group, of course, has its own educational and licensing requirements. The personnel system of our facility required that persons from each discipline be hired, evaluated, and supervised by a member of the discipline. Professional advancement, understandably, required adherence to the mission and goals of each discipline, thus making work from an ecological perspective secondary to the viewpoint of a particular discipline.

Limitations to Our Application of Ecosystems Work

Too Many Patients

As has been previously noted about an urban community mental health service with an uninsulated caseload (Kluger, 1970), we became inundated with more needy patients than we had the staff, time, and energy to treat. Our mandate was to offer services to all patients from our district. Our initial ideal was to provide continuity of care by having the therapist who first saw a patient at the time of crisis or walk-in keep that case for the entire course of treatment. Some clinicians accumulate caseloads of up to 60 to 70 clients (including long-term stabilized patients seen only every two to four weeks). We had no clear criteria or mechanism for discontinuing treatment for longer-term cases.

Clinicians with already full caseloads became intolerably overloaded with work when, in addition to their (per therapist) average of two to three new cases per week, they were expected to treat any of their own former patients who might return many months later with a new crisis. Their success as therapists was being rewarded with more work.

Because of the high volume of patients, it is often not feasible for us to make the extra effort required to reach out to family members and significant others in the patient's ecosystem. Therapists are sometimes relieved when a patient does not show up for an appointment. We found that as therapists become exhausted from dealing with a large number of crisis cases, which demand a great deal of time and emotional energy, a subtle incentive is created to keep their schedules filled with cooperative, "easier" patients for long periods of time. This can have the effect of inappropriately keeping some cases in treatment longer than their situation requires, and making some patients more dependent on us.

Similar to the utilization review procedures designed by third-party payers for hospital bed use, we have developed a case review system with standards for length of stay to weed out some long-stay patients in order to balance the way we use our limited treatment resources.

We have been able to maintain our original ideal of being immediately available for new and returning patients in crisis. After crisis stabilization, many cases are now reassigned to a therapist in our OPD. Sometimes a patient or family must wait as long as a month to see the new therapist, especially at busy times of the year or when we do not have a complete staff.

Our no-show rate at times has been as high as one-third of our appointments. For those patients whom we know are not able to keep regular appointments, we have developed a standby system, in which, like an airline trying to keep its seats filled, a clinician asks several patients to come in during a particular time period.

We have not yet been able to determine through a case review process what happens to patients who fail to return when we believe treatment is not yet over. We do not know how successful we are with those who intermittently use our service, as compared with patients who regularly keep appointments.

Diverse Patient Needs

As a community mental health service, we were funded to serve all persons in our catchment area who are in need of psychiatric care, whether or not they are receptive to involving their family and whether or not they have family members available. We quickly learned that despite our enthusiasm and consistency about viewing presenting problems in their family context, and our skills in a variety of family systems therapeutic approaches, it was not feasible to include the family in many cases.

Many of our patients' families are fragmented and overwhelmed by problems of poverty and their full participation in family treatment is often difficult. In both the day hospital and the OPD, many of the seriously and chronically mentally ill are living in residences or are isolated on their own. Given the limitations of staff time available for each case, contact and involvement with family members is viewed as either irrelevant, inefficient, or ineffective for some cases.

About 40 percent of our new OPD patients (including child cases) first come to us accompanied by a family member or significant other. In perhaps another 15 percent of cases, we succeed in getting the identified patient to return with appropriate family members by giving the patient a clear message that, "We can help you better if you will bring in other people involved in, or affected by, your problem." Of the 55 percent with whom we do have the opportunity to initially work with family members for crisis stabilization and evaluation sessions, only a fraction become ongoing family therapy treatment cases. Our statistics indicate an average of 20 percent of the entire OPD cases are being seen in ongoing family therapy (including multiple family groups) at any one time.

Owing to the various factors described earlier, most patients are seen not in families, but in individual treatment. However, ecosystems and family therapy concepts form the basis of the assessments and treatment. We have also accommodated the interests of staff members in developing varied approaches to treatment, and in so doing, have increased the modalities available to our patients. At various times, we have been able to offer neurolinguistic programming, stress-reduction techniques and hypnosis, acupuncture, and Ericksonian hyp-

notherapy. Clearly, our patients have benefited from the diversity of these approaches while the professional growth of the staff members is enhanced by
encouraging their creativity and the development of new skills.

A comphrensive group therapy program that includes special seminars and
supervision has been developed and is an important ongoing feature of our
overall program. We provide group treatment for more than 150 patients a year
in 15 different groups, including activity, socialization, parenting skills, and
insight-oriented, personal-growth groups. We have not yet achieved the hoped-
for goals of seeding the development of self-help groups for our patients.

Public Bureaucratic Systems

We found that a number of realities intrinsic to publicly funded and run
human service systems had a significant impact on our mental health program.

Fragmented Services

The Morissania mental health service is but one of many disconnected pieces
of the human service system in the Bronx community. For example, there is a
lack of coordination and continuity among the various components of the mental
health system, such as psychiatric emergency rooms, inpatient services, and
community programs. A basic requirement for quality services for the seriously
mentally ill is that such services be comprehensive, coordinated, and integrated,
(Bachrach, 1981). Similarly, income maintenance, special services for children,
the court system, and medical services are all separate systems that have little
contact with each other. A great deal of stress is created for poor families and
human service workers who must constantly strive to get and coordinate services
from these varied and disconnected systems in a way that meets their needs.

During the first few years of our program, we devoted a great deal of effort
to establishing liaisons with other relevant service providers in both the mental
health and the social service systems. For example, one of our clinicians made
weekly visits to the two city hospital emergency rooms and the state hospital's
wards serving our district in order to meet patients, arrange joint treatment
planning conferences, and so on. Despite our initial enthusiasm and the success
of these efforts, it became too costly of clinician time that had to be devoted to
reimbursable patient visits. In addition, the frequent change of personnel and
lack of commitment to this endeavor on the part of the other institutions made
it difficult to sustain.

Inadequacy of Resources

In our experience in New York City, poor people, the mentally ill, and the
human service workers devoted to providing services all suffer from the stresses
of a chronic shortage of financial resources, programs, and personnel. Our
health, mental health, and social services are chronically overwhelmed with
more needs than can be met.

In some years, the annual cycle of budget renewals has caused instability and tension in our program. A citywide chaotic process of threatened cuts and uncertainty about actual dollar amounts occurs that lasts several months into the new fiscal year. This has required periods of "freezing" vacant staff lines and, in some years, the threatened layoff of some staff.

Lack of Control

Similar to the feelings experienced by the poor in our society, we have difficulty sustaining a sense that anyone in the society at large really cares about, or understands, our problems. There is a sense of demoralization and powerlessness when we experience ourselves as subject to the larger political factors at the level of city or state government, or the ambition of politicians and administrators who can use the program as a tool for their own personal advance.

For example, in New York City, the city hospital system makes affiliation contracts for physicians and medical program leadership to be provided by a voluntary hospital or medical school—in our case, Montefiore Medical Center/Albert Einstein College of Medicine. These contracts are set up in such a way that there can be considerable ambiguity about the relative authority of the affiliation program chiefs of service and the city hospital administrators. Often, in response to citywide political conflicts between the city and the voluntary hospital system, struggles develop between the director of psychiatry and the city administrator over such issues as who will be hired or what levels of productivity are acceptable. When this occurs, a significant process of demoralization, increased sense of powerlessness, and loss of a sense of cohesion in the program result.

In our ten years of operation, we have experienced several cycles of instability and intense conflict stemming from the political/administrative context in which our program operates. This seems to be an inevitable reality of the organizational life of most public sector institutions.

As noted, many features of the fragmentation, crises, experience of powerlessness, and inadequacy of resources that characterize the context of our community mental health program are similar to those of the community and the families we serve! Moreover, in our society, psychiatry programs and the mentally ill, as well as poor people in general, are stigmatized. They are often viewed with contempt, blamed for their problems, and, it seems, only grudgingly given the resources they require.

CONCLUSION

We started out ten years ago to establish a new way of providing treatment in a poor community. We put together ideas from family and ecosystem treatment modalities that led to a nonblame competence model of treating our population. We viewed a large percentage of the presenting problems as temporary setbacks in the ability of our patients to cope. Using genograms and ecomaps to assess the strengths and resources from within the patient, family, and community, we then provided help in negotiating the agencies/institutions in the community. With the exception of the chronically mental ill, after crisis resolution we would end treatment with encouragement for patients to return if and when another crisis arose.

Critical to the success of this model was the multiracial/multiethnic interdisciplinary team that emphasized competence rather than hierarchy, sharing rather than competition. Both in this way, and in the way in which staff members joined together in resolving the patient/family problem, the teams reflected the extended families of our patients.

What happens to programs such as ours over time in the public mental health system? Innovations and changes in a human service delivery program are evolutionary. We cannot expect to create a totally new way of working while remaining connected to the realities of our context. The laws that regulate our clinics and license our professional practice, the schools and hospitals that train us, and our professional societies and the journals we read are all established institutions that determine the "culture" within which we think and behave. With respect to change through the generations, a new service organization such as the Morrisania program is really no different from a newly formed family. Both the system (clinic or family) and the individuals in it are the products of their particular history and cultural context.

Auerswald (1987), speaks to the difficulties inherent in maintaining an innovative systems-oriented treatment program. "To do therapeutic work without constant conflicts with colleagues, a site must be developed that consists of a community based health or mental health delivery system, designed to operate eco-systemically and staffed by people who can think eco-systemically. What makes this problem so difficult is that such programs are ecologically out of synchrony with the general society in which they evolve" (p. 325).

We have discussed above the problems we have experienced resulting from the social and economic influence of the larger community, the mental health service system, the mental health professional systems, and the internal administrative system of our own program.

In the American system of mental health care, there continues to be what can be characterized as two conflicting views of the mission of community mental health services. One holds that such services should offer traditional psychiatric care to low-income patients—that is, a medical model. The other view, a human services model, suggests that community mental health services should address the various social ills presumed to cause, or to aggravate, mental illness (Faulkner et al., 1982). These opposing views are seen as forming the basis for much of the interdisciplinary conflict and role confusion in community mental health (Boyts, 1985; Arce & Vergare, 1985).

It is our view that the mission of a community-based mental health service for the urban poor must embrace aspects of both of these models. The tensions and conflicts we have experienced in our efforts to carry this mission out do not dissuade us from our belief that systems clinical theory offers the best basis for achieving this integration.

A poor community, perhaps more than any other, requires institutional structures that are stable and able to support programs and staff. Such communities need talented and committed leadership from clinicians and administrators who have the executive skills necessary to manage the complex system in which the service exists. The program leaders must be able to bring clarity to an organization that can easily become chaotic and disorganized owing to the environment in which it functions.

When there are stability and clarity in a program with regard to its mission, goals, job functions, and accountability, the possibility of a multidisciplinary group succeeding in working ecosystemically is most likely to be implemented.

In assessing the results of our having established an ecosystemic community mental health service for the urban poor, we are aware that we were not able to accomplish or sustain many of our original ideals. However, we believe that what was achieved was significant. Our program has succeeded in affording services that take into account the importance of culture and family and whose providers understand the role of powerlessness and stress in the lives of the poor. A less judgemental and nonblaming clinical approach is carried out, using more than one treatment modality.

Applying Our Principles

Given the realities described, we have reaffirmed the importance of applying some of the following clinical principles to the workplace, as described earlier.

Emphasize Mutual Support and Networking

In dealing with the special stressors of working with the poor and mentally ill, it has been important to have a working environment in which our staff can share information and emotional support. Likewise, we have worked hard to develop an administrative style that provides a model for respecting difference while cooperating and resolving conflicts. Frequent parties, the mutual sharing of ethnic foods, and the maintenance of team cohesiveness have made work in this domestic war zone not only bearable, but exciting. Administrators who do not understand the special issues of dealing with our patient population have become uncomfortable with this different approach, and pressure continues to be exerted, that threatens the spirit of sharing and teamwork. This attitude requires constant sharing of information and advocacy work on our own behalf.

Recognize Strengths, Normalize the Problems

The stresses we experience are a normal aspect of delivering human services to the poor in public institutions. What we do achieve, often against great odds, needs special recognition and praise. Our sense of helplessness and demoralization is mitigated when we learn that others are in the same situation and have found ways to cope.

Encourage Growth and Change

Patients, families, staff members, programs, communities, and the entire service system all have their own cycles of development, crisis, and adaptation. A spirit of encouraging learning, growth, innovation, and change keeps us moving forward in trying new clinical interventions, redesigning aspects of the program, or teaching and advocating for our needs with other service providers, administrators, or politicians.

The work we do is stimulating, challenging, satisfying, often difficult, sometimes demoralizing, and never dull. The program has attracted, and continues to attract, many talented, dedicated, enthusiastic, and energetic people. We continue our work because we are convinced that what we do makes a difference in the lives of those we serve. We remain committed to providing quality care to the population of this community.

REFERENCES

Anderson, C. M. (1980). Family treatment of adult schizophrenic patients: A psychoeducational approach. *Schizophrenia Bulletin, 6*(3), 490–505.

Anderson, C. M., Reiss, D. J., & Hogarty, G. E. (1986). *Schizophrenia and the family*. New York: Guilford Press.

Arce, A. A., & Vergare, M. J. (1985). Psychiatrists and interprofessional role conflicts in community mental health centers. In *Community mental health centers and psychiatrists*, (pp. 51–68). Washington D.C.: The American Psychiatric Association and Rockville, Md.: The National Council of Community Mental Health Centers.

Auerswald, E. (1968). Interdisciplinary versus ecological approach. *Family Process, 7*, 202–215.

Auerswald, E. H. (1987). Epistemological confusion in family therapy and research. *Family Process, 26*(3). 317–330.

Bachrach, L. L. (1981). Continuity of care for chronic mental patients: A conceptual analysis. *American Journal of psychiatry, 138*, 1449–1456.

Boyts, H. (1985). Overview—Recruiting and retaining psychiatrists to work in community mental health centers: overcoming the obstacles. In *Community mental health centers and psychiatrists* (pp. 7–21). Washington, D.C.: The American Psychiatric Association, and Rockville, Md.: The National Council of Community Mental Health Centers.

Brown, D. B. (in press). Putting systems theory into service: The evolution of the Morrisania neighborhood family care center community mental health program. In Menfi, A. (Ed.), *Family therapy training and career development in the public sector*. New York: Brunner/Mazel.

Faulkner, L. R., Eaton, J. S., Jr., & Bloom, J. D. (1982). The CMHC as a setting for residency education. *Community Mental Health Journal, 18*, 3–10.

Feiner, J., & Brown, D. B. (1984). Psychiatric care of the urban poor: An ecological systems approach. *Einstein Quarterly Journal of Biological Medicine, 2*, 126–135.

Goldstein, S. J., & Dyche, L. (1983). Family therapy of the schizophrenic poor. In W. R. McFarlane (Ed.), *Family therapy in schizophrenia* (pp. 289–307). New York: Guilford Press.

Haley, J. (1975). Why a mental health clinic should avoid family therapy. *Journal of Marriage and Family Counselling, 1*, 3–13.

Kluger, J. M. (1970). The uninsulated caseload in a neighborhood mental health center. *American Journal of Psychiatry, 126*(10), 1430–1436.

McFarlane, W. R. (1983). Multiple family therapy in schizophrenia. In W. R. McFarlane (Ed.), *Family therapy in schizophrenia* (pp. 141–172). New York: Guilford Press.

Parnell, M., & Vanderkloot, J. (in press). Ghetto child. In L. Combrinck-Graham (Ed.), *Handbook of children in family therapy*. New York: Guilford Press.

Stack, C. B. (1974). *All our kin*. New York: Harper & Row.

12

AGING, POVERTY, AND THE FAMILY*

John H. Miner, Psy. D.

Paul S. was born in Boston in 1909, educated through high school, married and had three children, and worked for his entire life at Gillette as an inspector. He retired in 1974 with an adequate pension plan, Blue/CrossBlue Shield health insurance, Medex (a supplementary insurance plan offered through BC/BS), and Medicare. He owned his home and had paid off a good percentage of the mortgage. His assets totaled $60,000, which he held partly in bank savings accounts and partly in government bonds.

He suffered a stroke in 1981 and was hospitalized for six weeks. He was unable to regain all of his speech and full use of his right side. Home care was attempted for a year by his wife with help from homemaker and home health aide services, purchased from a community-based agency. Because of Mrs. S.'s increasing difficulties with providing personal care for him, as well as her own health problems, Mr. and Mrs. S. decided that he should enter a nursing home.

The family began to worry about finances as early as 1981, when home-care services had to be paid out-of-pocket, as they were not covered under the acute-care insurance and Medicare plans. Financial worries increased further after the nursing home placement, which, again, had to be paid by Mr. S. from his pension and assets, as neither BC/BS nor Medicare covered long-term care. Mrs. S. began to skimp on her own expenses and fretted over touching the nest egg her husband had saved. Nevertheless, she was forced to dip into it, and in time that reserve began to dwindle. She faced increasing worries about what to do when the assets were wiped out, and she dreaded the idea of having to sell the house. She felt ashamed that she could not somehow manage the finances better and guilty that her husband would think ill of her for losing his savings. These feelings she held inside.

The children were also worried. They feared that their mother was skimping on her own needs and deteriorating physically from worry over her husband. They felt helpless when approaching their mother, as she had become very reluctant to talk about herself and her worries. The family spirit, once so strong, had dissipated, and each member felt sad and lonely. Eventually, Mrs. S. reached a point of financial crisis: either she had to sell the house or default on nursing home payment. She called her son, who, in turn, called a lawyer for advice. The situation eventually was resolved satisfactorily. Details of how the resolution came about will be discussed later in this chapter.

SOCIAL AND POLITICAL IMPLICATIONS OF EXISTING HEALTH COVERAGE

It is evident from the example that people can be reduced to poverty over the course of a long-term illness. The range of people who are poor is thus broadened

*The author is indebted to Jane Lucke, protective service case worker for Somerville-Cambridge Elder Services, and Debra Wexler, social worker for Positive Aging Services at Massachusetts Mental Health Center, for sharing case material and clinical impressions drawn from their extensive experience with elderly families.

by the inevitable impoverishment involved in health care for the aged. People who had never been poor in their lives or had experienced poverty perhaps once, as during the Great Depression, are now reduced to an income level to which they are totally unaccustomed. This financial plight causes a great amount of stress for both the individual and the family.

Ultimately, as private resources are used up, the problem becomes a matter for government intervention through programs such as Medicaid, which is dedicated to health coverage for the poor. As it currently stands, Medicaid is the only insurance program that covers chronic illness and long-term nursing home placement. Within the existing system, a serious problem for families arises from the regulation requiring families to "spend down" to the poverty level in order to qualify for Medicaid coverage.† Thus, people like Mr. and Mrs. S. must undergo the ignominy, anxiety, and pain involved in losing much of what they had worked hard for their entire lives. Their plight is not unique or isolated. The growing numbers of elderly will increase the incidence of such occurrences multifold.

DEMOGRAPHIC AND SOCIAL TRENDS

The number of elderly people in the United States is growing at a faster rate than any other segment of the population. According to census reports and population projection studies (U.S. Bureau of the Census, 1983), the number of people over 65 was 26.8 million in 1982 (11.6 percent of the total U.S. population). By the year 2000, it is estimated that the number will increase slowly to 34.9 million (13.0 percent). By 2030, as the baby boom generation matures, the number of elderly will double. By 2080, there will be 73.1 million (23.5 percent) elderly people in the U.S.

The population aged 85 and over will grow even more rapidly than the 65-and-over group as a whole, assuming that the very old will benefit the most from future mortality improvements. At present, there are 2.4 million Americans over 85. Their numbers will double to 4.9 million by 2000, and reach 8.6 million in 2030 and 18.2 million in 2080.

The population of those aged 100 years and over is also growing substantially. At present, the centenarian population is about 32,000. By 2000, there could be 108,000; by 2030, 492,000; and by 2080, 1.9 million. Because of the increases in life expectancy, one-quarter of the elderly will be over 85 in 2080.

At the same time as the number of elderly individuals is expanding, demographic and social trends are changing American families (Aizenberg & Treas, 1985). A downward trend in fertility has decreased the size of the family and consequently reduced the number of available care givers for elderly family members. Further, the increase of women in the workforce outside the home

---

†Qualification regulations vary from state to state and from year to year. In Massachusetts, the 1987 limits were as follows: for a single person, income not over $455 a month, assets not exceeding $2,000; for a couple, $550 a month income, $3,000 in assets. Owned homes are exempt.

has reduced their availability as full-time care givers to the frail aged. The increased number of divorces probably also jeopardizes the ability of the family to sustain sick older relatives in the home. The mobility of the American family has further reduced the availability of some children as care givers for their parents due to geographic distance. Generational acceleration has made it possible to conceive four family generations in the time it formerly took to form three generations (Bengtson & DeTerre, 1980). Thus, aging families, comprised of the frail old-old (85 +) parent and the middle- or young-old (65 +) child are becoming more frequent. The likelihood that the young-old child may be frail and no longer working places limits on the amount of physical care and financial support the young-old child can give his or her parents (Torrey, 1985). These limits put the old-old at greater risk of using nursing homes for personal care. Moreover, the family is at greater financial risk, with fewer people actively earning an income.

All of these trends limit the ability of the family to maintain sick aged relatives in the home without professional assistance (Horowitz & Shindelman, 1983). If they choose to keep an aged relative at home, professional home-care support is expensive, and most of it must be paid out-of-pocket—which drains the family income. If they choose the nursing home route, that is even more expensive and leads to faster spend-down. Certainly, the complex and difficult choice of nursing home care involves more than economic considerations, and the reader might consult any of several sensitive articles in the subject (Brody & Spark, 1966; Cath, 1972; Brody, 1977; Tobin & Kulys, 1981). The discussion here is limited to the financial implications of health care in family dynamics.

ECONOMICS OF HEALTH CARE

In Mr. S.'s predicament, the income of a middle-class family was insufficient to meet the expenses of extended home health and/or nursing home care. In actual monetary terms, how much do these services cost, and, of the average, how much do the elderly spend on health care? How long might it take an average family to spend down to poverty level when paying for long-term services out-of-pocket?

The U.S. House of Representatives Select Committee on Aging has detailed per capita health expenses of the elderly. In 1977, the average amount spent on medical care by an older person was $712 (12.3 percent of total income). In 1980, it rose to $966 (12.7 percent), and to $1,526 (14.6 percent) in 1984. By 1990, it is estimated that personal health-care expenditures will average $2,583 (18.9 percent).

These averages do not reflect the high medical fees a family would have to pay for extended home-health or nursing home care. the 1987 rates for home-maker services in Massachusetts ran from $8.50 to $10 per hour. Home health aides (who give personal care) earned more, from $9.50 to $20 per hour, depending on the community. These figures average out to $12 an hour. It has been estimated that Alzheimer's patients require an average of 6.28 hours of homemaker or home health aide assistance per day (Hu, Huang, & Cartwright, 1986). Thus, the average daily home-care cost for an Alzheimer's victim could reach $75 (6.28 hours times $12) or $19,500 a year for weekday coverage. Alternatively, 1987 Level III nursing home fees vary between $65 to $85 per day, again depending on the community and the nursing home. Thus, a family might have to pay as much as $30,000 annually for that type of care.

Given these figures, the average family understandably cannot remain solvent for long. In a report to the House Select Committee, Branch, Friedman, and Socholitzky (1985) estimated how long it takes a family to reach poverty level (and Medicaid eligibility) when paying for long-term care. The results of their study are shown in Table 12.1.

The table presents the number of weeks it takes older people living in Massachusetts to become impoverished once they are either institutionalized or given home-care services for Alzheimer's disease. As the table indicates, the risk of spending down affects 75 percent of the older population within one year of institution of services. When one partner enters a nursing home, the remaining spouse also runs a risk of impoverishment. Home care is less costly, but it, too, presents financial risks, though at a slower pace.

These figures become even more dramatic and ominous if one assesses the estimated extent of nursing home use in times to come as the number of elderly increase. Prevalence rates for nursing home use by age are 1 to 2 percent for elderly 65 to 74, 5 to 6 percent for those 75 to 84, and approximately 22 percent for those over 85. It is further estimated that one in four of all people 65 years and older will enter a nursing home before their death (Branch, Friedman, & Socholitzky, 1985). Based on the prevalence of Alzheimer's disease alone, as many as 5 to 7 percent of people between 60 and 80 are at risk of needing either home care or nursing home care. Beyond this group are numerous others who will suffer from other debilitating diseases that require constant care.

From these data, one can see that the risk of becoming financially impoverished following institutionalization or after paying for home care affects the majority of elders, not just the low-income elderly. As most elderly are living on fixed incomes, and with medical costs rising drastically, the expenses involved

Table 12.1
Percent of Elderly Impoverished By Number of Weeks

Sample	Number of Weeks, %					
	0	13	26	39	52	104
Age 75+:						
Alone, in institution	7	46	59	66	72	85
Married, in institution	2	25	41	43	57	82
Married, at home	2	11	25	39	41	52
Age 66+:						
Alone, in institution	8	63	74	80	83	91
Married, in institution	4	37	47	53	57	80
Married, at home	4	16	33	39	47	55

in long-term care exceed life savings relatively quickly. This potential threat of poverty can affect older people and their families in myriad complex ways as will be presented.

REPERCUSSIONS OF ECONOMICS

Care giving for an elderly relative has an immense effect on the family. Some researchers have emphasized the positive effects of family support of elderly relatives (Brody, 1985; Cicirelli, 1981; Shanas, 1979). Others have focused on the negative aspects of the family relationships of the aged (Streib, 1972; Sussman, 1976; Zarit, Reever, & Bach-Peterson, 1980).

All of the investigators have cited some stress on the care giver as a natural consequence of the changed situation in which the child assumes more responsibility for the parent, and the parent becomes more dependent on the child. Family members who provide care to chronically impaired spouses or parents are more likely to suffer from a variety of stress-related problems, including substance use, depression, divorce, and psychosomatic illness (Cantor, 1983). Stress is experienced on both sides, however, and elderly family members are just as likely to be unhappy about changes in their level of independent functioning. Any number of emotional symptoms may appear: depression, withdrawal, irritability. Family conflict is common between parent and child.

When financial worries occur in addition to health problems, they greatly compound the stress and can exacerbate the symptoms and conflict. The threat of impoverishment awakens feelings of loss of power and control. Anger, frustration, and helplessness are characteristic responses to this financial change. For those who suffered poverty during the Great Depression, the possibility of becoming poor once again arouses even greater anxiety and fear.

The safety cushion of federal subsidy through Medicaid is no comfort to most elderly—indeed, many view it as anathema. The concept of going on welfare runs against the grain of many elderly, raised within the prevailing work ethic. They had worked hard for their money, and now they want to protect it, even if it means denying themselves necessities (including medical treatment). In clinical practice, it is often very hard to get elderly people to spend money on essentials for themselves. Rather, many choose to hoard. When ill health forces them to spend to save their lives, they and their families may experience a combination of painful feelings. In the interplay between the aged individual and the family, financial matters can become a critical, though often unspoken, issue.

With loss of health and subsequent reduction of income and assets, the aged person and his or her family face a crisis that, although may have been anticipated and feared, was usually not fully prepared for or discussed in detail. It is difficult for many families to discuss money matters when it comes to preserving the health and saving the life of one of their members. Families often feel that no expenses should be spared in providing continuing care for a sick parent. Limited family resources thus become dedicated to health care, once the insurance and Medicare run out. As we saw above, it does not take long to run through the lifetime savings of an older person in paying for such care.

The resulting impoverishment further taxes the individual's and family's capacity to cope. Strong feelings arise that can blur rational thinking. The ability to act as an integrated family and preserve customary behavior patterns is weakened—at least temporarily. With the coping capacities reduced, the patient and the family may lose track of their remaining strengths that would enable them to deal with the crisis in an active way. Rather, they may experience increased passivity and helplessness.

The financial crisis may create a tremendous problem for the individual and the family, but it can also provide them with the opportunity for further growth. Although their initial reactions may want scope, rationality, and satisfying effectiveness, most families can make restitutive attempts to regain some of their former stability. In the process of recovery, family members experience much affect critical to the restoration and continuing development of the family unit. If the therapist attends to the affect, it serves as an excellent guide to the family's stage of development.

ERIKSON & BEYOND: UNDERSTANDING THE CRISES OF AGING

Some of the feelings awakened by a pending financial crisis are evocative of those described by Erikson (1980) as critical to human development.‡ In summary, they are: (1) trust versus mistrust; (2) autonomy versus shame, doubt; (3) initiative versus guilt; (4) industry versus inferiority; (5) identity versus identity diffusion; (6) intimacy and solidarity versus isolation; (7) generativity versus self-absorption; (8) integrity versus despair. Erikson's theory applies quite relevantly to the crisis of the family at this stage. Converse to the standard biological formula, phylogeny can also recapitulate ontogeny: the family develops through crises in a progression similar to individual development. The family can become stuck at a particular point, weighed down by negative feelings, such as powerlessness, grief, anger, shame, self-doubt, inferiority, isolation, or disgust. At such times, many elderly feel that life might as well end, along with their health and money. Such situations often render families helpless in the face of such despair.

Initially, when confronted with both health problems and imminent poverty, an older person and the family may react with mistrust. The feeling may be externalized outside the family. For example, authorities such as the doctor or the government may be criticized and distrusted for taking all one's money. The same mistrust may be experienced toward family members. The elderly patient sometimes feels that he or she has been abandoned by the family, that there is no one to turn to for help or advice. This feeling of rejection or abandonment may be partly projection on the individual's part, in that the person may be experiencing considerable shame and self-doubt about his or her own performance and ability to manage. The critical self-evaluation and self-rejection he or

‡Of course, part of the experience can be a realistic response to geographical distance or children's other responsibilties that limit the extent to which they can be involved with their parents. In addition, the support system a person has built over the years may be also dwindling through illness and death.

she suffers may be directed outward at others in an irritable, angry way, as well as projected onto others, leading to a feeling of rejection by others.

The individual and the family may experience shame over having to take welfare money, and the individual is often further shamed by the new dependent position. Such shame appears closely tied to guilt. Some older persons do not wish to be a burden on others and feel guilty about making requests. Family members, in turn, may resent caretaking, from which they wish to be relieved in some way. The elder may feel guilty about using up the family estate and the children may resent the loss of their inheritance. These resentments and wishes commonly produce guilt. If the guilt is intense, it can severely restrict the patient and relatives from relating openly with one another.

The loss of assets and income can provoke feelings of inadequacy and inferiority. Sick old people often feel that they no longer are the persons they once were. This subjective attitude, to a large degree accurately derived from reality, further robs the older person of a sense of competency, usefulness, and effectiveness. Without the physical and financial resources he or she once had, the impoverished sick elder feels inadequate to cope with the taxing demands of the new situation. Family members, too, may feel inadequate to raise and discuss difficult financial issues with their parents. In most cases, they never before have had to deal with this type of problem with their parents. Moreover, their lack of clear-cut answers and solutions to the problem may inhibit them from actively addressing the issue. Like their sick parent, they feel useless and ineffective.

This experience of inadequacy and inferiority, when compared with former functioning as a family unit, may divest the family of its sense of identity. Roles and relationships are necessarily modified to meet the new financial and caregiving needs. They may prefer to avoid getting together as a family, which, in turn, leads to feelings of isolation from one another. Each family member may turn inward in sadness and dismay. In reaction to any financial or time demands, family members may become self-protective and self-absorbed. Frequently, it is left to one child (typically a son) to manage the financial affairs, with care giving left to a daughter. In extreme cases, the children may abdicate responsibility, leaving financial and medical care of their parent to state-run agencies or a lawyer, who may serve as conservator or guardian.

Faced with an unknown and frightening future, and with fewer physical, emotional, and financial resources, the poor elder may stagnate and pass each day merely waiting to die. Care providers and the family can become a target for displaced self-contempt and disgust, which renders care increasingly difficult. Hope shrinks.

Reactions vary from family to family. How people respond depends largely on available psychological resources. Some families are better able to band together and cope—ususally those that have past experience in coping with difficulties and that maintain a sense of control and choice over what they want to do. Others may need professional assistance, such as family therapy, to help them grow through their pain.

Growth comes through successful negotiation of each crisis. Thus, a sick, impoverished individual and family establish better terms with each other and achieve more trusting relationships through discussion and planning around health care. Open communication regarding feelings of concern and worry can set a common ground for the elder and the family to work together. In place of shame and doubt, a redefined sense of autonomy develops, based on a realistic acceptance of the new financial and physical limitations. The individual and the family can learn to maintain semiautonomy while working with government-financed support systems. They may even gain a pleasurable feeling of initiative and accomplishment in effectively and responsibly applying for appropriate government support. With more initiative, they usually feel less guilt and resentment and grow to appreciate one another as equal in worth despite differences in function and age. Initiative thus leads to feelings of effectiveness, usefulness, and productivity.

Although no longer exactly the persons or family they once were, family members can reenlist former coping mechanisms or find new ones to deal with their problems. In the process, they may redefine their identities in terms of new responsibilities and new relationships. If this occurs, the family functions more strongly and achieves integration once again. Rather than separating from one another in isolative, self-absorbed worry, the family members experience greater intimacy in solving problems together.

Ideally, this intimacy leads to a spirit of growth in which new family relations and resources are formed. Not only do family members feel closer reliance on one another, but care providers and friends can be incorporated into the family as an extended support network. Ultimately, the older person and the family can reach a level of integrity where they can accept the changes. This crisis has afforded them the opportunity to work out other latent family issues, allowing them better to accept one another and maintain a sense of dignity in the face of physical and economic threat. The crisis of ill health and impoverishment in old age can thus help the family reach a higher level of maturity and integrity than it might otherwise have attained.

SUGGESTIONS FOR FAMILIES AND FAMILY THERAPISTS

By far the best approach to issues of long-term care and finances is prevention before the crisis arises. This approach usually lies beyond the domain of the family therapist and in the hands of employers, personnel directors, family lawyers, insurance brokers, financial advisers, and—most important—the family itself. In terms of financial planning, family members should be advised to explore investment options§ as well as private long-term care insurance, which is an area just beginning to be developed (Friedman, 1986/87; Piktialis, 1986). If they have sufficient capital, they may investigate a retirement community that

§The magazine *Modern Maturity*, published bimonthly by the American Association of Retired Persons, is an excellent resource in this area. Each issue normally contains at least one article on financial planning. Families may write specific questions to the column "What Should I Do?" Back issues may also be consulted as a reference, although it is important to have up-to-date information, as tax laws, health insurance plans, and government policies change rapidly.

offers lifetime continuing care. Certainly, alternatives to nursing home placement, such as home care with the help of a visiting nurse program and a respite facility, may be considered.

On a broader basis extending beyond finances, family members should explore their preferences for long-term care, should a debilitating illness occur. Talking with friends who are facing or have faced a similar type of decision can provide added support and another perspective. Such discussions bring to light different family members' values and opinions about ethical choices that bear on future decision making. It is particularly important to ascertain the older person's wishes before any crisis, while he or she is still healthy and mentally sound. The family members can then meet those wishes as best they can, and, if the older person becomes incompetent, make any other decisions regarding care in keeping with what the person would have chosen for himself or herself.

If the individual and the family do choose nursing home care, the choice of which nursing home can be a difficult one, because quality of care may vary from one home to another. Beginning the decision-making process well in advance of crises allows the advantageous opportunity to visit several facilities and to evaluate which one seems best suited to the individual's needs and taste. It is important to look beyond the mere physical appearance of the building and to answer the following questions. What is the staff-to-resident ratio? Are the general spirit and tone warm, kind, and attentive to the individual? How active and varied is the activity program? What activities are available to the more impaired residents? Is physical therapy offered for rehabilitation? Is there a resident council to present resident wishes formally to administration? How receptive does the staff appear to be to family members? How appetizing is the food? It is also useful to discuss the benefits and drawbacks of the nursing home with a few of the residents.

All of this will probably sound alarmist and morbid to a family currently in good health. But, like making a will, it is better done in advance of crisis, when one can think calmly and rationally, with time to weigh various options.

Typically, however, the family enters therapy in crisis. Family therapy at that time can gain much impetus from the critical nature of the situation and the motivation of the family members to do work. Therapy can help the family discuss issues and feelings openly and in a focused way, find adaptive ways of coping, and make plans consonant with their wishes. The developmental stages described may be helpful in family work by providing direction and goals for moving from one stage to the next.‖ The therapist can help by offering information regarding various options. By encouraging the family to consider and make choices, the therapist returns to the family its natural power and freedom, so that it no longer feels helpless and passive, a mere recipient of what service agencies decide to provide. Although the therapist can advocate for the family for both financial assistance and health-care services, a question arises as to how much responsibility the therapist should take and how much the family should

---

‖See *The Family Life Cycle* by Carter and McGoldrick (1980) for another way of conceptualizing the normative stages of family development. Chapter 9, "The Family in Later Life," by Froma Walsh is particularly relevant and contains significant exposition and case material concerning major late-life crises, including "empty nest," retirement, widowhood, grandparenthood, illness, and dependency on one's children.

take. In general, families gain autonomy and energy if members mobilize to assume coordinated responsibility and activity in direct patient care, or, at least, in the choice of agency-provided services.

Studies have shown that families benefit immensely from support during times when an elderly sick person requires long-term care (Brody, 1985; Horowitz & Shindelman, 1983). Support services, especially those offering empathic understanding and emotional support, strengthen family care giving, giving the family a boost to continue operating under stress. The support can come from various sources, including church, neighbors, community groups, private agencies, or government-sponsored programs.

In the case of Mr. and Mrs. S., the support and counsel came from their lawyer.

> Worried about financing nursing home care for her husband, Mrs. S. went to see the family lawyer with her son. The lawyer advised Mrs. S. to pay off the principal on their mortgage, transfer the house into her name, and refinance to obtain money for everyday needs. The lawyer discovered also that Medicaid would permit her a minimal allowance for personal needs, as she had little income of her own.
>
> With a great feeling of relief, Mrs. S. felt better able to cope with her own affairs and to continue providing emotional support to her husband in the nursing home. She felt closer to her son, who had understood her problem and helped her. The other children felt relieved also, and began to approach their mother and father with less anxiety and reticence.

In cases where the issues are deeper and conflict more entrenched, family therapy is the treatment of choice. When used strategically at various points of crisis, therapy helped the following family change the ways they related to one another and made decisions.

> Mrs. W. was a 75-year-old, Irish-American widow, living alone on a fixed pension and small savings account in an apartment she and her husband had shared for 40 years. Recently, the building had been sold and the new landlord had raised the rent drastically. Mrs. W. wondered how she could afford to continue living there. In addition, multiple health problems—hypertension, congestive heart failure, and glaucoma—were preventing her from taking on the odd jobs of sewing, baby sitting, and housekeeping she had formerly done to supplement her income. Her three sons maintained some contact, but they were bitter about their mother's emotional remoteness throughout their childhood, and they had become remote from her. She depended much more on her daughter, who lived next door. The daughter resented her mother's increasing demands for attention and help.
>
> Mrs. W. was embittered by her children's avoidance of her, and she complained all the more, especially after the rent increase. Too proud to state her financial plight, she fretted about health worries, calling her doctor several times a month. He had already carried out a full physical examination. had prescribed appropriate medications, and now felt there was little more he could do for her. Concerned about how to respond to Mrs. W.'s continuing telephone calls, the physician contacted a social worker to evaluate the case and assist in treatment. He wondered if Mrs. W. would be better off in a nursing home.
>
> In meeting with Mrs. W., the social worker learned that she felt lonely, bereft of her husband and children. She expressed extreme anxiety about her future, especially her lack of money and her health problems. When asked abut the nursing home possibility, she was offended and became noticeably apprehensive and angry, saying that she would use up the little money her husband had left her. While she

talked with shame about her emotional needs of her children, she became more assertive and clear about her health problems, which she thought could be managed by house calls from her physician and daily monitoring by her daughter. Reluctantly, Mrs. W. agreed to the social worker's suggestion of a family meeting with all her children.

Over the course of three meetings, the children learned of her loneliness and anxiety about preserving their father's estate for their inheritance. Once expressed, her feelings for them began to soften their hard feelings toward her. The daughter admitted that she could not help her mother alone any more but needed assistance from her brothers or a visiting nurse. The brothers first excused themselves from helping, but eventually resolved to make weekly visits, each brother on a different day, which would expand the coverage time. They also offered to share in paying the rent.

This plan was effective for a year and a half, until Mrs. W. fell and broke her hip. She lived with her daughter for some time afterward, with continuing visits from her sons. Ultimately, the daughter felt that she could not adequately and safely care for her mother. Although they felt guilty about it, she and her brothers discussed transferring her to a nursing home. When Mrs. W. learned of their plan, she protested vehemently and denounced them as traitors who shirked their filial duties. Once again, the social worker was called in.

Several meetings were held to discuss various alternative plans. Mrs. W.'s doctor attended one of the meetings and concluded that, as the family could not afford long-term home care, nursing home placement (covered by Medicaid once Mrs. W. spent down) was ultimately the wisest course for the treatment of her worsening heart condition. Mrs. W. realized that her funds were dwindling and insufficient for the kind of home care she desired. Staying in her daughter's home would eventually entail more constant monitoring and care, requiring her daughter to quit her job. This situation would put her daughter's family at considerable financial risk. Reluctantly she agreed to go.

Mrs. W. was disappointed and guilty about not protecting her savings, but her children comforted her and reassured her that they did not need the money and would feel better if she used it herself for the best health care possible.

Family therapy was critical in the evolution of this family's growth and improved cohesiveness. Through their crises, they learned about one another, expressed their feelings directly, and made decisions based on mutual care and respect. The nursing home transition went more smoothly and Mrs. W. made a better adjustment than she might have without the preparatory joint decision making prompted by the family therapist.

ADDENDUM

The financial issues discussed in this chapter are in part an artifact of our present government policy concerning national health insurance for the elderly. They may be resolved through policy change. As this chapter is going to press, Congress is shaping new policy on coverage for initial catastrophic illness. Although the Congress recently (June, 1988) approved expansion of Medicare coverage for acute hospital care and prescription drugs, the legislation does not cover the more devastating financial threat of a prolonged nursing home stay. In the private sector, however, several insurance companies have assembled packages that provide continuing life-care coverage. Private facilities are being designed to offer continuity of care, where elderly can invest a sum in their early old age and be covered for the rest of their lives. The drawback to the private life-care plans is their expense, which is affordable only to those who have achieved house equity.

In the coming years, there will undoubtedly be many changes in health policies for older people. It will be interesting to see how society will adapt to meet the needs of the baby boom generation, creeping ever closer to old age.

REFERENCES

Aizenberg, R., & Treas, J. (1985). The family in late life: Psychosocial and demographic considerations. In J. Birren & K. W. Schaie (Eds.), *Handbook of the psychology of aging* (2nd ed.) (pp. 169–189). New York: Van Nostrand, Reinhold.

Bengtson, V. L., & DeTerre, E. (1980). Aging and family relations. *Marriage and Family Review, 3*, 51–76.

Branch, L., Friedman, D., & Socholitzky, E. (1985). A case study of financial risk from Massachusetts. Report to the U.S. House of Representatives Select Committee on Aging. (Comm. Pub. No. 99–538). Washington D.C.: U.S. Government Printing Office.

Brody, E. (1977). *Long term care of older people*. New York: Human Science Press.

Brody, E. (1985). Parent care as a normative family stress. *The Gerontologist, 25*, 19–29.

Brody, E., & Spark, G. (1966). Institutionalization of the aged: A family crisis. *Family Process, 5*, 76–90.

Cantor, M. (1983). Strain among caregivers: A study of the experience in the United States. *The Gerontologist, 23*, 597–604.

Carter, E. A., & McGoldrick, M. (1980). *The family life cycle: A framework for family therapy*. New York: Gardner Press.

Cath, S. H. (1972). The institutionalization of a parent: A nadir of life. *Journal of Geriatric Psychiatry, 5*, 25–46.

Cicirelli, V. (1981). *Helping elderly parents: The role of adult children*. Boston: Auburn House.

Erikson, E. (1980). *Identity and the life cycle*. New York: Norton. (Original work published 1959)

Friedman, D. J. (1986–87). Affordability of health care of the elderly in Massachusetts. *Massachusetts Journal of Community Health*, fall/winter, 20–27.

Horowitz, A., & Shindelman, L. W. (1983). Social and economic incentives for family caregivers. *Health Care Financing Review, 5*(2), 25–33.

Hu, T. W., Huang, L. F., & Cartwright, W. S. (1986). Evaluation of the costs of caring for the senile demented elderly: A pilot study. *The Gerontologist, 26*, 158–163.

Piktialis, D. (1986). Private long term care insurance: A partial solution? *American Journal of Alzheimer's Care and Related Disorders*, winter, 37–43.

Shanas, E. (1979). The family as a social support system in old age. *The Gerontologist, 19*, 169–174.

Streib, G. (1972). Older families and their troubles: Familial and social responses. *The Family Coordinator, 21*, 5–19.

Sussman, M. B. (1976). The family life of old people. In R. Binstock & E. Shanas (Eds.), *Handbook of aging and the social sciences* (pp. 218–243). New York: Van Nostrand, Reinhold.

Tobin, S., & Kulys, R. (1981). The family in the institutionalization of the elderly. *Journal of Social Issues, 37*, 145–157.

Torrey, B. B. (1985). Sharing increasing costs on declining income: The visible dilemma of the invisible aged. *Milbank Memorial Fund Quarterly, 63*(2), 377–394.

U.S. Bureau of the Census (1983). *Projections of the population of the United States, by age, sex, and race: 1983 to 2080*. (Current population reports, Series P-25, no. 952). Washington, D.C.: U.S. Department of Commerce.

Zarit, S., Reever, K., & Bach-Peterson, J. (1980). Relatives of impaired elderly: Correlates of feelings of burden. *The Gerontologist, 20*, 649–655.

Part IV
Forced Migration & Relocated Families

13

ISSUES AND METHODS OF TREATMENT FOR FAMILIES IN CULTURAL TRANSITION*

Judith Landau-Stanton, M.B., Ch.B., D.P.M.

Change is a natural feature of the world, affecting its physical properties, geography, and inhabitants. It is a topic that for years has occupied the minds of poets, song writers, and sociologists, among others. While the rapidity with which change takes place may vary from era to era, change is, nonetheless, a constant facet of human and societal development.

Although in many ways inevitable, societal change has rarely occurred without challenge from a segment of those affected. Within a given society, there usually are groups that cling to the safety of preexisting traditions and norms rather than accept the risk and loss of security accompanying the new or the unknown. That such groups emerge is probably in the nature of human social and political organization.

As a society is composed of subgroups that assume different positions (e.g., pro and con) vis-à-vis an evolving process of change, an extended family also is made up of such subgroups. In a sense, the family often isomorphically reflects forces within the larger society. It is a microcosm of the larger society. When such a family experiences major upheaval, for instance, when one of its contingents moves to a new environment or culture, the intrasystem conflict is intensified much as it would be if such were to occur within a larger social group. Under the stress of moving forward, the creaks and groans of the slowly advancing social organism become amplified and it may begin to lose its coordination. This asynchrony of either rates or directions of change among the subsystems inevitably leads to conflict. As the conflict arises from difficulties in negotiating transitions, we have called it *transitional conflict* (Landau, 1981, 1982).

*Portions of this chapter have been previously published in "Adolescents, Families, and Cultural Transition: A Treatment Model," in M. P. Mirkin and S. Koman (Eds.), *Handbook of adolescents and family therapy*, New York, Gardner Press, 1985, and are used here with permission. Earlier portions of the chapter appeared originally in "Therapy with Families in Cultural Transition" in M. Mc-Goldrick, J. K. Pearce and J. Giordano (Eds.), *Ethnicity and family therapy*, New York, Guilford Press, 1982, and are also used here with permission.

At such points of transitional conflict, intervention (i.e., repair or readjustment) may be indicated.

THE DEVELOPMENTAL PERSPECTIVE

The implications of change for individual mental health have long been recognized by students of human psychology. In great part, the connection between the two has been drawn by those working in the field of human development. They have come to recognize that the processes of change and development are inextricably linked.

Among the first to identify the connection among change, development, and mental health was Sigmund Freud. In particular, he stressed the importance of early childhood development in later emotional adaptation (Jones, 1953). Subsequently, Piaget (1958) pointed out the relevance of childhood cognitive processes for adult functioning. Erikson (1950), in his description of the "eight stages of man," outlined the important points of transition from childhood through to old age—a life cycle formulation. Kubler-Ross (1975) then carried such ideas to their end point in her work on death, terming it "the final stage of growth."

Broadening of the development perspective to include a family view of the life cycle occurred somewhat later than most of the individually oriented approaches to this topic. The first such work was sociologically based, and was presented by Reuben Hill and Evelyn Duvall to the National Conference of Family Life in May 1948, (Carter & McGoldrick, 1980). Subsequently, Scherz (1970) drew a comparison between the developmental tasks of the individual and those of the family. She noted that, much as the individual encounters tasks in developmental sequences that overlap and are frequently accompanied by stress, the family also moves through parallel sequential tasks and stress points.

The first explicit application of the family life-cycle paradigm to clinical operations was outlined by Haley (1973) in his book *Uncommon Therapy*, which married the techniques of Milton Erikson to a family life-cycle framework. Later, Sluzki (1979), writing on family migration, linked sound sociological thinking with the clinical implications for families undergoing changes in cultural context. Overall, then, one arm of the psychotherapy field has progressed from individual, through nuclear and extended family, to ecosystemic (Auerswald, 1968) and the-family-in-cultural-context notions.

CULTURAL TRANSITION

"Culture may be defined as the system of social institutions, ideologies, and values that characterize a particular social domain in its adaptation to the environment. It is also implicit in the concept that these traditions and beliefs are systematically transmitted to succeeding generations" (Hamburg, 1975, p. 387).

The rapidity of change in the modern world—and, more specifically, the threat of cultural migration—commonly leads to an increased intensity of cultural emphasis in a threatened group. It has frequently been surmised that the enormous cultural strength and constancy of the Jews and Poles were based on their being forced to return to the security of their traditional culture when dangers threatened their group existence.

The threat to the group varies greatly according to the pattern of cultural transition. In some ways, it would appear that the particular ethnicity is less important than the process by which the ethnic group or family is molded with its new context. Where the migration is within the same country, the change may be limited to loss of family support systems and alteration of the level of urbanization. When outside influences are responsible for altering an existing culture within the home country, there is more likely to be a certain amount of group and family support as the changes impinge on the community as a whole (Landau, 1982). Where a new country is chosen, an entirely new value system and language may have to be contended with, as well as the loss of family support systems and the change in urbanization levels.

The ease with which a family, individual, or group undertakes and resolves the transition process is also greatly influenced by the level of choice that determined the decision. Forced migration is far more likely to result in transitional conflict than is a move or change by choice. The forced migrant population has all the same issues and adjustments to face, but, in addition, frequently has to deal with the guilt of leaving relatives and friends behind. These migrants often are left with the awful guilt of the survivor, nightmares about leaving loved ones to torture and death, and the realization that they either cannot ever return or, if they do, that the homeland will never be the same. Frequently, photographs and other memorabilia are lost in the escape, and, all too often, contact with loved ones is disrupted. Many migrating to foreign lands lose not only their cultural identity, family, and sense of belonging, but work or professional identity as well.

Migration may involve many families from a particular country, region, or culture, or it may be an isolated experience for a single family; more frequently, it falls between the two extremes (Sluzki, 1979). The resources needed for handling the transition process are obviously vastly different in each case, as in the difference between forced and elected migration. It is, therefore, useful to ascertain the transitional history of the migrant group before drawing conclusions as to the stresses affecting any individual family. A working knowledge of the group's developmental history and social and cultural norms will help the therapist avoid misinterpreting the family process—such as viewing a family-environment conflict as primarily arising from conflicts within the nuclear family.

The period of time through which change occurs is perhaps the most crucial factor affecting adaptation. Where change occurs over many generations, the adjustment may be scarcely noticeable, and may, in fact, be too gradual to be seen in the space of one lifetime, as in the case of rural Africa (Landau & Griffiths, 1981). By contrast, families undergoing cultural migration may face the stresses of both rapid industrialization and urbanization. These are often accompanied by attitudinal changes, mass media inundation, alteration in dependency patterns, gender role confusion, and increasing occupational demands, in addition to the pressures inherent in entering a new culture.

The factors determining the facility with which each family resolves issues of transition are both intrinsic and extrinsic to the family unit. If the resources of the family itself and the support systems of the community around it are adequate, and, more particularly, if the other families in that social group are at a similar stage, problems of acculturation are more likely to be satisfactorily resolved—the family adapts positively (Landau, Griffiths & Mason, 1981). If, such resources are not available, the family may encounter a severe crisis—a transitional conflict. If unresolved, this conflict may lead to symptomatology.

Factors Affecting Cultural Transition

Some important factors affecting cultural transition include the following:

Reasons for migration and realization of goals

Cultural migration occurs for diverse reasons—for instance, to escape political harassment or the dangers of war. It may be a fleeing from famine and over-population or the founding of a penal colony. It may serve in the search for personal fulfillment and betterment of the fortunes of the family. It may even result from a search for diamonds or gold or the glory of pioneering and excitement of adventure. Or the move may be an attempt to resolve continuing family problems. A major consideration in the adjustment of the family is the extent to which its original expectations of the migration compare to its reality.

Availability of support systems

The support systems in the community play an important role in determining the facility with which each family resolves transitional issues. If other families in the social group are at a similar stage of transition, the problems are more likely to be satisfactorily resolved. The attitude of the family of origin and its health and resources are also major determinants in the system's adaptation. Another major factor is the readiness of the receiving community to integrate the new arrivals, as well as the availability of resources to aid in their adjustment.

The structure of the family

The structure of the family is an important factor in its adaptation to its new environment. The natural development of the family as a sociological unit follows a pattern from extended to nuclear family and from nuclear to newly emergent family forms beyond the nuclear family (Landau & Griffiths, 1981). Migration moves the family along this pathway at a more precipitous rate than such factors as urbanization and industrialization. An individual, or a small nuclear unit, moving away from a close traditional extended family into a new culture where nuclear independence is expected, is likely to feel severely threatened. There is a sudden lack of extended family support at a time when it is most needed. The new isolated unit is also, for the first time, responsible for making and maintaining its own set of rules, which, in view of the new situation and its strange demands, need to be different from those previously maintained and administered by the hierarchy of the extended family (Landau et al., 1981).

Degree of harmony between cultures

The relative stress of migration is in part determined both by the country and culture of origin and by the country and culture of adoption. A decision to emigrate from the Far East or East Asia is likely to be taken by an entire nuclear family, frequently accompanied by one or more members of the extended family, if this is possible. If a member needs to emigrate alone the rest of the family generally tries to follow. A man from the Western world, by contrast, is far more likely to move alone, followed at most by his immediate family if he has acquired one, or, if a bachelor, by his creating a nuclear family in the country of adoption. An immigrant from the Middle East may choose either of these alternatives but, if emigrating alone, often retains far closer links with his family and country of origin than his Western counterpart.

As an example, a Hindu family leaving India in search of greater opportunities in the United States or Great Britain will experience a dramatic transition from the security of a close traditional extended family to the isolation of a nuclear family. It will also be confronted by the totally foreign values of a country with vastly different culture, language, religion, and life-style.

In contrast, the young Anglo-Saxon bachelor emigrating from Great Britain to Australia or South Africa may have minor difficulty in finding a group with which he can identify. His problems with language relate to accent only; his religion is no hindrance to the adjustment process; and his family of origin is more likely to accept his decision without question or threat of permanent mourning. In addition, his facilities for revisiting Great Britain are great, and the stress of cultural migration slight.

When, however, a young Greek or Portuguese decides to leave his homeland in search of financial improvement and educational opportunities for his children the bereavement is intense. He may well decide to emigrate alone, send for his wife and children later, when possible, and spend the rest of his life in sad exile supporting both his family in the homeland and his nuclear family in the country of adoption. He may face both his own difficulties in the process of adaptation and the misery of lack of acceptance by the citizens of his new home. The same applies to East Asians and Afghans fleeing for their lives and Russians and Poles escaping political persecution.

The clash between the cultures can also be drastically heightened when issues of prejudice arise. These are generally based upon such factors as ethnic or racial differences, competition and fear of job security, the threat that there will be a takeover by the new and different group, and the dread that the host children will be adversely influenced by the new group's customs and value system. Hence, the more similar the immigrant group, the less is the threat and the better is the the reception.

Incorporation of transition as a developmental stage

Severe crises frequently result from the lack of resolution of transitional issues. The family's healthy adaptation to transitions may be viewed as a successful negotiation of a developmental stage of the family's growth in society, and unresolved transitional conflict may be regarded as leading to dysfunction in the same sense that the unresolved stages of a family's life cycle may result in dysfunction in the system.

Changes Associated with Cultural Transition

The visible markers of a family's ethnic background are its language, religion, education, and life-style. A family in cultural transition often must confront change in all of these areas.

Language

Language is an important vehicle of culture and tradition, and is, therefore, a major factor in the adaptation to a new cultural environment. The average youth living in a new culture regards it as modern and westernized to drop the vernacular. There are many immigrant families of three or four generations in which the older generations are unable to communicate with the young people because they have no language in common. This leads inevitably to severe transgenerational conflict and the threatened disruption of family integrity and bonding. Unfortunately, it is not uncommon for the first- and second-generation youth to equate the speaking of the traditional language with lack of education. This increases the transgenerational conflict, and also, in some instances, leads to peer group conflict, on the one side by those who despise all things traditional and on the other by those who regard the aspiration to the new country's ideals as shameful and disloyal to their own identity. For immigrants who do their best to assimilate there are frequently the problems of nonacceptance because of strange accents or foreign word order usage.

Religion

Religious practices exert a strong influence on families in cultural migration, the older generations tending to adhere to the traditional and the youth being forced to choose between identification with their families or with their peers. In some groups, such as Muslim, Jewish, and Greek orthodox, schools are provided for religious education after ordinary school hours. Failure to attend these schools results in severe conflict with parents and religious peers. Attendance, however, may result in the children being excluded from extracurricular sport and ordinary social activities with nonsectarian peers. These problems often lead to poor religious identification and severe transgenerational conflict.

Education

Schooling is a factor that frequently provokes further stress in families in cultural migration. It is not uncommon for the parents of an immigrant family to learn to rely heavily on the better education and adaptation of their offspring, resulting in enormous stress on the functional boundaries of the family. Further transgenerational problems are induced by the parents' feeling of inferiority vis-à-vis their offspring and peers. Education of the children is often a major reason for the migration itself, and the parents are left feeling confused and ambivalent about the result. The children, in turn, may be ashamed of their parent's deficiencies, and so the problems are multiplied. In addition, adults who had had good jobs or professions may find that their qualifications do not transfer to the new situation because of the question of degrees, licenses, or language. They then find themselves coping not only with lack of self-esteem and satisfaction, but with their children's advancing beyond them.

Life-style

Major adjustments in life-style are frequently necessary and generally take a couple of generations to be adequately resolved. Migrants are prepared for the confrontation with a new language but are rarely aware of the enormous adjustments that are necessary in their daily living. The type of employment available in the adoptive region may be entirely different from that previously experienced. It may, at best, only appear strange because of the new environment and the attitudes toward foreign colleagues. A man used to leisurely work in Mediterranean olive groves or vineyards needs to make an enormous adjustment to the long hours and customers' demands of a busy cafe. A move from a socialist work environment may create great difficulty in adjustment to a capitalist system.

Apart from the enormous adjustments that may be necessary on the part of the breadwinner(s), the changes in daily living affect every member of the family. Leisure activities and mode of social contact are likely to be very different; an Italian or Greek family used to sitting in the village square in the evening is likely to become progressively more isolated in a Western city. Transgenerational conflict is easily precipitated by the differential rate at which the younger and older groups adopt new behavioral standards and customs.

It may be clear that many variables determine whether the transition is negotiated with relative ease or with extreme difficulty. The contrasting cases may illustrate:†

Case A. James Clarke,‡ aged 28 years, decided to emigrate from England, where his family had resided for many generations. He was convinced that, for a steam fitter, South Africa offered better work opportunities and a higher standard of living. He and his wife, Anne, and their two sons, Michael, aged five years, and John, aged three years, had lived in a different city from both families of origin for some years. Contact had been limited to letters and telephone calls to celebrate major events or to discuss family illness. Visits had been occasional. Both sets of parents were very pleased with the young couple's drive and ambition and encouraged the venture.

On arrival in South Africa, the family rapidly found friends and neighbors with whom they could communicate and identify. The only obvious difference between

---

†Cases involving forced migration and exile are presented in the Chapters 14 and 17 and reflect the enormous difficulty of transition under those conditions.

‡The names of all families described in this text have been changed to maintain confidentiality.

them and their new companions was that of accent. Mr. Clarke was easily accepted at work as his attitudes were very similar to those of his colleagues and he was more than happy to join them at the local pub on a Friday night. The Clarkes accompanied their neighbors to the local branch of the Anglican church, and within a few months regarded themselves as well settled. They made plans to save for a future trip "home" and were very well satisfied with their new position, as were both families of origin.

Case B. For Luis da Costa, the move from Portugal to South Africa was not nearly as easy. At the age of 32, he decided to emigrate in search of financial improvement and educational opportunities for his children, hoping also to be able to offer his parents better support than he had been able to manage in Portugal. He arrived in Capetown with a smattering of English, less education than most South Africans of equivalent socioeconomic position, and very little idea of what to expect in his new country. It was his first parting from a very close traditional extended family, and he was desperately lonely, as well as feeling very guilty about his parents' opposition in his decision and their prolonged mourning caused by his departure and the imminent loss of their grandchildren.

After a year had elapsed, he had saved sufficient money to send for his wife and four children, who ranged in age from 11 to three years. Far from life becoming easier, his problems seems to intensify. Mrs. Da Costa showed no enthusiasm for learning English, would not go shopping alone, and was desperately homesick. The children rapidly learned the language and how to use the local currency, and, within a short time, were trying to teach their mother how to behave in her new environment. They were ashamed of her and her unacceptability to their new friends.

Mr. Da Costa's response to his children's reactions was to increase discipline and restrict their contact with their peers, as he felt they were being adversely influenced. He emphasized the importance of their education and drove them to achieve good marks at school. As the rebellion of the children increased, so did the confusion about the correct standards of behavior, and the family system became severely dysfunctional. Both Mr. and Mrs. Da Costa missed their large extended family desperately and felt overwhelmed by the enormity of the problems that they were forced to tackle without assistance.

Family Reactions Associated with Transitional Conflict

As noted earlier, where the stresses are extreme and the support systems and health of the family insufficient, the family may become dysfunctional. When family members adjust at different rates, the system is severely stressed and transitional conflict may occur; this can be manifested in several forms.

Isolation

Isolation is a paramount risk of the migrant family. Fear of the new situation and a longing for the safe and familiar may cause the family to remain separate from its new environment. Differences in language, education, religion, and life-style accentuate the difficulties of adjustment, and where a large, close, extended family has been left behind, the stress of isolation may lead to severe problems of acculturation. Isolation may also be perpetuated by the well-established cultural groups in the adopted country, which often see the new family as "strange" (and exclude it).

Enmeshment

The threat of the new culture, fear that the family's young people will be lost to it, and the family's unacceptability in its new environment may lead the system to fortify its boundaries with the outside world. The family that continues to impose strict traditional values on its members and retains its religion and language is forced to strengthen family bonds in an attempt to cope with the unprecedented stress confronting it. If problems arise, the family is not in a position to make use of the helping facilities of its new community, nor is it able to adapt to new demands. Under stress, the family closes ranks and becomes progressively more enmeshed.

Disengagement

In certain instances, individuals in the family become isolated as they no longer accept the family's values and life-style. This leaves them very vulnerable in their new environment. In other cases, the whole family is immobilized, which precipitates the loosening of boundaries to the point of disengagement, ultimately increasing the vulnerability of all its members.

Transitional conflict

The most significant transitional stress occurs when a family member or several members move more rapidly than the others along the transitional pathway. They adapt to the new environment while others remain resistant to the process of change and struggle, often out of loyalty to home and extended family, to retain the culture at all costs. As this movement is curvilinear or oscillatory, it may appear that there is not only a differential rate of adjustment, but also a discrepancy in direction. The resultant conflict of direction and pace precipitates severe problems within the family system. *Recognition of transitional conflict is the key to helping families in cultural transition*. For example, severe sibling rivalry may, on careful assessment, be found to be based on adaptation conflicts. When one spouse is an immigrant or has immigrant parents, the presentation of marital difficulties may signal adaptational stress. The attitudes of an immigrant grandparent may be in serious conflict with those of an adolescent grandchild who presents with behavior disturbance or drug addiction. The resultant conflict may eventuate in severe problems within the family. Such transitional conflict is rarely presented directly, and very thorough investigative methods must be employed.

> **Case C.** Andreas Papadopoulos, aged 14, experienced severe schooling difficulties, and the family was referred for therapy.§ At the initial home visit, it was apparent that his parents and maternal grandparents were rigidly traditional, as were his three older sisters. His brother, 18-year-old Philotheos, however, spoke excellent English and had made a reasonable adjustment to the new way of life, except that he and his parents argued continually. Mr. and Mrs. Papadopoulos, threatened by the potential loss of their older son, had responded by attempting

§The author was the therapist in all the cases described in this chapter.

to close the family's boundaries; they refused to allow friends to visit the house as they were bitterly opposed to outside influences. They rigidly enforced Greek tradition and religion.

Andreas was caught in an impossible bind. To please his parents, he had to achieve well at school, but to do this, he had to adapt to the new culture and make friends with his peers, thereby risking alienation from his parents. He had to choose between conflict with his grandparents, parents, and sisters, or with his much admired older brother and peers. Each member of the family was caught in the transitional conflict of the system.

TRANSITIONAL THERAPY WITH FAMILIES IN CULTURAL TRANSITION

The range of cultures confronting the family therapist is vast, and the challenge of acquiring a working knowledge of each group's developmental history and norms is overwhelming. An attempt by any therapist to understand the values, traditions, and language of all immigrant groups, though ideal, is far from practical. Consequently, the therapist may be aided by conceptual schemata and operational principles that allow him or her to be as effective as possible across a wide range of families and ethnic groups. In essence, a therapist can proceed by combining these concepts and principles with the specific cultural information provided by a given family. It is assumed that the family knows more about itself and its culture than the therapist ever could. The therapeutic system is, therefore, composed of two subsystems of "experts"—the family, including as many members of the extended family and friendship circle as possible (experts on its structure, history, culture, and goals for change), and the therapist, aided by the community network where appropriate (experts on the theory and means for bringing about change). The referring person(s) or agency(ies) are generally included as a part of the therapist's subsystem. The remainder of this chapter will deal with the melding of these two areas of expertise.

There have been several approaches to developing a culture-free family therapy. The members of the Milan group (Selvini-Palazzoli, Boscolo, Cecchin, and Prata) have devised a form of therapy that they believe cuts across cultural differences through recognition of elements universal to family systems (G. Cecchin, personal communication, Nov. 1980). Andolfi (1979), too, has a technique of using a common language as a therapeutic tool. Our own approach takes its direction from a combined assessment of both (1) the relevant migration and acculturation stresses on the family, and (2) the presence of the kind of typical transition problems described above.

The therapeutic methods presented below were developed more or less independently. However, the techniques, principles, and thinking often include what we later learned were structural, strategic, and experiential features (Landau, in press).

Analysis of the System

Upon encountering a symptomatic person and his or her family, it is important to establish whether transitional conflict is occurring, and also whether this is relevant to the problems presented to the therapist. Not all immigrants and their families are in need of therapy, and the therapist must take care not to overinterpret the cultural phenomena present. Many families negotiate the acculturation process with minimal difficulty if the factors affecting adaptation are favorable. However, many families experience differential rates of transition among their subsystems, inevitably leading to transitional conflict. In this case, therapy is usually indicated.

The transitional techniques outlined below—transitional mapping, link therapy, and transitional sculpting (previously termed "dual sculpting"; Landau, 1982)—may be used either as the total focus of therapy or as part of an overall therapeutic plan. They are used for both diagnostic and therapeutic purposes. In treating families and systems, the distinctions between diagnosis and treatment is blurred. Any intervention has diagnostic value as the therapist observes the response to it. Any diagnostic action, by its nature, conveys a message from therapist to family, and is, therefore, an intervention (Haley, 1970).

Transitional Mapping

Mapping has become a relatively standard practice in both individual and family therapy. It is extremely useful both as a positive reframing of the problem and as a method for assessing cultural transition. Sluzki (1979), working with migrant families, states categorically that "in the course of the first interview, the therapist should establish which phase of the process of migration the family is currently in and how they have dealt with the vicissitudes of previous phases" (p. 389). A comprehensive map should extend beyond that of the individual's and family's life cycle to include the transitional position of the multigenerational family within its social and cultural context. This differential map should include the position of each individual and the extended family as a whole in life cycle stages, cultural origin, family form, and current status relative to other family members and the community, and, where relevant, political and social factors across both previous and current contexts. It should also include the degree of ease or difficulty with which continuity is maintained with the previous context. By helping the family map the continuity between past and present, the therapist is able to help it clarify choices for the future. A more detailed explanation of the technique, with illustrations, appears in Landau, 1982. Factors aiding or hindering adaptation should be considered, as should the rates of adaptation of family members and the system as a whole. Whenever differential rates of adaptation are found, the influence of transitional conflict may be presumed and appropriate therapy instituted.

Case D. Anna Como, aged 29, was referred by her general practitioner for treatment of a severe depression. The family map elicited from Mr. and Mrs. Como and their 10-year-old son, Reno, at the initial family interview revealed that the family move had been instigated by Mr. Como, who had persuaded his wife that there was more opportunity for motor mechanics in South Africa than in Italy. He had adapted extremely well to the move and was anxious for his wife to become more independent both of him and of her own family.

Mrs. Como's family of origin was a traditional one, of close extended patriarchal structure. Mrs. Como's emigration was the first rupture in her family's stable pattern. The general practitioner had noticed that Mrs. Como was most depressed when her mother from Italy visited her in South Africa and when Mrs. Como visited Italy. Her parents' response to her depression had been an immediate invitation for the young family to return home.

During the initial interview, there were signs of marital conflict. Further evidence of dysfunction in the system was the recent change in Reno. His marks at school had deteriorated, and he had lost interest in sporting activities. His position on the map had changed; where previously he had been adjusting well to his new environment, he was now spending more and more time with his parents, not speaking English to his father unless ordered to do so, and spending almost none of his leisure time with his peers. Mrs. Como's only social contacts were at the Italian Club. The family was becoming progressively more enmeshed.

The mapping showed that Mrs. Como was trying, unsuccessfully, to negotiate both separation from her traditional extended family and acculturation, whereas Mr. Como had successfully negotiated the transition already. Reno, too, was caught in the system's transitional conflict, which had caused decompensation at multiple levels.

Link Therapy

It is commonly the experience of migrant families to move from close traditional extended families into new situations where nuclear independence is either expected or made inevitable by geographic isolation or political cutoff from the country of origin. As noted earlier, when some members acculturate more rapidly than others, transitional conflict develops. Under such circumstances, a therapist faces two dilemmas: (1) whether to attempt to reverse the direction of transition or whether the extended family should be pressured into accepting the inevitability of the transition, and (2) whether to take control of the family's direction or allow the family to determine its own direction.

Traditional extended families tend to resolve their own emotional difficulties themselves through prescriptions that are dictated by their culture—usually without recourse to outside agencies (Landau & Griffiths, 1981). A therapeutic decision to work with the more traditional members of the system, therefore, would imply acceptance of their set of values and would lead ultimately to abdication by the therapist. Conversely, a decision to work with the most acculturated member would indicate acceptance of the new set of values. The choice of which family members to involve in therapy can, therefore, artificially determine the transitional direction taken by the therapy. It is thus necessary to establish methods of selection that will avoid artificial momentum but that will enable the family to resolve the transitional conflict, thereby facilitating further growth and development.

In our initial work we tried network therapy as devised by Ross V. Speck in the mid-1960s (Speck & Attneave, 1973). We found, however, that it frequently failed in the face or resistance from the rigid hierarchical members of the extended family. An additional problem in working with these families was that many of them came from the lower-income group and could not afford therapy, or could not all afford or arrange to be at therapy sessions together. There was, therefore, a real need to use brief, strategic intervention wherever possible.

The principle of working with the extended network applies whether one is actually working with the entire network, which we frequently do, or whether one is working with a part of the network from a systems perspective. It became apparent to us that a single family member could be used to provide the *link* between the family therapist and the rigid structure of the extended family, as extended families commonly deny the therapist adequate entry (Landau, 1981). This method allows us to avoid the issue of defining therapy as "family therapy," in that the whole family does not have to be present at one time. For example, many Greek, Indian, African, Vietnamese, Laotian, and Iranian families cannot tolerate discussion between parents in the presence of their children in the typical mode of conventional family therapy. By using link therapy, families that would not otherwise become involved in therapy may be treated. It is also an expedient form of therapy, using only one therapist and, for the greater part of the therapy, only one family member.

Link therapy involves the training and coaching of a family member to function as a therapist to his or her own family system (Landau, 1981, in press). During an initial family network assessment, this family member (link therapist) is selected and goes back alone into the family to initiate interventions with the continued guidance and supervision of the family therapist. The link therapist is coached to assist the family in resolving its transitional conflict in a direction of the link therapist's choice.

Selection of the link therapist

The link therapist needs to be both acceptable to and effective with the family, as well as available and amenable to the family therapist. In a patriarchal system, the most effective link would frequently be a man of some seniority, such as an uncle or older son.‖

The therapist should avoid the temptation to select the most acculturated member of the family whose life-style and values most closely approach the therapist's. Selection of either the most traditional or the most acculturated member would give artificial momentum to the direction of resolution of the transitional conflict.

The person initially seeking therapy is usually either an acculturated family member or an entrenched traditional member. In each case, the motivation is clear, and agreement to work with either would predetermine the transitional direction taken. Instead, we have found that the most effective link therapist is a family member whose position has not yet been resolved, one who, caught in the system's transitional conflict, is in the process of cultural transition. This

‖The link therapist is hereafter referred to by male pronouns because a male is most commonly selected for this role. Female link therapists, however, are not uncommonly selected, as is a mixed co-therapy pair.

person is generally not the complainant, and may even be a peripheral member of the family.

Since our initial use of the link technique in transitional extended families, we have used it successfully for other transitional situations, one of the prime areas being that of adolescence. Here the adolescent functions as link. By investing the adolescent with a specific role in the therapy, one stabilizes the adolescent's typically mercurial view of himself or herself as alternating between omnipotence and impotence. By allowing and encouraging him or her to be the link, one avoids suspicion of the coalition between therapist and parent, or parents, that he so readily presumes to be present. Other instances in which it is a useful adjunct is in cases of transgenerational conflict, marital conflict, and blended families, and in transitional nuclear families where therapy with other family members is not appropriate or where they are not available.

Negotiation and logistics of the contract†

The initial negotiation occurs during the first consultation or home visit when the link therapist is selected. This initial session preferably involves as many members of the extended network as possible as well as the referring person(s). The immediate and extended family members are automatically included, as well as neighbors, friends, and members of community groups, schools, churches, and agencies who are likely to be able to assist the family in any way, or are invested in the family's well-being. The wider the group participating in the selection of the link therapist, the more successful the therapy is bound to be.

In instances where the network works well together and has no problems with the intrusion of the therapeutic system, therapy may continue in this form without the use of a link therapist. In fact, it is at the network session that the decision can best be made as to whether to proceed with network therapy, or whether to select a link therapist. If network therapy continues, the entire system is involved in the brief therapy and the "family subsystem" takes responsibility for the direction of change. This form of network therapy differs from that of Speck and Attneave (1973) in that the entire network (or as many members as possible) is present throughout the therapy and takes primary responsibility for it—generally four to eight sessions. The therapist explains to the family that there seem to be many difficulties because family members appear to want the family to go in different directions. Some members may want only the traditional language spoken, and others choose only the new one; some may want to live in nuclear units, and others are trying to keep the extended family together. Some members may be grieving the loss of the old, and others are rushing to embrace the new. Some may have wanted, or chosen, to leave the old country, and others may have preferred to stay. The areas of conflict are simplified in order to illustrate the directional and temporal discrepancy to the family so that they can arrive at mutual goals for change.

---

†As many of these families are patriarchal, the male pronoun has been used to refer to the link therapist. Women, however, are generally selected in matriarchal systems and also frequently function as therapists in patriarchies.

When it is apparent that network therapy is not appropriate, or feasible, the extended network participates in the selection of the link therapist. The link therapist is invited to attend an appointment with the family therapist in order to talk about what is happening in the family and to determine whether the therapist might be able to assist him in helping the family to sort out its difficulties. It is usually a great relief to the link therapist to feel that he is regarded as competent, an aspect that is stressed during the initial invitation.

is regarded as competent, an aspect that is stressed during the initial invitation.

Arrangements for payment are worked out by having the link therapist ask the family, "How shall we pay for this?" Allowing him to negotiate the issue with his family is further confirmation of his competence. In private practice, fees may be covered by medical insurance. Where the family does not fall into this category, the link therapist decides how the clinic fee (usually nominal) will be met.

During the first link session, a contract is negotiated for the link therapist to attend four to six sessions with the family therapist over a period of six to eight weeks. Preceding each appointment with the family therapist, the link therapist is encouraged to conduct an extended family network session, of at least one or two hours. Arrangements are also made for a family network interview including the therapist three to six months later.

Coaching of the link therapist

Coaching commences during the first session with the link therapist. The object of coaching is to supervise the link therapist's work with the family. He needs to be encouraged to decide the direction of resolution of the family's transitional conflict. To do this, he needs to feel that he is invested with sufficient authority to create change. There is an ambivalent message implicit in this that needs to be reconciled before work can begin.

The coach must work out how to supervise while investing the link therapist with confidence and authority. We have found that the most effective method is to take the one-down position, using a lot of gentle humor to make the process enjoyable and to diminish the therapist's authority. Positive encouragement and reframing are used liberally in order to elevate the link therapist. Discussion and supervision are kept as simple and clear as possible. The link therapist is encouraged to meet with individuals and subsystems of his family, in addition to the extended network sessions, so that he has a clear sense of where to head by the time of the larger session. Link therapists are very creative and their network sessions have occurred at picnics, family reunions, the beach, and other sites very different from those generally selected by therapists.

> **Case E.** The following extracts from first and second link sessions with the Naidoo family are taken from a case discussed briefly in an earlier paper (Landau, 1981). The Naidoo family emigrated from India, a patriarchal society with strict definitions of family roles based upon gender.
>
> The therapy with such families as the Naidoo family poses many problems for the modern therapist, particularly one with firm ideas about social change and the rights of women. One of the inherent tenets of the link therapy model is that of noninterference in the family value system. All previous therapies with the Naidoo

family had failed because the counselors had imposed their ideas and values on the family. The moral issue raised is whether it is the responsibility of the therapist to make families "better" according to the therapist's own cultural norms, personal beliefs, or whether responsibility ends at successful termination of symptoms.

The Naidoo family was referred to a university clinic by a local social welfare agency as a multiproblem, low-income family. Many of the family members had been treated off and on for a number of years by the agency and various other mental health and alcoholism clinics. The 11 Naidoo children ranged in age from four to 24 years old. The three oldest were all married sons living in the family home. The fourth was a married daughter, the only one living away. Following her were four girls (ages 18, 16, 14, and 12), a boy of nine, a girl of six, and a four-year-old boy.

The major presenting problems were the serious acting-out behavior of the adolescent daughters, one of whom (the 16-year-old) had recently produced an illegitimate child and was abusing marijuana, and the severe alcoholism of the two oldest sons. In addition, the daughters-in-law had severe ongoing problems with their mother-in-law, which resulted in their frequently deserting the family home, with or without their husbands. The Naidoos, as prescribed by their culture, believed that Mr. Naidoo's authority had been usurped by his wife and he relied on severe asthma attacks to retain some modicum of control.

The initial extended family network assessment session was held in the home. Over two dozen family members were present, including both parents, nine of the 11 children, several daughters-in-law, a number of grandchildren, and some cousins, as well as the social worker from the local agency who had referred the case. The multiplicity and severity of the problems, the checkered therapeutic history, and the complex logistics required to gather this clan together on a regular basis indicated that link therapy might be an appropriate option.

The third son, Ganesh (aged 22), had been absent from the initial interview, and also appeared to have the least difficulty moving in and out of the traditional extended family home. He was the only son with steady, gainful employment. He had never needed therapy. As the most transitional and peripheral member, he was invited, with the family's consent, to be the link therapist. His older brother, who was adamant about sons having their own homes, had little sympathy with the traditional values, and had clearly completed the transition, was not a suitable choice for link therapist.

At the first link session, discussion revolved around the family difficulties:
Therapist: What have the problems been in the family?
Ganesh: I've had no problems.
Therapist: This is the main reason I wanted to meet you. It seems that the rest of the family has had much difficulty and that you hadn't, so I thought maybe you would be prepared to help me help the other members of the family. How would you feel about doing that?
Ganesh: Okay.

Ganesh then discussed his feelings about being the brother with the greatest strength and the one best able to control his wife. However, he sounded daunted by the magnitude of the family's problems.
Ganesh: Too many problems, too many! It's difficult to stay calm because everyone shouts and swears and there is too much corruption because of my mother letting the girls do just what they want.
Therapist: Who is the boss of the house?
Ganesh: The head of the house is my father.
Therapist: And does he manage?
Ganesh: I don't think so.
Therapist: Can your father tell your mother what to do?
Ganesh: No, she never listens. (Chuckles.)
Therapist: How would you like to change things in the family?
Ganesh: Married ones should live separately.

Ganesh then outlined his ideas and goals. He wanted the family to progress to a point where there was looser bonding of the extended and nuclear units (the constellation most frequently found en route to nuclearization).

Therapist: How can we best help the rest of the family?

Ganesh: We have regular meetings and discuss like now and I go back to them and help my father stop the women from winning all the time.

At the second link interview, two weeks, later Ganesh explained:

Ganesh: I spoke to my father and saw that it wouldn't work so I called my uncle down and we chatted. I told him of all the carrying on at home and of the corruption. He has a lot of strength and he said that he would help me run the house the right way.

Therapist: How are you going to tell the rest of the family?

Ganesh: My uncle told them and my father is very glad because my mother will listen to him.

Therapist: Do you think that things in the family will work out?

Ganesh: Of course. My uncle gave them all lectures about how to behave, especially the girls. My mother is scared of my uncle, and she was silent as soon as he came. She listened to every word.

Therapist: So you are happy about things now?

Ganesh: Yes, things are coming straight now.

To the therapist's amazement, Ganesh had elected to call in a traditional authority figure to reestablish the hierarchy of the extended family. Ganesh canceled all further link meetings, and at a follow-up home visit three months later, the therapist was told that there were no further problems. It was difficult to believe that there was no further dysfunction of the system. What was evident, however, was that the return of the family to its traditional extended form prevented the necessity for outside intervention, as problems were once more resolved according to strict traditional prescription within the boundaries of the family system. As will be discussed later, when a family returns to its traditional form, there are risks of further crises of cultural transition and resolution of conflict may be temporary.

However, in the case of the Naidoo family, follow-up after several years showed a maintenance of the daughters' health and asymptomatology, while the family was gradually moving along the transitional pathway toward acculturation. The family's values and relationships were progressively becoming more attuned to the culture around them, women were gaining authority and independence and no problems were evident. The principle remains that, in this particular therapy mode, synchrony in the family has to take priority over, and precede, synchrony with the larger context. The accent is on family synchrony. Once this has occurred the family can proceed to acculturate or continue to function without transitional conflict or crisis, but at a pace acceptable to all.‡

Case F. The course of therapy was very different with the Casalviere family. It had been referred for treatment because of the children's bad behavior. Ten-year-old Fabrizio was acting out at school. He was "untidy, rude, and constantly getting into fights." His father had given the teachers permission to discipline the boy as was necessary, but they were not able to achieve much change in his behavior. In addition, Felice, 14 years old, was refusing to speak Italian and becoming very insolent to her parents and grandparents.

At the initial family interview, it was discovered that Luigi Casalviere, an engineer, aged 36, and his wife, Tiziana, a housewife, aged 34, had immigrated to South Africa with their children (Felice, Fabrizio, and Fabbiola, aged eight) five years previously. Luigi's parents remained in Italy but Tiziana's parents, Mr. and Mrs. Girone, had joined the family in South Africa 11 months before the referral. The additional member of the housefold was Luigi's brother, Aldo, a 30-year-old bachelor who had arrived shortly after his brother.

---

‡*Ed. Note:* One concern is whether Mrs. Naidoo stopped voicing her ideas and leadership because of her fear of the uncle. In that case, the functioning of the rest of the family may be pitted against the well being of the mother.

The interview was very strained, with Mr. Girone keeping tight control of all that was said. He kept reiterating that "everything's fine in this house," and made the therapist feel like an unwelcome intruder. Aldo was very polite and obviously intent on not upsetting Mr. Girone. Luigi made some hard comments about his son, Fabrizio, and seemed less awed by the situation.

Luigi had apparently made a large circle of friends, which he shared with Aldo and with whom he was spending increasing amounts of time away from home. His job was going well, and he could not see that there were any problems apart from his children's behavior. Tiziana was relatively silent but looked especially unhappy when Luigi's friends were discussed. She also remarked that the children were forgetting both their Italian and their religion, and that their respect for their grandparents had deteriorated. The latter was stated with an accusing look at her husband. It was evident that the traditional members of the family would sabotage therapy, if given the chance, so the link technique was selected.

Aldo was the most suitable link therapist: he was acceptable to the traditional members of the family, was ready to work with the therapist, and was in the process of making decisions about his transitional position. The family agreed, rather reluctantly, to allow him to attend the first link session one week later if something could be done about the children.

During the first session, Aldo expressed his doubts about carrying any weight with Mr. and Mrs. Girone, but said he felt competent to talk to the younger members of the family.

Aldo: The kids are good kids, they listen to their uncle most of the time, and my brother—well, he's okay. But her parents—everything old is good; they don't want to hear.

Therapist: I don't know. They seemed pretty fond of you when I saw you all together.

Aldo: Mmm.

The therapist encouraged him to look at how well he got on with the old people, how they shared a sense of humor, and how they all lost patience with Luigi at times. Aldo gradually became aware that he might have some ability to guide their opinions, certainly far more than the therapist—who shared a good laugh with him about that!

Aldo felt that the solution to the family's confusion and conflict was for everybody to learn English better, "but not forget to speak Italian ever," and for Luigi to "make more fuss over Tiziana and take her out more with his friends—she doesn't know them and makes a big noise all the time. If they go out more, she won't be hearing her mother all the time and then she won't give Luigi such a hard time." He also felt that the children should spend more time with their schoolmates and be more involved in sports.

Aldo undertook to spend at least two hours a week discussing the plans with the family. With some gentle guidance, he agreed that he should work with Tiziana and her parents before "interfering" in his brother's marriage. He decided to encourage Mr. and Mrs. Girone to get out of the house more and planned to take them to the Italian Club.

At the fifth link session, seven weeks after the first consultation, Aldo reported that the situation at home had improved considerably. Tiziana was even speaking English to the children on occasion, and Aldo felt that she was not so much under her father's control. Aldo still felt that Luigi ought to take his wife out more, and that they were not getting along well enough. He felt, however, that he would like to continue working without the therapist's supervision, and an arrangement was made for a family meeting three months later. The therapist felt that if resolution of the cultural transitional conflict continued and there were still problems in Luigi's marriage, conventional marital therapy could be considered.

The second family consultation was markedly different from the first. Mr. Girone allowed Aldo to say almost as much as he himself, and there appeared to be far less tension (possibly because the therapist was no longer a total stranger). The most significant change was Tiziana's bright appearance and her active participation in the session. Aldo felt that no further help was required at that stage, but he promised to contact the therapist if he felt it was needed in the future.

The school reported a noticeable change for the better in Fabrizio's behavior and the parents stated that the problems with Felice and Fabrizio had abated. At telephone follow-up six months later, the school principal stated that all the children were doing fine and that there had been no further difficulties.

The link therapists in transitional families generally elect to move the family along the natural direction of cultural transition, but this is not inevitable. Some choose to return the family to its traditional form, as did Ganesh. Where this occurs, resolution of conflict tends to be temporary and is superseded by further crises of cultural transition until the natural direction is pursued (Landau, 1981). When the natural direction is followed, as in the case of the Casalviere family, successful resolution of problems is far more likely to result.

Link therapy may be used in any situation of cultural transition where access to the family as a whole is not feasible or appropriate. It may be used for adolescent difficulties within a family, for a child who presents with problems at school, or for any instance of cultural transgenerational conflict. In one family where the traditional family members remained in Germany, the son-in-law was sent to do the link work on an intensive basis. He achieved satisfactory resolution of the directional conflict, and the South African part of the family system improved. It may also be used in cases of transitional conflict not related to culture. This may be utilizing the entire link method or partial link therapy.

We might wonder how this approach differs from that developed by Bowen (1978). The two approaches are similar in that they both employ the coaching of one person and both relate to the total family system. One difference is that the Bowen method emphasizes the dynamics within the multigenerational family system, whereas the link approach stresses a broader system involving both the multigenerational family and its socioanthropological context. There are three major operational distinctions, however:

1. The Bowen approach aims at differentiating the individual from his family system, whereas the link therapy technique is more problem focused and trains a family member to be the therapist to his own family system.

2. The tendency with the Bowen approach is to work with the index patient or the person appearing for therapy with a complaint either about himself or herself or about other family members. In contrast, link therapy involves scanning the family system and *selecting a change agent*. This change agent is rarely the presenting person. Thus an intermediate step is inserted into the process whereby the therapist attempts to analyze (e.g., map) the total system in order to determine both where the members and subsystems lie along the transitional pathway and who might be the most appropriate link therapist. Incidentally, this method also avoids the family's de facto self-selection process of nominating a symptomatic member, or a member most "upset" by the problem, to be seen; the decision as to where (and with whom) to intervene is removed from the family, along with its possibly homeostatic—or "no change"—trappings, and is instead made by the therapist.

3. Link therapy is a much more concentrated paradigm, aimed at rapid

resolution and change over a brief period of time. A Bowen therapist might meet for sessions monthly or even yearly, whereas the link model usually involves four to six sessions over a period of six to eight weeks, with a follow-up session three to six months later.

Transitional Sculpting

The technique of transitional (or "dual") sculpting was developed for use in families where members in transitional conflict are amenable to and available for therapy. Should the families of, for example, a married couple (i.e., the two sculptors) not be amenable to, or available for, the session—as frequently happens in cases of severe cultural conflict—students, colleagues, or clinic staff may be used to simulate family members.

Transitional sculpting has grown out of the original sculpting technique pioneered and developed by such therapists as Virginia Satir, David Kantor, Fred and Bunny Duhl, and Peggy Papp (Duhl, Kantor, & Duhl, 1973). Hoffman (1981) summarizes the use of sculpting as follows:

> To elicit major coalition formations and homeostatic sequences, so that old patterns can be perceived and played out different. . . . It can also be used by members of a family in therapy as a geospatial metaphor for various aspects of a relationship system: closeness/distance; splits and alignments; the experience of being one up to one down in reference to another. (p. 250)

Transitional sculpting differs from other sculpting in that we use a sculptor from each of the two families (or the two parts of the family) in cultural conflict and assist them in negotiating a joining of the two. Transitional sculpting provides a visual and experiential joining of past to present and this continuity allows experimentation with future directions. Recognition is given to the larger system of the family in its cultural community. The method is thus an invaluable tool for working with families in cultural transition.

In the case of a couple in marital therapy, each member of the couple would sculpt his and her family of origin. In the case of intergenerational conflict, either a member from each generation might be invited to sculpt his or her view of the family, or, as with an identified marital problem, the two parents might be the sculptors. In other words, with adolescent-parent conflict, the adolescent could be one of the sculptors and a parent the other, or both parents might sculpt. Table 13-1 outlines the various steps.

In transitional sculpting, one of the two family members selected as sculptors chooses to sculpt first while the other watches. The sculpting may be either in tableau form (as though posed for a family photograph) or in action (with members moving towards and away from each other to explicate the movement of changing family coalitions), according to the preference of the sculptor. The initial sculpting is nonverbal and as true to life as possible. Once the sculpture is complete, the therapist suggests that the sculptor move into fantasy and alter the sculpture according to his or her own personal desires. The therapist as mentor encourages as much change as possible at this stage. When real family members are used, their reactions to both the original sculpture and the changes

Table 13-1
The Procedure of Transitional Sculpting: Sculptors A and B

1. *A* sculpts	True to life: then according to fantasy	*B* observes
2. *B* sculpts	True to life: then according to fantasy	*A* observes
3. *A* moves into *B*'s sculpture	True to life: then according to *A*'s fantasy	*B* observes
B moves into *A*'s sculpture	True to life: then according to *B*'s fantasy	*A* observes
4. *A* and *B* sculpt their own positions relative to each other		
5. *A* and *B* create	The transitional sculpt: reassemble original sculptures and negotiate joining of the two	

are gently discussed. The procedure is then reversed, with the first sculptor becoming the observer while the previous observer sculpts his or her own family or subsystem.

When both sculptors have completed realistic and fantasy sculptings, they are asked to reassemble their original sculptures. Each sculptor, in turn, is then asked to move into the other's sculpture in the position or role of the original sculptor to experience the feeling created by the other. After discussing their reactions, they are encouraged to make alterations with which they feel comfortable. Each then returns to his or her own sculpture to experience the changes brought about, and again their reactions are discussed. Each is usually able to go much further in fantasy in the other's sculpture than in his or her own, and a depth of experience and insight not found in individual sculpting results.

It is frequently useful at this stage to ask the two sculptors to sculpt, without words, their position relative to each other. Brief discussions may follow this, but the positioning is nonverbal and opportunity for negotiation is not given at this stage.

The final stage of the actual transitional sculpting is then started, with the sculptors being asked to negotiate the joining of their two original sculptures. They are given permission to exclude peripheral members of their families, if this is appropriate. Often a great deal can be achieved during this final phase.

As the sculptors struggle to impose the transitional directions of their choice and become ultimately aware of the opposing forces, a profound level of insight is often achieved. Family members learn to accommodate and compromise, and are also given the opportunity to be creative.

Because the technique of transitional sculpting is a very powerful tool, attention must be paid to the debriefing period, which is critical. Participants are encouraged to discuss and share their experiences of the session. We have found it useful to have audiovisual recordings for this purpose. We have also found it necessary that the initial discussion about the sculpting experience occur during the same therapy session as the sculpting, although it naturally continues beyond this into subsequent therapy sessions.

Eight-year-old Basil Wald was doing very badly at school, and his father was requested to call at the school. Mr. Wald, an accountant, aged 33, whose parents were Jewish immigrants from central Europe, was alarmed to hear that Basil's behavior was intolerable to the teachers and pupils alike, that he was distractible during lessons and violent during breaks, and would have to be removed from the school if matters did not rapidly improve. The school counselor referred Basil and his parents to the family therapist.

At the first family consultation, attended by Mr. and Mrs. Wald and their two sons, Basil and Julian (aged three months), it became evident that the family was on the point of dissolution. There had been underlying, scarcely suppressed, marital strife for many years, which had come to a head with the birth of Julian. Mr. Wald regarded his wife, a dedicated physiotherapist, aged 30, as far too independent, a hopeless cook (particularly when compared with his mother, whose main purpose in life was baking and cooking for the family), a careless mother, and an undemonstrative wife, who chose to share nothing of her life, verbal or practical, with her husband. Mrs. Wald, the daughter of Irish immigrants, felt that there were no further sacrifices she could make for her husband and his family. Despite her conversion to Judaism, she had never felt accepted by her husband's family. She did not understand his need for her to give up her job and could not bear his continual demands for public displays of affection and verbalization of every minor situation. It was evident to the therapist that Basil's behavioral disturbance was symptomatic of a stressed parental system and a decision was taken to commence work on the marriage.

As Basil's problems were the only topic of common interest currently shared by his parents, structural intervention seemed appropriate. However, on the transitional map, the cultural conflict was readily apparent, and it was felt that this needed to be resolved before therapy could proceed further. The cultures of Mr. and Mrs. Wald's parents were very different, as were the needs of the couple, neither of whom seemed aware of the origins of their difficulties. As the therapist felt that the transitional conflict was primary to the problems that the family system was experiencing, a decision was made to use transitional sculpting.

Neither of the families of Mr. or Mrs. Wald could be appropriately included in the therapy session, and so a group of family therapy trainees was invited to participate in the sculpting. The therapist chose to exclude the children from the session as the major business was between the parents.

Mr. Wald was invited to be the first sculptor. He was instructed, with as little use of language as possible, to select people from the group to represent the members of this three-generational family of origin. He was invited to arrange the members of his surrogate family as he saw them in relationship to each other, making use of space and movement wherever possible, but not speaking other than to inform the therapist of the identity of each member. Mr. Wald arranged his family in a busy domestic scene with his mother actively involved in food preparation in the kitchen, his father reading the newspaper, but observing the family's activities over the top of it from time to time, and he and his siblings comfortably arranged around the dining room table, each busily involved in some separate activity but with intermittent, marked interest in each other. His youngest sister moved repeatedly to the kitchen to participate in mother's activities. Mr. Wald placed his grandparents in a nearby room.

The therapist then asked Mr. Wald to move into fantasy and to alter the family in any way he wanted, pretending that any change was feasible. Mr. Wald's only alteration of the scene was to ensure that his older brother took a greater interest in his writing, discussing it with him at regular intervals. Despite considerable encouragement from the therapist, he was unable to introduce further changes.

Mrs. Wald, when asked to experience her husband's family as he had arranged it, felt severely constricted and immediately moved both the paternal grandparents, who had been sitting quietly in what appeared to be the living room, away from the sculpture. She informed the therapist that they had both been deceased for a considerable time and decided that it was high time that they were truly buried, as she felt that their influence over the family was iniquitous. The paternal grandparents had died before her husband was born. She further separated the children, moving the married members of the family away. Her last move was to seat her mother-in-law on a chair near her father-in-law.

When Mr. Wald was asked how he felt about his wife's fantasy, he appeared delighted with the burial of his grandparents but found it extremely difficult to take the disruption of the sibling generation. He also enjoyed the proximity of his mother and father, and expressed surprise that he had felt unable to institute the necessary change. Mrs. Wald was able, by her fantasy, to help Mr. Wald create changes that he would never have considered.

Mrs. Wald then proceeded to choose and arrange her own family members. The scene was one of amazing activity. Her father paced restlessly up and down, two of her brothers rushed in and out of the tableau with alarming speed, and her mother repeatedly turned toward her father in supplication and then away in despair. Her younger sister lay on the carpet, apparently engrossed in a book, and Mrs. Wald sat at a table involved with her sewing.

When asked to move into fantasy, Mrs. Wald brought one brother back into the family and banished the other. She placed her father firmly in a chair with the newspaper and seated her mother nearby. She tried tentatively to make them touch but was unable to sustain the contact and returned her father's hand to his newspaper.

Mr. Wald, given free reign with his wife's family, reintroduced the missing brother and formed a cozy domestic scene with which Mrs. Wald felt extremely uncomfortable.

The couple was then asked to show the therapist, nonverbally, where they now were in relationship to each other. Not surprisingly, they placed themselves at opposite ends of the room and, despite Mrs. Wald's attempts to reach her husband, they remained distant from each other. The therapist realized that her hypothesis that the couple had never really negotiated a marriage was correct; they had never received parental blessing for the marriage (Stanton, 1981). She then requested that the couple, using words where necessary, attempt to negotiate with their parents the joining of their two families of origin. They each made vain attempts to introduce their fathers and gave up; they had more success with their mothers, and none at all in a joint arrangement of the family. Despite a repeated compression move towards families of origin, the couple was not able to get any closer (Stanton, 1984).

The situation was gently interpreted during the session, and the interpretation was continued in the debriefing process. Mr. and Mrs. Wald spent two more sessions working through the video material with the therapist. After considerable debate, they decided they were prepared to put in the work necessary for continuation of the marriage and committed themselves to marital therapy.

During the ensuing six months, structural family therapy (Minuchin, 1974) was employed in order to stabilize the intergenerational boundary. This was accompanied by marital therapy for the couple as well as compression back to families of origin. As the couple spent more time with their parents they became freer to court each other. The situation improved remarkably. Basil's behavior at school continued to settle and his marks became progressively better. The therapist considered using Mr. Wald as a link therapist with his family of origin, but this proved unnecessary as the family opened its ranks to accept Mrs. Wald once the marital situation had improved.

SUMMARY

This chapter has examined some of the specific effects of migration on the family system. It will be evident from the discussion that the larger system of the family in its community must be considered, and that a knowledge of culture, tradition, reason for migration and ethnicity is vital in understanding adolescents and families in cultural transition.

Case studies were used to illustrate the necessity for careful examination of families in order to locate their phase of cultural transition and the presence of conflict. Cultural conflict is usually most intense between parents who retain their traditional values and their children who move more quickly to the values of the new culture. It is all too easy for the therapist to presume that the new or dominant culture of a society must be right for everybody and that the nuclear family structure, or the therapist's own, is the only correct paradigm. Families should be allowed and encouraged to make their own choices, facilitated by the therapist where intervention is appropriate.

The key to treating families in cultural transition is to recognize that their problems arise because different family subsystems adapt at different rates. This notion underlines the framework presented here—a framework that cuts across many dimensions of family functioning, transcends ethnic boundaries, and provides a blueprint for systemic change. The particular therapeutic mode used—for example, link therapy or transitional sculpting—is less important than adherence to this conceptual paradigm. Transitional therapy clarifies the differential rates of adaptation and facilitates the family's resolution of transitional conflict.

REFERENCES

Andolfi, M. (1979). *Family therapy: An interactional approach.* New York: Plenum.

Auerswald, E. H. (1968). Interdisciplinary versus ecological approach. *Family Process, 7,* 202–215.

Bowen, M. (1978). *Family therapy in clinical practice.* New York: Jason Aronson.

Carter, E. A., & McGoldrick, M. (Eds.) (1980). *The family life cycle.* New York: Gardner Press.

Duhl, F. J., Dantor, D., & Duhl, B. S. (1973). Learning, space and action in family therapy: A primer of sculpture. In D. Bloch (Ed.), *Techniques of family psychotherapy.* New York: Grune & Stratton.

Erikson, E. H. (1950). *Childhood and society.* New York: Norton.

Erikson, E. H. (1975). *Life history and the historical moment.* New York: Norton.

Haley, J. (1970). Approaches to family therapy. *International Journal of Psychiatry, 9,* 223–242.

Haley, J. (1973). *Uncommon therapy.* New York: Norton.

Hamburg, B. A. (1975). Social change and the problems of youth. In S. Arieti (Ed.), *American handbook of psychiatry* (2nd ed.). New York: Basic Books.

Hoffman, L. (1981). *Foundations of family therapy.* New York: Basic Books.

Jones, E. (1953). *The life and work of Sigmund Freud.* London: Hogarth Press.

Kubler-Ross, E. (1975). *Death: The final stage of growth.* Englewood Cliffs, N.J.: Prentice-Hall.

Landau, J. (1981). Link therapy as a family therapy technique for transitional extended families. *Psychotherapeia, 7*(4), 382–390.

Landau, J. (1982). Therapy with families in cultural transition. In M. McGoldrick, J. K. Pearce, & J. Giordano (Eds.). *Ethnicity and family therapy*. New York: Guilford Press.

Landau, J., & Griffiths, J. A. (1981). The South African family in transition: Therapeutic and training implications. *Journal of Marital and Family Therapy, 7*(3), 339–344.

Landau, J., Griffiths, J. A., & Mason, J. (1981). The extended family in transition: Clinical implications. *Psychotherapeia, 7*(4), 370–381. Republished in F. Kaslow (Ed.), *The international book of family therapy*. New York: Brunner/Mazel, 1982.

Minuchin, S. (1974). *Families and family therapy*. Cambridge, Mass.: Harvard University Press.

Piaget, J. (1958). *The growth of logical thinking from childhood to adolescence* (translated by A. Parsons and S. Seagrin). New York: Basic Books.

Scherz, F. H. (1970). Theory and practice of family therapy. In R. W. Roberts & R. H. Nee (Eds.), *Theories of social casework*. Chicago: University of Chicago Press.

Sluzki, C. E. (1979). Migration and family conflict. *Family Process, 18*(4), 379–390.

Speck, R. V., & Attneave, C. L. (1973). *Family networks*. New York: Pantheon.

Stanton, M. D. (1981). Marital therapy from a structural/strategic viewpoint. In G. P. Sholevar (Ed.), *The handbook of marriage and marital therapy*. Jamaica, NY: S. P. Medical and Scientific Books.

Stanton, M. D. (1984). Fusion, compression, diversion, and the workings of paradox: A theory of therapeutic/systemic change. *Family Process, 23*(2), 135–167.

14

UNDERSTANDING AND TREATING LATIN AMERICAN TORTURE SURVIVORS*

Michelle Ritterman, Ph.D.,
and a contribution by
Richard Simon, Ph.D.

For most of us, the three-minute clips we see on the evening news about wars and struggles in other countries manage to inform us of the state of the world while keeping everything at a safe distance. The suffering we see in bits and pieces on the news has no psychological reality for us as we sit comfortably in our living rooms. How are we to comprehend the misery of people whose everyday world is so much harsher and more perilous than the world we know?

Over the past several years, as a member of a group offering medical and psychological assistance to Latin American survivors of social violence, the first author has had a chance to observe close-up the tactics repressive regimes use to keep their citizens in line. The actions of politically repressive regimes resemble a twisted, upside-down version of what we try to accomplish in therapy. Like many therapists, such regimes deal in trance, but the spells they weave constrict people's worlds rather than enlarge them. While therapists help individuals develop their inner resources and strengthen their relationships with family and society, repressive regimes work in the opposite direction, demoralizing individuals, families, and communities in order to make them easier to control.

When we look at the practice of therapy entirely within the context of our everyday routines, it seems like an apolitical activity, a job like any other. But examining how the processes of human influence can be hideously distorted heightens our awareness of values to which we are committed as therapists. By showing us the mirror opposite of what we strive to do, the atrocities around the world define more clearly our own task.

*This chapter is an expansion of an article printed in the January 1987 issue of the *Networker*.

WHAT IS TORTURE?

Most of us have grown up thinking of torture as a medieval relic, a practice abolished throughout western Europe by the 19th century. But, in fact, torture is currently used as an instrument of state policy in over one-third of the countries of the world (Amnesty International, 1984). In the countries that employ it—whether capitalist or communist—torture is justified as a means of protection from *them*, that is, any group seen as a threat to the state. In Argentina, *them* started off as Jews and a spectrum of leftists, and eventually included anyone sustaining a liberal, human rights ideology. In El Salvador, anyone who serves the poor is called a "subversive" and considered fair game for any type of repression. In the Soviet Union, political dissidents are subject to abuse. In Chile, torturers are told, "Our country has a cancer in it. It is your job to remove it." In such societies the torturer is taught that his work is an act of patriotism.

Dr. Inge Kemp Genefke, (1984), director of the first international Rehabilitation Center for Torture (RCT), observes: "The purpose of torture is not primarily to extract information . . . it is to destroy the victim's personality, to break down, to create guilt and shame, to assure that he will never again be a leader."

In societies around the world, torture and social pacification consultants are recruited from the ranks of therapists and physicians. Sophisticated ideas about the connections among individuals, families, and their communities are used to advance the power of the state. However, in torture these ideas are used to narrow the range of mental states accessible to the victim, so that fearlessness will be erased by terror, enthusiasm by "readiness for the worst," hopefulness by numbness or resignation, and commitment to a humane cause by contempt for humanity. Ultimately, torture aims to make the external world seem inhospitable and to place fear and mistrust in the forefront of both waking and dreaming consciousness. In other words, torture is the reverse of everything that psychotherapy stands for.

Countertherapy

The case of 29-year-old Carlos demonstrates the awful force of this form of destructive countertherapy. Six years ago, right after finishing medical school, Carlos returned to his hometown in the El Salvador countryside. Two colleagues came with him to set up the first rudimentary health services for that area. He knew he was at risk because many medical and mental health professionals serving peasants had already been called "guerilla sympathizers" and killed.

Sure enough, the three young doctors were arrested, "detained," and interrogated by the military. For a month, without any explanation, the physicians were regularly tortured with electric shocks and were forced to watch each other being humiliated, insulted, and beaten. Sadistic suggestions were given during this time, such as, "You will remember your friend's face only as you see it now for the rest of your life." Recognizing Carlos' compassion and wish to serve others, his torturers used his own morality to break him down. The torturers refer to this approach as a "personality reversal" process. Whatever a person cares about is used to produce apathy in the person; whatever the person embraces is used to produce phobias; whatever the person loves is used to produce hatred.

"Here, you are a doctor, now fix your friends," the torturer told him, as Carlos was forced to watch his companions tortured to death. This step of producing helplessness in conjunction with a feeling of responsibility locked Carlos into a kind of immobilizing spell. Because his family was able to find out where he was and to contact a relative with a high rank in the military, Carlos survived and was eventually released, but in such bad condition that he had to crawl from prison to a bus stop.

When I met with Carlos in California months later, he was still incapable of saying he was a doctor. "I am a refugee," he said, massaging the still-seeping electric shock wound in his left ankle. With tears in his eyes he said, "That is all I am. That is all I will ever be. They tortured my friends to death before my eyes. I can't forget their faces. I could do nothing. I can never be a doctor again."

For Carlos, a sense of responsibility for his friends' fate had been soldered together in the heat of terror with the pain of his own torture by means of such intermittent suggestions as, "You will never again be a healer," "How shameful and dirty you are," "Look how you let your friends die." In the aftermath of this strategic abuse, Carlos' previous identity was now alien to him.

Instilling Paranoia

Trying to minimize observable evidence of abuse, torturers sometimes use only psychological methods. Such was the situation in the case of Patricia Jonas, whom I interviewed in the women's prison in Santiago, Chile in April 1986. Patricia's known psychiatric problems became the focus for her torturers' efforts to disorganize her personality.

Patricia was a graduate student in engineering and a recognized artistic talent. As a supporter of Allende, she was considered an enemy of the state of Chile. When her friends got in trouble with the police, she was brought by 20 armed guards of the Chilean police to incommunicado detention and held there for over ten days. Her captors acted jovial, even comical around her, mocking her and then humiliating her, intermittently betraying her trust.

They convinced her while she was hooded that the audio tape materials they played were nighttime television news coverage of her children being killed in a shootout with the police. Using injections of psychoactive drugs, they convinced her that her mother was an agent of the Chilean secret police. They made her reveal anything of interest about her friends, and then forced her to repeat, "I did not tell you anything," in an effort to intensify her uncertainty about what was real and what imaginary.

Three months after her systematic brainwashing, she was still unable to recognize her children and was positive her mother was a government agent. Having lost any ability to trust, she ran around her cell, her eyes demented with paranoia. When I met with her in prison, I asked her to tell me her story. Her voice was flat and affectless, as if she were in trance:

> They picked me up and took me to a car. Perhaps it was the CNI [information police] . . . perhaps they were my friends. They brought me to a room and took off my wig [her hair had fallen out during Pinochet's violent coup] and said I look like Kojak. But I am convinced they did not intend to hurt me. They took off all my clothes and put on something like overalls and put a hood over my head. [Her shoulders, arms, and hands are trembling uncontrollably.] Then they left me on a concrete bed without food or water for about ten days. I wondered where they had gone. But I was totally calm.

I asked her how she managed to feel like that in the hands of the police:

> Perhaps the lady does not know what I mean by the word "calm." By calm, I mean that when they turned on the television news report covering the murder of my sons by the police, when they convinced me my own mother was an agent, when I heard the children and women screaming all the time in the rooms next door and down the hall . . . I was a bit afraid. [She gestures, as if wiping away a tear.] But . . . I was also totally calm . . . I was many things.

Patricia's children won't come see her anymore. According to her mother, a woman in her 50s with grief written all over her face, Patricia's father cannot bear to see her either: "He does not know her, she is so different. He cries and can't stop when he sees what has been done to her."

The Breakdown of Community

But torture doesn't work only on individuals like Carlos and Patricia. It is often just as carefully orchestrated to break down whole families, and even communities. The goal is to squelch any possibility of organized protest against the status quo. In the public jail in Chile, I spoke with Carlos Garcia, a political prisoner condemned to death; that is, he could be executed within 48 hours of notice. Part of Carlos' torture included hearing his wife and new baby tortured for ten days. The baby, who was scarred and badly burned, was so traumatized that she did not recognize her mother for three months after the secret police returned them to their home. The torture of his baby was used not only to break Garcia down, but also to destructure his family and to terrorize his entire community by providing a public example of the ultimate horror of torture. It was a message to anyone stepping out of line with the state that the consequence of their action might be the most anguishing of possibilities.

Another goal of torture is both to isolate the survivor from his or her family and to make the larger community fear association with the family, thus eliminating any social support for those tagged as enemies of the state. In Chile, for example, several days after I left, police raided homes in the poor community of La Victoria, which had been designated as the kind of area that fosters protest against the state. The police destroyed everything they could, and seemingly arbitrarily seized people to be tortured. The torture in these cases was against "the poor" rather than against those with an ideological commitment. Likewise, when the corpse of a Salvadoran mother is left mutilated in front of her house, its purpose is to terrorize not only her children, but her entire community.

Both family-oriented and community-directed torture overload kin bonds with excessive intensity, and replace love and trust with feelings of terror, guilt, helplessness, and shame. For the state, torture is most "effective" when it turns family and community against the survivor instead of against the torturers. It is not uncommon for the spouses of tortured activists to say, "Why have you brought this on yourself? On us? If you loved me you would put me before politics." The parents of torture survivors have been known to collude with the state by rejecting their own children and breaking up their families: "If you stay here, they'll come after us."

The return of a torture victim to a family can be overwhelming for everyone. A wife may have so much trouble coping with her own grief and anxiety and dealing with her spouse's altered personality that she can barely fulfill her role as wife and mother. And her response may, in turn, foster the survivor's feelings of guilt and shame. A vicious cycle is set in place, substituting for, or even erasing, the bonds that once defined family life. Other families in the community fear association with the threatened family. Through terror, forced emigration, and other secondary aspects of torture, even centuries-old communities can be broken down.

After such experiences, what can therapy offer to people subject to the tyrannies of social repression? According to many experts in this area,† psychotherapists trained to work with torture victims have much to offer. Therapy can help some survivors restore a sense of hope and dignity within weeks. It can reduce many of the pervasive aftereffects of torture—headaches, depression, extreme anxiety, irritability, intrusive thoughts, flashbacks, fatigue, phobias, concentration and memory problems, sleep and sexual difficulties—within a few months.

Torture typically locks its victims into a trancelike state, in which a narrow range of affects, a few overwhelming memories, and a sense of mistrust keep immediate contacts at a distance. Initially, the therapeutic relationship instills trust and helps the person, in a safe context, become progressively desensitized to the trauma of torture. Ultimately, the goal is to restore their fundamental sense of human dignity. Power must be placed in the hands of the victim to overcome the overwhelming suspiciousness that follows the experience of torture. The therapist serves as client advocate, consultant, and supporter during this process.

Allowing survivors to recall and retell—in safety—how they experienced each part of their brutalization is an important part of the desensitization process. Most experts‡ agree that promoting the normal expression of the affect—which had been prevented at the time of torture—produces a profound release. The "regression" or turning back, however, is kept brief and therapy returns as soon as possible to a focus on daily, pragmatic concerns.

The main goal of the progressive desensitization is to prevent survivors from either totally denying what has happened to them or from having unpredictable

---

†The reports by experts are based on personal communications (1984) with Dr. Inge Kemp Genefke, director of the first international torture treatment center in Denmark; Drs. Paz Rojas and Mario Inunzio, who treat torture victims in Chile; Tato Torres, director of La Posada, a San Francisco clinic treating survivors; and Dr. Jose Quiroga, a Chilean in exile who has taken testimony from hundreds of Chileans and Salvadorans.

‡The experts cited are listed in the preceding footnote.

rages or homicidal and suicidal impulses. For example, one man was taken in custody by the police in a rage after seeing his cousin shot to death in a fight about a parking space. This bizarre and terrifying event was similar enough to his experience of being tortured that it triggered his psychological disorganization. (Tato Torres, Personal Communication 1985).** Helping people monitor how much remembering and forgetting they can handle helps prevent this kind of unpredictable response to old memories.

To protect themselves psychologically, many torture victims dissociate from the experience. One man described it as "the mind hears and sees what is around it, but it is so busy keeping the body alive there is no energy to respond." Behavior like this is reminiscent of what Ernest Hilgrad identified in his trance research as a "hidden observer." In Hilgard's study, hypnotized subjects who submerged their hands in ice cold water did not feel pain although some part of them was fully aware of what was happening. Similarly, torture victims generally seem to be aware of a sense of terror and rage, but these feelings are witnessed rather than experienced. While maintaining this kind of psychological detachment can be a necessary survival tactic for torture victims, it may become a problem following their release. Until their "hidden observer" testifies and begins to cry out against and denounce their own torture, the spell of their trauma often remains in place, waiting to be catalyzed again.

FORCED EXILE

In their effort to stifle internal dissent and assert control over their populations, threatened regimes have found ways to move beyond directing repression at just individuals and families. In many countries, whole communities have become the target of their government's attempts to assert authority at any cost. In El Salvador, for example, 25 percent of the population has either been displaced inside the country or forced to leave it. It is as if the military had decided that to get rid of the fish (the guerillas), one must eliminate the water (the populace). When they believe that an area provides too much support to the government's enemies, the military will order an evacuation or conduct, what the El Salvadorans call, a "guinda." Survivors of a guinda return to find all their possessions destroyed—every utensil broken, their cattle killed, and all their crops and huts burned. The military calls these actions "clean-up" jobs.

If torture says, "I will render your inner self uninhabitable," the strategic displacement of a population says, "We will render your community uninhabitable and assault your basic sense of cultural identity." In a matter of hours, a way of life evolved over many generations can be shattered and a community's feeling of shared destiny devastated. Even if the remains of a community are collected, the new arrangement will never replace the old. Where familiarity once gave hope, a profound sense of loss pervades the life of the survivors. This deep experience of collective pain becomes incorporated into the new community, defining people's underlying view of the possibilities of their lives.

The most extreme form of displacement is being forced to leave one's homeland. Sometimes, as we hear of the terrible oppression people around the world face, we may wonder if it would not be easier for them just to leave. We might expect that people whose life has been threatened will find some relief just by being away from immediate danger. The reality is, of course, far more complicated. Paula, an El Salvadorean with whom I I spoke in a refugee camp in Costa Rica, who had fled her country with her mother and four children, said, "In El Salvador, I didn't have enough food, but at least I had my hut to live in. I knew my way. Even though I just lost my husband to the repression in El Salvador and I could have died, I want to return there."

The stress of leaving their familiar life behind facing the uncertainties of a new one overwhelm many exiles. Paula was suffering headaches and memory losses. Her sense of responsibility for her mother and small children was almost more than she could tolerate. Living in a strange, new environment, confronting a relentless flow of challenges each day, she would find herself staring off into space for great stretches of time and afterward she would be unable to remember what she was thinking. She felt she could not afford any more loss of control over her circumstances.

Pervasive Ambivalence

With the safety net of community torn away, exiles often find their life dominated by a kind of pervasive ambivalence. The war without is reproduced in a war within. Consider the case of Maria, a psychologist who had run afoul of the El Salvadorean military and was suspected of being a subversive. After receiving an anonymous telephoned death threat, she decided to leave El Salvador. Here is how she describes her departure:

> On Christmas day, my husband, four children, and I boarded the airplane in San Salvador for Costa Rica. We were told that take-off would be delayed for an hour. I thought I would die of an anxiety attack for fear I would be taken from the plane and "disappeared." Although I felt total release as the plane carried me toward Costa Rica, looking out over my country, as it got smaller and smaller filled me with an overwhelming sense of loss.

For Maria and millions like her, intense ambivalence about leaving their native country becomes part of family life in the new country. If children adjust too quickly or too well to the new circumstances, parents fear they are "allowing them to forget their homeland and their true cultural identity. At the same time, they want their children to feel at home in the adopted country. While in exile, many exist as if they are "on hold," living as if they were "neither here or there." The question becomes how to keep allegiance to the old country alive without letting grief preclude healthy adjustment into the new. But ambivalence pervades all relationships. Maria describes how their exile has shaped her relationship with her husband, Ricardo:

> Sometimes Ricardo and I are so full of grief we forget to notice the children. We don't even realize how depressed we've become. Sometimes I lock myself in the bathroom and cry because I know Ricardo is at his maximum grief and I'm afraid I'll break his spirit with mine.

Phillipe was an El Salvadorean doctor working in a Costa Rican refugee camp who also had been driven from his country by the military. Because he continued to work to build a rudimentory health-care system from exile, he still would not communicate with his family back in El Salvador without fearing for repraisal against them. One morning while I was on a visit to a refugee camp, I saw him pacing back and forth. "What's going on?" I asked him jokingly. "You look like a man expecting a baby."

"Last night I started really missing my children and my mother," he told me. "I couldn't stand it anymore. So I called my mother and I found out my father died two months ago. I never knew. There has been no way for me to have any communication with my family that I thought was safe, not even on the phone. I couldn't really say anything to her. I couldn't tell her where I was. I couldn't tell her what I was doing." Then Phillipe took out his wallet and showed me a little wrinkled piece of paper. With tears in his eyes, he said, "The last time I was in San Salvador, I went to see my children. On the doorstep of their mother's house that morning, the death squads had placed a cadaver. That was over three years ago. I never saw them since. This is the last letter I got from my daughter." In it, she begs him "Please, daddy, don't ever forget us." She also includes a poem:

> There is a man who loves the truth.
> Everybody loves this man because he speaks only the truth.
> But because he speaks the truth, he cannot see his children.
> Oh, this man, he is my father.

Protecting Others from Grief

Those who live in an exile community struggle to protect those around them from their own grief. Anna is a Nicaraguan woman who is a member of a community of 400 persons who fled as a group to avoid massacre in El Salvador and were granted ownership of a plot of land. Every day, she and two or three other women prepare the tortillas and one cup of beans per person, which is the staple of the diet of the community. The civil war had cut her off from her national roots, and also separated her from her two sons, who were unwilling to leave the country. She was constantly worried about them. "Worry is all over the community," she told me. Most people had lost somebody before the "guinda" or had left somebody, and everyone missed their homeland. As we talked, she ground her fist into the hollow of her stomach with the same motion she knuckled cornmeal and water against the smoothed oval stone. She was so frail, it seemed her fist would come out through her back.

"Why do you do that?" I asked.

"It hurts, it hurts me," she said.

"Is there anything that makes it hurt less?"

"Yes sometimes I have cried . . . but we do not do this."

She was explaining to me not only a Salvadorean value, but also the way exiles around the world, even those living in the same community, experience their isolation from one another. Just as Maria hid from Ricardo to keep her supply of tears from flooding the household, so Anna contained her tears from dampening the community spirit.

"Isn't the water in the creek below the water of God?" I asked her.

"Yes, of course," she smiled sadly.

"And that water must flow to remain fresh. Isn't that why you move that big rock away after you wash the clothes there and let the children play there? And, aren't tears water? Then tears, too, are the water of God, and, in the dark of night, they may flow also, to cleanse and purify."

Like all Salvadoreans I met, Anna truly appreciated that a North American cared about her plight. But it remained unclear what to do with feelings automatically awakened by repression and how to find ways for the community to share pain without becoming only a culture of pain. Until these questions could be answered, crying in private might be the only way to help relieve excess pain.

THE FAMILY'S ROLE IN HEALING

Family therapists working with the survivors of torture must evaluate the advantages and disadvantages of involving families in their therapy. If bringing in family members will lead to blaming the survivor or touching off political antagonisms, caution must be used in how best to involve them. The secondary effect of the torture on the family may be harder for the person to deal with than the torture itself.

Generally, however, family support makes a very significant difference in the success of therapy. Sometimes a family is invited in a session to return to their memory of when the torture survivor was arrested in order to highlight how the family's like and attitude towards the world changed in the interim. One family became so paranoid after a son's arrest that they began guarding the windows and, for the next month, did not leave their home before dark. Their deeply entrenched suspiciousness was rooted in this first assault against them. Only by sharing this moment of fear again in the safety of the therapeutic relationship were they able to begin to challenge their social isolation. (Tato Torres, Personnel Communication, 1985).

As with any tragic loss—like the death of a child—the patterns developed in response to the immediate trauma can crystallize, leading to future problems in the marriage or between other siblings. It is important to identify and challenge these patterns and help survivors tell their stories to their families, to overcome both the family's fear of hearing them and the survivor's fear of talking about the awful things done to them. This process helps the individual become part of the family again. It also progressively desensitizes the family to the terror. Torture becomes a shared family problem. The torture is let out of the dark box of the individual's memories. In the light of day, it begins to be seen for what it is—a social violation of a community.

One young Salvadoran exile living in the United States had lapsed into repeated fits of violence after hearing that the military had killed his father.

Although they had not expressed it directly, his two uncles, with whom the young man lived, felt their nephew had caused his own torture by foolishly opposing the military government. Once the therapist, Tato Torres, enabled the nephew to describe his experience to them, their whole reaction changed. Later, the therapist helped them set up a symbolic funeral for the father at a Bay area church. In building stronger bonds between this young man and his relatives, the therapy offered an antidote to the nephew's guilt and isolation. The young man was also encouraged to increase phone contacts to relatives in exile in Guatemala, giving him a position of increased centrality and purpose in maintaining connections between the remnants of his kin system.

The family members of torture victims sometimes need individual attention, such as a wife overloaded with grief or a child manifesting symptoms. A child of one torture survivor became socially aggressive and eneuretic, but after one session with a pediatrician, her symptom was gone for good. "Who made your Daddy get tortured?," asked the pediatrician. "I did," the girl explained. "Some relatives told me so." After she was assured by her parents that it was untrue, her symptoms cleared up. Obviously, in other cases, symptoms will persist longer, but issues of responsibility and culpability are worth looking into as soon as the family is ready.

Healing and Community

To counter the social isolation and the social demotion of the survivor, most therapies of torture victims include some form of public testimony. Initially, the victim tells his story to a tape recorder—as the "neutral" listener or recipient. This gives the survivor complete control over the event. The tape is then typed up and the transcript can be used for social and political purposes—from helping the survivor personally get asylum, to supporting broader human rights work, to providing the basis for speeches to religious or other concerned groups. In this way, the survivor is hierarchically elevated over the torturer and also permitted some revenge, as part of the natural healing process.

Whatever the therapy used, treatment entails establishing relationships in which one respectfully helps survivors remember what happened to them and recognize techniques employed upon them. In this way, persons who had been reduced to a preverbal, disorganized state, give voice to precisely what was done to them. In their testimony to family and society, they take control over the terrible experience and shame their torturers. The victim is elevated above the torturer who transgressed the victim's humanity. Therapy transforms what has turned inward, becoming a private, festering, self-absorbed process, into a public event of shared social concern. In this way the spell of "I am damaged" can be challenged in the context of a new message: "The social process dominating me was and is deranged."

The successfully treated survivor can never simply return to being the person he or she was before torture. Torture of the kind we have examined, like many traumas, changes a person. Although unsettling thoughts will continue to recur, total anxiety need not pervade the survivor's life. Guilt may persist, but it is not the dominant or sole state of which the person is capable. Research shows that the loss of a child is always recalled with intensity, which, to observers at least, looks like that of a fresh loss. Torture may affect a person on that level—the wound, the loss, is always there. But life goes on around it. And as one young torture survivor put it, "The business of being alive is related to the necessity of overcoming those experiences."

HELPING EXILES

Exiles need help in finding ways to share and transform their sorrow. For the therapists who work with them, it is important not to operate from a pathology model. Whatever mode of therapy that is applied, it is crucial to ensure that individuals and families do not mistake their pain for an indication that something is wrong with them.

One of the things that must be addressed is how to bear pain, sometimes of a genocidal proportion. It is helpful to read diaries of Holocaust survivors, and of those who did not survive, if only to deepen our sensitivity to the depth of losses at hand. Etty Hillesum (1981), two years before she was killed in Aushweitz, wrote:

> You must be able to bear your sorrow, even if it seems to crush you, you will be able to stand up again . . . and your sorrow must become an integral part of yourself, part of your body and your soul if everyone bears his grief honestly and courageously, the sorrow that now fills the world will abate. (p. 100)

The exile often needs help to find a livable view of his or her suffering. As part of learning to bear pain is learning how to share it, catharsis is a vehicle for further problem solving among exiles.

One theme I used in working with an exile group is a metaphor of mobilizing oneself. Just as one must "mobilize one's troops" in combat, one must mobilize, discipline, and organize one's "inner troops" (feeling, memories, ideas) to fight the struggle for survival in exile. Deadening of the senses through repression or displacement only serves the repressive regime. People who fail to mobilize, who no longer care about things like social justice, can be contained more easily by the prevailing order. Grieving for what is lost and finding even simple things to do to, at least bear witness to the old life that has been stolen, helps people "mobilize their inner troops."

In one group I led, some people thought they would plant a tree in honor of someone back home they loved, others decided to compose yet another song of resistance, create a painting, or write a poem. Still others dedicated themselves to working with political causes. These may seem like small gestures, but it is important to realize that rushing to quick solutions to nearly exhausting problems may lead to disappointment and failure.

It is also important to help people distinguish between conflicts caused by social repression and those that are related to other issues. One man in the exile group explained that he had been divorced shortly before he fled. Empathically,

I asked whether the terror had affected his marriage. "No," he smiled, "just a bad marriage!" Another couple had been torn apart by their flight. The wife had not wanted to leave even though their courtyard had become an open graveyard where buzzards fed on the bodies of relatives killed by the military. When this mother of eight arrived in Costa Rica, however, she became involved in serving the exile community and attained a social status she had never had before, The husband, a hard-working farmer, was suddenly transformed into a useless cipher. In the two years of exile, he turned to alcohol and became abusive. They needed help to separate their marital differences from the terror that had exacerbated their troubles.

Culture differences also pose a challenge. When we were thinking of uniquely Salvadoran ways to solve a marital conflict role played in the seminar, one woman, formerly an English teacher, told me of her priest's technique. A woman complained that every day when her husband would come home from work, he would yell at her. Then she would yell at him, and a brawl would ensue. The priest asked her to wait a moment. He returned with a bottle of "holy water." "Go home. Fifteen minutes before your husband is to come from work, fill your mouth with holy water, hold it in your mouth for 30 minutes, and may God be with you." She did. The priest did not hear from her for a month. When she returned, she was desperate. "Didn't the holy water help?" the priest asked. "Yes, Father," she said. "Once I have a mouth full of holy water, he immediately calms down. But please, I ran out, and I am afraid it will all start up again." With exiles especially, we can be more effective if we find out about existing approaches within their own culture and religion.

The field of psychotherapy has realized that what goes on in people's heads reflects family difficulties and even economic difficulties. Now we are faced with the responsibility of going even further and looking at the immediate effects of a country's political climate on people's fantasies, trances, and family relationships. As therapists, we can help some survivors of state violence by encouraging family members to be supportive and helping them find community resources. But millions of cases will not get to us, leaving people like Patricia Jonas and her family endangered beyond clinical repair.

REFERENCES

Amnesty International (1984). *Torture in the 80's*, Bath, England: Titman Press.
Genefke, I. (1984), Personal communication.
Hillesum, E. (1981). *An Interrupted life: The diaries of Etty Hillesum, 1941–1943* (translation). New York: Washington Square Press.

**Torres, T. (1985), Personnel Communications.

15

LEGACY OF SLAVERY: THE EXPERIENCE OF BLACK FAMILIES IN AMERICA*

Elaine Pinderhughes, M.S.W.

Dilemma, duality, contradiction, confusion, entrapment, craziness, schizophrenic existence—such are the words that have been used to characterize the reality of Black people's experience in America since slavery. Not long ago, a social work student in a class exploring how to work with Black families asked in desperation, "How can I help Black families when I feel so helpless myself?" On another occasion, a well-known family therapist made the comment: "The problem in working with Black families is that the therapists feel incompetent because they get as overwhelmed as the families." "Black" does, indeed, mean another level of complexity.

I learned that the hard way. I worked for seven years at a well-known child guidance clinic where using a White middle-class model, I worked with clients who were White middle-class and poor. Even though I was Black. I did not think seriously about how it was different to work with Black families. I sealed it off in order to do my work. As it got to be the late 1960s and I was forced, along with others, to think about it, to consider what Blackness was, and what Black meant, I decided to take a job at another child guidance center in the Black community.

I learned the hard way the differences in working with Black families—the stress it can involve, the exhaustion one can feel. I experienced all of those consequences: confusion, dilemma, contradiction, entrapment, and craziness. And I have been struggling ever since to process what became an unforgettably painful experience for me.

*In this discussion, "Black" families will refer to families of African descent whose ancestors were slaves. This term will be used interchangeably with "Afro-Americans."

ISSUES FACING PRACTITIONERS: BLACK CULTURE AND THE SOCIETAL PROJECTION PROCESS

Looking back, I would describe this exhaustion I felt, this helplessness the student felt, the sense of being overwhelmed that the family therapist felt, as related to the fact that training has failed to prepare practitioners in two vital areas: conceptualizing Black culture and understanding societal projection.

Black Culture

Our efforts to help Black families were seriously hampered by the fact that we did not even consider Black culture as an issue. Culture in general was almost universally ignored at that time, so that in the field of mental health there was little effort expended to define and understand it. What has now become clear is that efforts to work with families must take into account the fact that culture which is manifest in peoples' values, norms, behavioral practices and ways of living represents people's adaptation to the political, economic, and social realities they face (Navarro, 1980). Understanding these realities and the culture developed is critical because the goal of helping families must include assistance in coping with these realities. As a Black person, I certainly had some ideas about what Black culture was, but I soon discovered that my perceptions, which had developed as a result of growing up in Washington, D.C., did not apply to all Blacks. Instead, my perceptions applied only to those who, like me, were middle class and had lived a substantial part of their lives behind the walls of segregation. In some ways, too, my perceptions had validity only as my personal experience.

Since my perception of what constitutes Black culture was too narrow, I turned to the experts. To my amazement, I found little agreement among them. It was hard to find two experts who agreed on a definition of Black culture. I learned there were very good reasons for this enigma. First of all, the notion of ethnicity is a complex one. But understanding Black culture and Black as ethnic involves yet another level of complexity. Blacks are the only ethnic group whose cultural designation in this country centers completely on race. Caucasians or White ethnics are identified mainly by nationality (e.g., Irish-American) or religion. Even other people of color, such as Asians, are referred to as hyphenated Americans, for example Chinese-American. Only American Black people are referred to by race. Furthermore, race is a biological, not a cultural, designation, but as a result of experiences in our society, race has taken on a cultural meaning.

The dynamics of race in American culture have operated such that stereotyping based on biological differences has become the basis for status assignment and the erection of societal structures that have created a power differential between Whites and people of color. These social structures, which become a significant part of the realities faced by people of color, affect their life chances, life-styles, and quality of life, and those of Whites as well. Over time, the effects of the social structure not only compound and exaggerate biological differences but also lead to the creation of coping responses that acquire cultural meaning. For the culture of American Blacks, whose beginnings and ongoing reality in this country have been unique, the dynamics of race have had great significance. This uniqueness is manifest in the joke that Afro-Americans are the only ethnic group that was invited to come to America, and also had ships ready to escort them and a reception committee with jobs waiting upon arrival. The invitation, the escort, the reception, and the subsequent occupational "opportunities" occurred under conditions of extreme force and were engineered for the benefit of persons other than Afro-Americans. The powerlessness that has characterized these beginnings in America has continued to dominate their lives, becoming interwoven into the social fabric of America as institutionalized racism as well as a critical factor in the responses of Blacks to racism.

In trying to conceptualize Black culture as a response to the societal realities faced by people, I learned that historians disagree about the reality and consequences of slavery, the first condition of powerlessness that greeted the ancestors of Afro-Americans upon their arrival. Although these conditions varied and were dependent on many factors, the following have been identified as significant to the powerlessness that characterized slavery (Billingsley, 1968):

1. The disengagement from African cultural roots.
2. The deliberate separation of persons with the same tribal connections.
3. Massive disruption of previous cultural forms and substitution of slave practices that were cruel and inhuman, including:
   a. View of the slave as chattel, inferior, childlike, and worthy of degredation.
   b. The lack of protection for marriage.
   c. The breakup of the family during slave sales.
   d. Denial to the male of his traditional role as protector and provider for his family.
   e. Sexual abuse of the woman and use of her as breeder.
   f. Demand of absolute control and obedience, including control over all communication.
   g. Legal prohibition against education.
   h. Forced training to be dependent, submissive, and fearful of the master, and to regard self as inferior.

After emancipation, the socioeconomic conditions in America continued to reinforce social, political, and economic powerlessness for most Afro-americans. Data show, however, that despite the threat to family life that slavery had posed, 90 percent of all Afro-American children were born in wedlock (Staples, 1978). Struggling to build a better life, Afro-Americans created and strengthened support systems such as the extended family, the church, lodges, fraternities, neighborhood associations, and other forms of mutual aid societies (Franklin, 1967). However, they were persistently frustrated and undermined in these attempts by the racism and repression of the late 19th and early 20th centuries, which have been identified by some historians as the "most explicitly racist era of American history" (Staples, 1978). In competition for jobs and other resources with the large numbers of White ethnics now pouring into the country, Afro-

Americans were neither supported nor protected by the American social system. Instead, they were deprived of opportunities for education, employment, and other resources. These resources were available to most White ethnics and thus facilitated their full participation in the mainstream. Moreover, the attempts of Afro-Americans to protest these injustices and to advocate for their rights were met by violence and reprisals (Comer, 1972). Economic survival was precarious and large numbers of uneducated and unskilled Blacks sought to eke out an existence as servants sharecroppers, laborers, and strike breakers.

In the 20th century, another level of powerlessness was introduced by the destructive forces of urbanization and industrialization that have pushed large numbers of Afri-Americans into urban centers to seek a better life and some measure of economic independence. Here, their major structure for survival, the extended and nuclear family, has been profoundly threatened as evidenced in the increase in broken families, one-parent families, male-female antagonisms, violence, and child abuse, alcoholism, and drug abuse.

The stress of the ongoing economic, social, and political powerlessness that has characterized reality for Afro-Americans has been magnified by its systemic nature: denial of access to resources reduces the opportunity for acquisition of skills and employment and threatens the opportunity to develop self-esteem and to function adequately in the family role. The consequent poverty and strain on family role cause problems in individual growth and development. Poverty and other resultant problems in individual functioning stress the community system, which is the expected source of support for individuals and families. The community system is stressed by poverty and problems in individual functioning at the same time that it has fewer resources (schools, jobs, housing), thus becoming disorganized, a breeder of crime and other social pathology, and itself a creator of powerlessness (Soloman, 1976). It is important to understand tht the skills and strengths needed to cope with these political, economic, and social forces are dependent upon those very political, economic, and social forces that cause the powerlessness.

Societal Projection Process

The systemic nature of societal victimization has been noted by Bowen (1978) in his discussion of the societal projection process. This process enables one group in society, the benefactors, to perceive and treat another group as inferior and incompetent. Through the use of projection upon the victims, the benefactors are able to relieve tension and reduce anxiety in themselves. Bowen lists among the victims of the societal porojection process minorities, mental patients, alcoholics, criminals, and the poor. He notes:

> These groups fit the best criteria for long-term anxiety-relieving projection. They are vulnerable to become the pitiful objects of the benevolent, oversympathetic segment of society that improves its functioning at the expense of the pitiful. Just as the least adequate child in a family can become more impaired when he becomes an object of pity and oversympathetic help from the family, so can the lowest segment of society be chronically impaired by the very attention designed to help. No matter how good the principle behind such programs, it is essentially impossible

to implement them without the built-in complications of the projection process. Such programs attract workers who are oversympathetic with less fortunate people. They automatically put the recipients in a "one down" inferior position and they either keep them there or get angry at them. (pp. 444–445)

I thus hypothesize that Afro-Americans, as victims of the societal projection process, have been trapped in positions of relative powerlessness where, confined and prevented from full participation in the mainstream, they have served as a balancing mechanism for the American social system. In this role, they have provided stability for Whites, who, as beneficiaries of the projection process, have been able to channel the larger system's tension, conflict, contradiction, and confusion away from their communities and into that of the victims. For confirmation, we need only look at inner-city barrio or ghetto communities. Residents are forced to struggle with poverty, drugs, crime, and inadequacy, disorganization, or absence of necessary services while suburbia enjoys relative safety, peace, tranquility, and organization. The cultural response to living with the consequent conflict, contradition, confusion, and powerlessness inherent in this position has been a major factor in the individual and family functioning of Afro-Americans.

Defining Black Culture

Experts disagree as to the nature as well as the source of Afro-American culture. Some assert it has been heavily influenced by African values and cultural practices. They point to the folk beliefs and the emphasis on family, high spirituality, art, and music. The practices that *have* endured have persisted under conditions of cultural and psychological cutoff. Charles Pinderhughes demonstrated the enigma of Black culture in a rather dramatic fashion through an experiment he conducted at a conference for cross-cultural training in psychiatry:* He asked everyone in the group to stand up. He then directed everyone who was White to go to one side of the room, those who were Black to the other side, and others to the rear. There were 30 Whites, 30 Blacks, and nine Asians. Then he asked all who knew the country, language, and religion of their ancestors to sit down. All nine Asians sat down. Twenty-eight of the 30 Whites sat down. Only four of the 30 Blacks sat down. He then took out a card and read two hypthoses:

1. The only Blacks who would sit down would be from Africa or the Caribbean, or would be members of the Haley or Vaughn families (who have traced their ancestry back to Africa).
2. The only Whites who would not sit down would be orphans.

He found that of the four Blacks who sat down, two were West Indians from the Caribbean and two were members of the Vaughn family. Of the two Whites who remained standing, both knew the country, language, and religion of one parent but not the other: One person's father had died while the person was an infant and the other, born out of wedlock, knew nothing of his father.

While the debate concerning the survival of African values and practices in the culture of American Blacks continues, exercises such as this one dramatically demonstrate the cutoff for persons who, with rare exceptions, know little or nothing about their ancestors or ethnic origins.

The cutoff from African roots, along with other conditions mentioned above, have been critical factors in the cultural adaptations developed by Blacks. The current emphasis on Blackness is an effort to reinforce, reclaim, or revise African cultural practices such as affiliation and collectivity as well as an effort to identify the valiant and positive attempts to deal with the fragmentation and lack of cohesiveness that have been so typical of their entrapment. Variability in both experience and adaptive strategies have prevented the development of consolidated effects to alter the oppression and entrapment experienced by Blacks.

I saw, then, three sources of Black culture: (1) African cultural practices that may have survived, (2) American culture, and (3) responses developed to cope with the victim system—societal projection process. All of these cultural systems, with different value orientations that Blacks share in differing combinations, account for the complexity and diversity found among them and for the conflict in values that plagues them. The solutions to value conflict which are recommended by experts have not been available to Blacks. They include: (1) identifying exclusively with one's own ethnic subculture and remaining isolated from the American mainstream; (2) becoming completely "Americanized," and thus renouncing the subculture by joining the "melting pot"; or (3) integrating the two options (Papajohn & Spiegel, 1975). But identification for Blacks is *not* a matter of choice because they are *never* completely admitted to Americanization and cannot easily assume an identity that is *not validated* by others (White Americans) who share it. They are left with two options: (1) to remain isolated from the mainstream (where cultural prescriptions are based on African residuals and victim system adaptations—a choice of many), or (2) to *exist in a state of biculturality*, which means relating to both cultures but being unable to integrate them. This foot-in-both-worlds approach means that Blacks remain permanently in a condition that is only transitory for White ethnics. Numerous authors have identified and discussed this nearly universal adaptation of Afro-Americans. It has been viewed as a state of affairs that can sometimes take an extensive toll in the form of conflict or create amazing strength (Knowles & Previtt, 1969). Biculturality is identified as a primary coping mechanism for warding off the inconsistency, injustice, and oppression of the "victim" system, resulting in a "psychological unity for the adequately functioning individual" (Chestang, 1972). It is only one of the mechanisms adopted by Black families to cope with the powerlessness, contradition, and confusion of being tension relievers and anxiety relievers in the society projection process.

With some recognition of the complexities that characterize the reality of Black culture, and of the societal projection process as the context for my work as a family therapist. I began better to understand how that process maintains my Black clients in a one-down position where they function as stabilizers and circuit breakers for the tension, conflict, contradictions and confusion that have existed within the larger social system. I also began to better understand my fatigue and exhaustion and the sense of powerlessness that grips us as practitioners, when, in treating Black families, we also become enmeshed in the systemic process that has so entrapped them. And I could see further that the situation had profound implications for my clients and for me as both beneficiary (i.e., middle class) and victim (Black and female).

UNDERSTANDING POWER DYNAMICS AS A CRITICAL FACTOR IN CULTURAL PROCESS: IMPLICATIONS FOR TREATMENT

Things become somewhat clearer when I begin to see that the victim system projection process that entraps my client and me is really a one-down, one-up power system. Work with Black families is thus conceptualized as empowerment to cope with this one-down position. Enpowerment means being able to manage the stress of this position, find ways to turn that powerlessness into power, and to achieve some reasonable control over their destiny—relative freedom from this position of entrapment.

Conceptualization and Definition of Power Dynamics

In using this formulation, some basic notions about power in general must be kept in mind. I define power as the ability to exert influence for one's own benefit on the forces that affect one's life space. Powerlessness is the inability to exert such influence. While power is a dirty word which people avoid thinking about it operates on all the levels of human functioning. There is power in terms of (1) status—social role and racial status, class status, ethnic status, gender status; (2) individual function, that is, a sense of mastery and a sense of control over one's own behavior; and (3) interactive behavior, that is, dominance, submission, and so forth. Power, or powerlessness on any one of these levels can reinforce its existence on any other. At the same time, a sense of power is vital to mental health. "A feeling of controlling one's destiny to some reasonable extent is the essential, psychological component of all aspects of life" (Basch, 1975, p. 419). A sense of power thus becomes a major issue in mental health. Powerlessness is painful; no one wants to be powerless and everyone seeks to defend against it by behavior that brings a sense of power (McClelland, 1975).

In using a power dynamics formulation of treatment, I have to keep in mind that since culture is a response to the political, economic, and social realities Blacks have faced, their responses (values, social roles, norms, family sytles, etc.) have represented efforts to get a sense of power. This understanding of culture and power allows appreciation for the creativity and complexity involved in their responses and of the rich and varied subtleties and nuances of responses (Pinderhughes, in press; Green, 1982). At the same time, we must recognize that some of these behaviors, while bringing a momentary sense of power, create a greater sense of powerlessness at a later point or in another aspect of functioning. These ideas can be used in work with Black families to help them grow and deal with their paradoxical position. It is first helpful to identify what is needed to cope with these realities faced by Black people and to clarify the kind of functioning they need to have. This information will provide guidelines for treatment.

Defining Healthy Black Families

Healthy Black families have been described by numerous experts. Hill (1972) described them as having: high achievement orientation, strong kinship bonds, high work orientation, flexibility in roles, and strong, religious orientation. In terms of family structure and functioning, healthy Black families have strong, flexible boundaries; values that support cooperation and negotiation and at the same time facilitate toughness and strength. Structure and process are marked by a high degree of organization and self-differentiation in members, effective leadership, the ability to communicate clearly and to negotiate, the ability to tolerate differences in values and perceptions among members and to function biculturally, as well as the capacity to build and use strong support systems such as the extended family. Development of these characteristics is the goal in my effort to empower Black familes. Some families have been able to develop these characteristics and to secure for themselves the external and internal resources needed to maintain them. What becomes clear, however, is that these mechanisms are in constant jeopardy of being undermined as their existence is dependent upon the very forces that they must struggle against.

The flexibility of a family's boundaries is critical. Families need connection to the outside world, to other systems that are nourishing and protective. Thus, an isolated Black family is in real trouble. We know that any isolated family is in trouble because every family needs support and cultural connectedness. However, when a Black family is disconnected, it not only is without supports, but it is at the mercy of systemic forces—racism and oppression. For such families, racism and oppression constitute another level of powerlessness that is not there for White families. Not only must the outside systems be supportive to enable management of the stress of their position, but the boundaries of the family must be flexible enough to let in supplies that are nutritive and to keep out noxious influences. As the family closes off to protect itself from noxious external influences, it becomes vulnerable to rigidity, so that even if there is a source of support, the family cannot use it. The opposite effect can also occur when the family, in its struggle to extract some nurturance the environment, maintains boundaries that are too open so that there is no discrimination of noxious forces and no protection against them. As social workers, we are all familiar with such families who have numerous human service workers moving freely in and out of their midst.

Thus, rigidity in function, where boundaries are either overly open or closed, represent an attempt to get needed supplies and to cope with environmental failures (and thus the powerlessness, contradiction, confusion, etc.). But overly open or closed boundaries, solutions though they may be, can lead to other problems as they reinforce vulnerability in the family's internal structure and process: with rules, roles, communication, and so on. The systemic nature of family dynamics is such that a problem in one component of family structure and process can cause problems in the functioning of any other. Thus, for example, rigid boundaries, that cause isolation of the family can cause problems with rules, roles, communication, affect relationships, and the like. Guerin and Pendagast (1976) discuss the way in which isolation affects emotional processes within the family, creating fused relationships:

> It is important to document social and familial isolation because it can create an emotional cocoon that intensifies emotional processes in the nuclear family, and significantly limits the relationships available to dissipate anxiety and emotional duties. (p. 452)

We must also recognize that although the values of cooperation, togetherness, and affiliation that many Black families adopt facilitate the cohesive functioning necessary to cope with a hostile outside world, they can have the opposite effect if they become exaggerated under stress and lead to lack of autonomy and poor self-differentiation. At the same time, very different values may also embraced: strength, cunning, toughness, struggle, winning. The competitive stance, one-up behavior, and emphasis on winning that can stem from these behaviors can be understood as critical strategies to deal with realities faced by Black families.

For Black people winning means not being powerless and trapped. In the attempt to solve problems and create a sense of power, the family's emphasis on struggle, toughness, and the like, can create other problems such as the tendency toward ongoing struggles and escalating conflict in relationships that can interfere with the development of the needed harmony, sensitivity, and vulnerability. Thus as noted earlier, other problems in the family's structure and process are reinforced. Struggle and toughness also conflict with values of affiliativeness and cooperation. These contradictory sets of values again reflect the contradictory and paradoxical position of Blacks in the American social system.

Moreover, when a family has been excessively victimized, family members may adopt values that emphasize autonomy (e.g., doing it oneself, going it alone), which is adaptive to coping with powerlessness and achieving a sense of power but is maladaptive for enhancing cooperation and cohesiveness. This autonomy does not stem from the American values of individualsm and independence but from a sense of aloneness and a feeling that there is no help anywhere. Aponte (1976) identified these dynamics and demonstrated appropriate solutions in a case where he was working with a mother and several teenagers and latency-aged children, one of whom was the identified client who had been referred for "acting out in school." Aponte began by asking what was going on in the family. He learned that the mother worked hard all day, then came home to clean, and do other household tasks. Showing his empathy for her predicament, he let her know that it sounded overwhelming and asked why her children did not help her. She responded that she had tried to get them to, but they would not. He then asked her to show him how she asked them to help her and found that she did not know how to ask. Her experience in growing up had been extremely depressing. Alone, isolated, without supports, she had learned to function by doing everything herself. This autonomy had been adaptive for her at that time but meant she did not expect or know how to acquire help from her children or others. The remainder of the treatment involved showing her how to delegate responsibility to the teenagers, who, in turn, delegated tasks to the younger ones. He also coached the mother on how to approach the school on behalf of one of the teenagers who was about to drop out. The mother expected not to be heard or respected and felt that she did not have the skills to intervene. Aponte described this family's structure as underorganized. Rigid and stuck in developmental arrest as a result of the stresses upon them, this family had never developed the differentiation and organization needed to cope with stress. In our interventions, we must respect the behaviors clients have used as having been adaptive but teach them other behaviors that will not be as costly.

Issues with power and conflict are another problematic aspect of family structure and process. Although healthy Black families are known to have a high proportion of egalitarian relationships, it is my contention that such families also have strong supports and other mechanisms supporting this function. I hypothesize that the victim societal projection process system creates responses that support nonegalitarian relationships. We have already seen how developing harmonious relationships can be jeopardized by exaggerated emphasis on struggle, toughness, and power, and how this reinforces conflicts. One widely recognized way of managing conflict is the strategy of dominance-submission. Bowen (1978) states:

> One of the commonest mechanisms is one in which the two pseudo-selves fuse into a common self, one going up a pseudo-self to merger and the other gaining a higher level of functioning of self from their merger. This avoids conflict and permits more closeness. The dominant one who gains self is often not aware of the problems of the adaptive one who gives in. (p. 476)

But dominance-submission, as Bowen points out, also makes one vulnerable to lowered self-differentiation, and hence lessens the ability to cope with stress.

There are other complex and confusing coping behaviors utilized by persons whose realities have been characterized by contradictions and powerlessness. They may try to gain a sense of power by embracing, in an exaggerated way, the negative stereotypes of themselves, as being a superstud, supercrazy, or superdependent. The powerlessness one may feel is neutralized by taking the initiative to exaggerate the stereotype. I remember a client who feigned being dumb. Although the results of her psychological testing indicated above-average intelligence, she embraced the stereotype of stupidity to an extreme. My efforts to encourage her to change her behavior met with failure and I found that I had a headache after every session. In acting dumb, she not only was taking the initiative, but she also created a sense of powerlessness in me. There is often little appreciation of these dynamics and the adaptive nature of this behavior. McClelland (1975) suggests that dependency can be a way of getting close to the source of power.

> They are dependent because it makes them feel strong to be near a source of strength. Strictly speaking, there is no such thing as a need for dependency, a need to feel weak and dependent; what is sometimes described as a need for dependency is the act of being dependent or weak, which has as its goal feeling strong. (p. 15)

A sense of power at all costs is the goal. One mother jokingly described how she had handled her irritation at her son's rebelliousness. She counseled him that if he was going to be a sonofabitch, he should be the best there is. Her jesting message to get a sense of power at all costs was taken literally: he became a drug addict, and eventually died from an overdose. Once again, strategies devised to get a sense of power can lead to more problems: powerlessness, imprisonment, addiction, and being a slave to drugs.

Put-downs and power behavior can become a way of life for persons who have been extremely victimized. One mother told her social worker: "Easter's coming. And when they get all dressed up they get uppity and have to get a beating before the day is over."

This mother's oversensitivity to power behavior in her children was such that any assertion was interpreted as "uppityness" that must be eradicated. The problems this stance creates for self-esteem and a positive sense of self for the children (and for the mother) are obvious.

These are ways to manage the intense rage that stems from the sense of powerlessness. But when these behaviors are rigidly embraced, which often happens in the struggle of Blacks to deal with their paradoxical position, interpersonal conflict is reinforced along with an inability to be tender, vulnerable, or sensitive.

Deception is another behavior that can be confusing to others but is used to get a sense of power. This is a strategy that has been used by the Irish (McGoldrick, 1985) and other groups with extensive experience of oppression. Black people have used deception in communication since the days of slavery. Their use of a patois that outsiders do not understand is well documented. Less clear is the strategy of changing meanings and turning things around. For example, "bad" means good and "nigger," a term signifying degradation, is often used to indicate affection. This achieves power because initiative has been taken to alter its generally accepted negative meaning, thus undermining the powerlessness and entrapment its generally accepted usage had brought.

Middle-Class Families

A conceptualization of the effects of the societal projection victim system upon middle-class families must take into account the fact that most have more resources, knowledge, and skill in developing coping strategies than do the Afro-American poor. However, they do not completely escape the victim system and their family life may be significantly different from that of White middle-class families. Harris (1980) notes the following characteristics of Afro-American middle-class families: They are strongly oriented to self-determination, to empowerment in such areas as education and employment policies; they have a strong sense of identity as Afro-Americans and identify with such American values as achievement and competition. Tending to be nuclear rather than extended, usually composed of no more than four or five persons, they "interact with and are influenced by both the Afro-American community and wider society," which leads to a duality in values and life-styles. Harris continues:

This difference in life-style between the Black comunity in which Black families are rooted psychologically, regardless of where they reside physically, and the wider society, in which they must also participate, places an extremely heavy demand on the Black family in effort to adapt to both systems. (p. 171).

In coping with their paradoxical position in the social system, they have relied heavily on social support systems, such as extended family, friends, church, clubs, and other activities that provide a sense of belonging and a sense of protection. They have also developed other adaptive responses which include flexible roles, egalitarian decision making, ambitious striving, and encouragement of children to achieve. But when under stress, they, too, are liable to rigidity or disorganization. Moreover, attempts to cope with the stressors can lead to exaggerated behavior where "hard work can easily slip into driven dedication, strength into abuse of power, persistence into stubbornness, flexibility into inconsistency and caution into immobilization" (Pinderhughes, 1986, p. 59).

Intense, exchaustive efforts must often be exerted to maintain middle-class status, which partly accounts for the prevalence of health problems among middle-class Blacks. Awareness of the significance of education in the maintenance of their position creates high anxiety about their children's performance in school, the adequacy of the school, and so on. Their task is formidable: raising children to be cautious and strong in a hostile environment; maintaining loving, caring relationships marked by tenderness, sensitivity, and the ability to be vulnerable in the face of stressors that could evoke power behavior; and functioning with competence as providers and protectors in the face of ongoing undermining of these roles.

Most vulnerable to conflict is the male-female relationship where defensive maneuvers to deal with powerlessness and acquire a sense of power can have disastrous consequences. Rapidly rising rates of divorce and one-parent families among this group have caused one expert to declare: "The very survival of the Black family is being threatened and the survival of Black children is becoming more and more doubtful" (Rodgers-Rose, 1980, p. 40). Disruption in their protective support systems also cause Afro-American middle-class families to experience great difficulties (Harris & Balpogal, 1980; MacAdoo, 1971). Thus, a move to a different locality or the nonavailability of support for whatever reason leaves the family isolated and more vulnerable. Common among this group is relocation due to educational and economic opportunities. MacAdoo (1978) discusses the strain on the newly arrived middle-class nuclear family where achievement may stress ties with the extended family and old support systems. The newly arrived family may be pressured by having to provide resources for those "left behind" or may feel forced to engage in an emotional cutoff to protect itself.

As noted earlier, a major issue for middle-class families is biculturality. In this context the middle-class adolescent's task of establishing a clear sense of adult identity is compounded by the paradoxes, contradictions, and dualities that the victim system has created. The family is clearly at risk and vulnerable to struggles, stress, and problematic solutions if there is not enough external support, or if the family leadership is not unusually strong, wise, and flexible.

CLINICAL STRATEGIES

As earlier stated, healthy families have supportive networks, and the structure to utilize these supports, are cohesive and experience relative harmony among its members, utilize conflict-resolving mechanisms, and have flexible roles, clear rules, and clear communication. I have also shown how Black families' positions as tension reducers and anxiety reducers in the larger social system have created cultural responses to the ensuing powerlessness that jeopardize the ability of Black families to acquire and maintain healthy functioning. These characteristics of a healthy family, however, will guide treatment strategies so as to empower the family to reach these goals.

The magnitude of the task cannot be underestimated. The systemic process has resulted in a sense of entrapment that is characterized by powerlessness on a number of levels that reinforce one another. The family is locked into the rigid systems that have created their rigid respones, both of which will present formidable resistance to change.

Empowerment begins by teaching the family about power dynamics in terms of both external systems and the family. We can help them sort out what belongs to the system and what belongs to the family, thus preventing their assuming blame for systemic influences but taking responsibility for how they may collude in their own powerlessness. In terms of the family itself, intervention can focus on any component of structure and function. The critical need for connections to the outside world, to other systems that are nourishing and protective, means that it is mandatory to make sure that external supplies are there. This involves working with systems outside the family to ensure the availability and appropriateness of the supplier. Natural networks, such as the extended family, the church, and fraternal groups, should be given priority as they are culturally consistent. In their absence or failure (such as in the case of severely pathological extended families where the systems are hopelessly locked into destructive structure and function), other systems, such as social services, support groups, and treatment groups, can become involved. Harry Aponte (1976) has emphasized the importance of organizing all services from an ecological perspective, meaning that there is a fit rather than a conflict between the family's needs and the services provided. In this way, there is certainty that these services work for the benefit of the family rather than placing added or conflicting burdens upon an already stressed system. This work needs to take place in the context of agencies that support helpers and that make serious commitments at the highest level to organizing, streamlining, and coordinating services with other agencies.

A Department of Social Services (DSS) social worker was working with a single mother in her children in therapy. The condition for return of the two children, who had been taken from her, was that she change her passive, permissive stance with her children and learn to set limits. Angry at the worker, she insisted she did not understand what she had to do to get her children back. She became demanding and threatening to the worker, who felt helpless and trapped as an enforcer in the system. The DSS worker joined with the social worker at the day-care center to reach the mother and begin to model good care and limit setting. This strategy changed the DSS worker's image of herself as helpless and of the mother as hopeless. The key here was connecting the client to a nourishing resource that neutralized the powerlessness of the worker and the distrust of the client.

The work is time consuming and arduous, as the supports available are often not helpful but instead are destructive, inadequate, or nonexistent. Thus, extra effort on the part of the clinician is required to ensure that the supports are there and appropriately nutritive. Nothing is more demoralizing for a therapist than to be expected to assist with problems for which there are no solutions because services are unavailable or inadequate. This may account for the "burnout" and depression identified by Aponte (1976) as a risk for helpers, as well as the helplessness cited by the students and family therapist noted earlier. They, too, become trapped in the conflict and contradictions. Treatment must recognize the adaptability of the maneuvers, which families use and must help a family to see that its problems are the result, in part, of a natural wish for power and strength. Being strong is a critical attribute in Black families *that needs validation*. We must convey that we recognize the cleverness, adaptability, strength, and resilience these mechanisms represent. The task becomes that of developing other ways of interacting. New ways are introduced by such comments as: "This is not always helpful," "Another way is to . . . ," and "You have a choice." Choice is critical to developing a more effective sense of power.

We must help them understand their behaviors, which are based on their determination to have a sense of power: using reaction formation and being oppositional, passive-aggressive, stubborn, manipulative, and attacking are all behaviors calculated to cope with a sense of powerlessness. But although these behaviors do create a sense of power and make them feel strong in this way, they also make for the problems discussed earlier. We try to help our clients see that these behaviors program them to react instead of act. This means that they cannot make decisions, choices, take leadership, and so on, if they are preoccupied with reactions to another's initiative rather than with behaving in accordance with their own goals and beliefs. This does not facilitate the strong and positive sense of self needed to cope with their realities.

The task is to help them see what they are doing and why they are doing it, and to identify the adaptive as well as maladaptive aspects of their efforts to get a sense of power. This strategy enables clients to feel respected in a total way—respected for their struggle and adaptability, but realistically warned of the price they pay. For example, a teenager who is responding to his sense of powerlessness as a Black and as an adolescent by being late for class and talking back can be told that talking back may be his way of expressing his strength but that this way of being strong does not prepare him for being a competent student. An underfunctioning father whose response to systemic stress has been to reduce his role can be told that while backing off may be his way of reducing stress in the family, a sign of his caring and wish to make things better for the family, his family needs him.

One useful strategy is that of sharing perspectives, that is, discussing how family members perceive a given situation, what may be the values that guide their behaviors, and the beliefs they hold. We can ask the family members to discuss their beliefs, values, the meaning of being Black, and so on. We can help them explain themselves to each other, clarifying their perceptions about the ambiguity contradiction, ambivalence, and dual identity of Blacks in this society. We can ask what rules and goals they want to have in the family. By sharing the confusion and ambiguities in the roles Blacks have to assume, they will be more able to communicate without blaming, denying, and putting down. For example, one client commented, "Hearing about the craziness Blacks have to live with helped me understand why mother was so hard on me." For him another level of complexity became clear. In asking people to process their beliefs in the presence of one another, we can expect not to have agreement or sameness in perspective, but agreement on the twoness, the ambiguity, the contradiction. That may be the best that can be expected because conflict is such a pervasive factor in their realities. But sharing and recognizing differences can be helpful because all of these mechanisms are a result of having to balance the social system, being perpetually a part of two subsystems—African and American—and of being trapped in the consequences of the societal projection process. Developing tolerance for conflicting values and perspectives can enhance the ability to manage conflict, negotiate, compromise, and work together. It cuts down on the conflict that stems from the need for sameness that is a consequence of fusion.

My Preparation for Client Empowerment

What should a clinician do to be ready to deal with these issues? What did I do? Although I am Black and have had to deal with a certain degree of powerlessness, it has not been the same as that which entraps many clients. I first had to understand conceptually not only how power dynamics operate and how to help clients use power constructively in their lives, but how to apply these ideas to myself. The power dynamics that operate in the clinical encounter mean that I am in an interactive process where I, as a clinician, am endowed with power from that role whereas my client experiences powerlessness because he or she has failed to solve his or her problem. My identity as middle class in interaction with poor Black clients compounds this power differential. My knowledge of power dynamics helps me to understand that a sense of power is, for me, as for everyone, critical. Also, as with everyone, I am vulnerable to using this compounded power in the clinical encounter to relieve anxiety I may experience as a result of powerlessness elsewhere in my life (Pinderhughes, 1983). I, therefore, must guard against exploiting my clients to benefit myself. All clinicians, service providers, and helpers must examine themselves as beneficiaries in the societal projection process a role that they may use to benefit themselves at the expense of their clients.

The White Therapist

For White clinicians, there is another level of power that is connected with being White, and the way in which that may influence their behavior with Black clients. In a process I have developed for learning cultural sensitivity people examine their experiences in relation to ethnicity, race, and other areas of difference in order to discover how they have reacted to having or lacking power (Pinderhughes, 1989). What has become clear is that many Whites have never thought about what it means to be White, are resistant to confronting it, and use many avoidance strategies, including a focus on their ethnicity. Upon further examination, feelings related to great discomfort are identified, such as guilt, fear, anger, shame, embarrassment, and pain.

Avoidance and ignorance of the meaning of White identity will hamper the White helper in efforts to engage Black clients and to help them cope with their realities, which are so intertwined with their identity as Blacks. Moreover, fosters the use of defensiveness and projection. Guilt and other feelings distort perception and push Whites to behave in ways that relieve their own consequent discomfort. Such responses along with other personal need can press Whites to misinterpret, misunderstand, and misbehave in the clinical encounter. A female psychiatric resident shared her fantasy of wanting to take her Black patient home, not so that she could take care of the patient but so that the patient could take care of her. Another faced resentment at seeing a Black woman driving a Mercedes (which he hoped to own someday) instead of the stereotypic Cadillac. A third discussed his anger at the distrust he encountered in a Black colleague. Having worked for civil rights, he felt hurt that she did not automatically credit his efforts. Furthermore, he did not consider himself "like other Whites," (i.e., prejudiced), and resented being lumped with them. Since he did not view their response as an adaptive mechanism, he too early diagnosed distrust and paranoia in his patients. Gibbs (1984) describes research showing that Blacks take a longer time to focus on treatment goals because they focus first on the therapist and the relationship. What this young resident also needed to learn was that deciding what is pathological for Blacks and what has been adaptive takes time, careful thinking, and checking out.

Acknowledging one's feelings about being White is important so that they can be controlled and not interfere with the goals of the treatment. It is important that White people be able to admit, "I feel lucky, glad I'm not Black," but such responses must never be projected since Blacks, like all people, must value their identity. Whites, too, need to have this feeling of value about themselves. Many Whites, especially those who are sensitive and caring, do not, and there is reluctance to confront this threat to self-esteem. As one colleague said, in refusing to explore the meaning of being White, "I'm not going to talk about it because I feel bad about too many things and I am not going to feel bad about being White." A positive sense of the meaning of being White is critical not only for effectively assisting Blacks, but also for one's own self-esteem. Discovering what would be involved in acquiring this positive sense as a White should be a priority.

For some people, refusing to confront the meaning of being White means wanting to hold on to the power imbalance that exists in society, wanting to keep the beneficiary position in the societal projection process. This, too, must be confronted since effective work with Black families means a change in this imbalance which has been syntonic for Whites. Successful outcome will help Blacks escape from their entrapment as systems balancers and tension relievers and will assist them to experience the sense of power they need to function constructively as peers who are equal partners in this society.

In summary, application of concepts related to the dynamics of culture, power, powerlessness, and systems process to the experience of Black American families informs us about their position in the societal projection process and their cultural responses to that position. It also clarifies treatment goals and the stance of the therapist who is a participant in this societal process from which he or she seeks to free clients.

REFERENCES

Aponte, H. (1976). Underorganization in the poor family. In P. Guerin (Ed.), *Family therapy theory and practice*. New York: Gardner Press.

Basch, M. (1975). Toward a theory that encompasses depression: A revision of existing causal hypotheses. In E. J. Anthony & T. Benedek (Eds.), *Depression and human existence*. Boston: Little Brown.

Billingsley, A. (1968). *Black families in White America*. Englewood Cliffs, N.J.: Prentice-Hall.

Bowen, M. (1978). *Family therapy in clinical practice*. New York: Jason Aronson.

Chestang, L. (1972). Character development in a hostile environment. *Occasional Paper*, no. 3. Chicago: School of Social Service Administration, University of Chicago.

Comer, J. (1972). *Beyond Black and White*. New York: Quandrangle Books.

Franklin, J. (1962). *From slavery to freedom*. New York: Alfred Knopf.

Gibbs, J. (1985). Establishing a treatment relationship with Black clients: Interpersonal vs. instrumental strategies. In *Advances in clinical social work*. Silver Spring, Md.: National Association of Social Workders.

Green, J. (1982). *Cultural awareness in the human sciences*. Englewood Cliffs, N.J.: Prentice-Hall.

Guerin, P. & Pendagast, E. (1976). "Evaluation of family system and genogram," in Guerin, ed., Family Therapy Theory and Practice New York: Gardner Press.

Harris, O., & Balpogal, P. (1980), Intervening with the Black family. In C. Janzen & O. Harris (Eds.), *Family treatment and social work practice*. Itasca, Ill.: F. E. Peacock.

Hill, R. (1972). *The strengths in Black families*. New York: Emerson Hall.

Knowles, L., & Prewitt, R. (1969). *Institutional racism*. Englewood Cliffs, N.J.: Prentice-Hall.

MacAdoo, H. (1978). The impact of upward mobility of kin-help patterns and reciprocal obligations in Black families. *Journal of Marriage and the Family, 40*(4), 761–776.

McClelland, D. (1975). *The inner experience*. New York: Wiley.

McGoldrick, M. (1985). Presentation on ethnicity and family therapy for the Coastal Community Counseling Center of Braintree.

Navarro, V. (1980). Panel on culture and health. Symposium on Cross-Cultural and Transcultural Issues. In *Health care*. San Francisco: University of California.

Papajohn, J., & Spiegel, J. (1975). *Transactions in families*. San Francisco: Jossey-Bass.

Pinderhughes, E. (1982). Family functioning of Afro-Americans. *Social Work, 27*(1), 91–96.

Pinderhughes, E. (1983). Empowerment for our clients and for ourselves. *Social Work, 64*(6), 331–338.

Pinderhughes, E. (1986). Minority women: A nodal Position in the functioning of the social system. In M. Ault-Riche (Ed.), *Women and family therapy*. Rockville, Md.: Aspens Systems.

Pinderhughes, E. (1989). *Teaching cultural sensitivity: Ethnicity, race and power at the cross-cultural treatment interface*. New York: Free Press.

Rodgers-Rose, L. F. (1980). *The Black woman*. Beverly Hills, Calif.: Sage Publications.

Solomon, B. (1976). *Black empowerment*. New York: Columbia University Press.

Staples, R. (1978). *Black family life and development in mental health: A challenge to the Black community*, L. Gary (Ed.). Washington, D.C.: Institute for Urban Affairs.

16

HOLOCAUST TRAUMA AND IMAGERY: THE SYSTEMIC TRANSMISSION INTO THE SECOND GENERATION

Faye L. Snider, M.S.W.

For a long time, I have been interested in the question of how it is that Holocaust imagery appears in the dreams, personal writings, and response to day-to-day events in many of my clients, none of whom themselves were alive during World War II. I begin this chapter with a writing from a client's journal. Her name is Fern. Her father just barely escaped Hitler's death machine, while his sister, her husband, two nephews, and many relatives did not. My hope is that her words and images will capture your heart and mind and give you the courage to proceed with the journey of this chapter.

> March 16, 1986: There are thousands, probably hundreds of thousands, of people all over the world who have thoughts and images and nightmares like the ones I have—but we each will have to face our own and come to terms with the responsibility and the legacy left to us by those people who were victims of the world's insanity. Their lives must have meaning and their deaths must teach us something about them, about the world, and about ourselves.
>
> My father was another kind of victim of that insanity. I can picture him as a little boy in another world. I can picture him as a man, as my father, with a faraway pain in his eyes—that struggle to let me know him, to know me—yet to keep himself protected from the closeness. The silence was deafening. I hated it. The silence made me angry and lonely and very, very scared. The silence he created left no opportunity for growth. It stifled him. It frightened me and created a world of depression and fear in which I grew up and took with me even when I no longer lived in his home. His face spoke of sadness and anger and guilt, but the silence won out. As I write, I can begin to feel and "hear" the screams of silence inside my head. I don't want to continue this and yet I'm afraid not to. Something has to make these screams and nightmares come to an end.
>
> I wish I could talk to my grandmother. My aunt described her as a strong-willed, proud woman. I see her in my mind. I see her with her daughter, her son, her grandsons, and several others whose faces I can't distinguish. I see them sitting

in their home in Lithuania. I feel a warmth I so rarely feel. I see them on a Friday night—smells of a Sabbath eve—and sounds of a poor, but emotionally rich family. I dream about them often, but that dream always becomes a nightmare. How did they die? I have so many images—of ovens, of open graves, of screams and pain, of barbed wire, so many scenes of open graves with hundreds of bodies and then faces of grandmother, my aunts and uncles and cousins. . . . They're staring at me, wanting me to help them. They're dead. No, they're not . . . I can't reach them. . . . Why couldn't I help them? It's only a dream. I have to keep myself in the present. But the present is my father. What is he trying to say to me? He always was "saying" something in his silence.

In most of the second-generation survivors I have worked with in the past six years, the patterns and themes of fear, profound loss, and unsafety such as Fern described are ever present. Moreover, it is significant that the majority of these clients came from silent families where the past was not openly discussed. In the therapeutic work, death-ridden, fearful, painful images spring forth in poems, dream states, and journals. Often, there are panic reactions to daily events that invariably represent secret or repressed family events.

From this work, I experienced the notion of "psychic osmosis," or the unconscious transmission of traumatic imagery and patterns of psychic denial from one generation to another. Fern richly describes this process as she observed her father's silent suffering. It is as if she sat in the theater of her family, watching a silent movie without the subtitles. Her father, the main actor, experienced his own remembrances as flashing internal pictures, while his heart was mournfully silent. Fern sensed the pain around these events, existentially feeling the importance of the loss as an explanation of her father's past. Her struggle to define reality is apparent; and in so doing, she plays her own version of the family imagery in a random and detached kaleidoscope. Events and feelings from the present become confused with images and fears from the past, as she struggles with her own connection to it. Imagery of the Holocaust is inexplicably present, a matter of course that is implicit, and rarely explicit.

It is the purpose of this chapter to show that the event of the trauma of the Nazi Holocaust triggered a multisystemic pattern of psychic reactivity that, to this day, is effecting the adjustment of the world community, and in particular the second generation, at multiple levels. One of the most profound reactions to this level of trauma is that of denial caused by numbing. Healthy denial allows the traumatized individual to organize defenses and move through the traumatic event. In the absence of the opportunity to abreact and deal with the terror, habituated numbing can set in. According to Robert J. Lifton, who studied the traumatized victims of Hiroshima (1968), the Buffalo Creek disaster (1976), and Vietnam (1973), this habituated pattern of psychic numbing can limit psychological flexibility and adaptability.

Trauma is generally defined as a terrifying and life-threatening event in which the individual is caught unaware. The stimulus of the surrounding event(s) is compelling. Most often, there is little or no choice of action available to the individual. Having no opportunity to anticipate, the person is caught unaware. Anxiety, fear, and internal emotional flooding take over. To cope, the psyche regulates the emotional flood by building a dam or a wall, depending upon the nature and degree of the trauma. Those who build a dam have a regulated flow of energy to fuel their strategies for managing the trauma. Those who build a wall feel cut off from hope, and thus the energy for aggressive coping and action is blocked. The individual is subsumed by the events of the trauma and must accommodate and go along in order to survive.

When we apply this phenomenon to families, we know that each generation teaches the next generation its version of life in its behaviors, actions, words, and reactions to daily events. This process is called transmission; and the transmission from generation to generation is called the systemic transmission process, or the flow of information from one part of a system to another. In this case, the systemic transmission is from the first generation of survivors to their progeny. Therapists who treat victims of the Nazi Holocaust need to be aware of the possibility of the intergenerational transmission of the trauma response. At any point, we can be sitting in our office and come upon a genogram in which a generation of a family has been wiped out by the misfortune of being within the boundaries of the Nazi death machine. Our ability to explore, comprehend, integrate, and manage the fact of that experience with the family will depend upon our own pattern of adaptation and response, as well as our awareness of how this level of trauma and loss affects the individual and those immediately involved.

Even now, as some of you begin to explore your curiosity about this topic, you may notice your mind struggling with random thoughts and wanderings that appear as distractions. Words such as Holocaust, Nazi death machine, or trauma may trigger tricks of the mind to dissuade you from facing the topic and its content. I am aware of my own interest and curiosity about this information. Yet, at times, I have difficulty focusing and holding my concentration. As I write, I often experience a curious restlessness and a pull to be elsewhere. These responses are symptomatic of what I call anticipatory trauma anxiety, an automatic defensive phenomenon that protects the psyche from the possibility of frightening thoughts and ideas when facing information that stimulates life-threatening images. Part of my purpose in writing this chapter is to provide the information and awareness through which therapists can better counter their denial and psychic-numbing reactivity and thus be more present and available for the client's need to process very difficult imagery.

THE HOLOCAUST AS TRAUMA

The Working Group to revise the third edition of the *Diagnostic and Statistical Manual of Mental Disorders* (1985) of the American Psychological Association offers the following definition of trauma: "An event that is outside the range of usual human experience and that is psychologically traumatic—e.g., a serious threat to one's life or personal/physical integrity, destruction of one's home or community, seeing another person who is mutilated, dying, or dead, or the victim of physical violence" (p. 6). The event of the Nazi Holocaust faced by mankind and, in particular, its victims with information and a level of horror for which there was no precedent. Robert Lifton's (1979) interest in the effects of massive trauma has led to a description of the adaptive patterns which the mind of the survivor undergoes so as to cope with the unbearable. He defines a survivor as "one who has come into contact with death in some bodily or psychic fashion and has remained alive" (p. 169). In various writings, he has articulated five distinct, yet interconnected, survival patterns: (1) death imprint and related death anxiety, (2) death guilt, (3) psychic numbing, (4) conflicts over nurturing and contagion, and (5) struggles with meaning or formulation. Let us look in more depth at what Lifton can teach us about the victim's response to trauma.

Death Imprint and Related Death Anxiety

At some time in our lives, we all have been faced with the possibility of a traumatic event. One that I vividly recall from my adult life took place at age 23. It was a winter day and there was snow on the ground. Marv, my husband, and I were driving home from work on a country road we traveled daily. Suddenly, the car hit a snow-covered ice patch and swerved out of control. In that moment, my life seemed in suspended motion: The car made a 180-degree turn, and landed on an embankment faced in the opposite direction. I remember feeling as if I were awakening and coming to life again. I was tremulous with the fear of what might have been had there been another car coming in the opposite direction. This is what Lifton (1979) calls the "death imprint or the radical intrusion of an image—feeling of threat or end to life" (p. 169).

Lifton states that the degree of unacceptability of death—be it in its prematurity, grotesqueness, or absurdity—is important. In the experience, the individual calls upon all his or her resources regarding death and its meaning. Thus, in the moments following our near accident, Marv and I anxiously spoke of death and how it was for us. We found ourselves reviewing sudden losses in our families. We compared ourselves to others whose families had experienced painful and sudden death. In that moment, we came to understand that any individual who is suddenly faced with the threat of death will have difficulty with assimilating the overwhelming feelings. After awhile, I calmed down. Yet, the images and feelings can still be recalled these many years later. According to Lifton, the degree and level of anxiety are determined by the suddenness of the event, how extreme or protracted it is in its impact, and whether or not it is associated with the terror of premature, unacceptable death. Thus, I can imagine that if the death threat had been protracted or prolonged by actual physical hurt or if others around me had been hurt or killed, I would not so easily have come to terms with it.

Lifton and Olson's (1976) research on the adaptation and adjustment of the victims of the man-made flood disaster in Buffalo Creek, W.V., in 1971, is particularly instructive. In less than one hour, 125 people were killed and nearly 5,000 made homeless. Imagine living in a quiet community by a creek. For several days, it has been raining. Suddenly, you hear a roar. It is a new sound. You wonder what it is. As you wonder, it gets louder and louder; and then you see it—a 30-foot jet-black mass of water sweeping down the creek and coming right toward your home. If you don't act, death is imminent. Yet, there is little time to think or to act. We can pause to wonder: how many of those 125 individuals who died had no choice but to die; or how many had a moment's choice, but remained frozen and immobilized by the terror of death, and thus could not act.

Equally important here are the aftereffects of trauma. What Lifton and Olsen (1976) learned was that the traumatic event was only the beginning of a series of adaptive responses, much as it was with survivors of the Holocaust and Hiroshima. Every aspect of normal community life was wiped out within a half hour. The death imprint and its association with rain and the possibility of flooding and total disaster were firmly imbedded in those 5,000 surivors, as well as those in surrounding communities. In the words of one survivor, we can clearly see the emergence of the roots of the psychic transmission process:

> When it rained hard last week, it was like the past came out again. I took the family down to the cellar and (at times like this) I just know the whole flood is going to come back . . . it's like you might step out of the trailer and get caught in something. (p. 2)

Lore Shelley (1983), in her doctoral dissertation, offers in-depth data on the psyche's struggle to come to terms with the phenomenon of massive trauma as she deals with the death imprint and death anxiety triggered by the Holocaust. Her study consists of 485 respondents, most of whom had been in Auschwitz or its satellite camps. Some 75.7 percent of her sample agreed with the statement: "Even if my life proceeds normally during the day, there still are the nights with their dreams and nightmares," and 40.4 percent agreed with, "Every night I am back in camp, I really never left it." Death anxiety can take on different forms and symbols, as is shown by the 72.2 percent of the sample who agreed with the statement: "Some rather harmless events can be anxiety provoking for me; for example, the sight of a uniform, a knock at the door, dogs barking, smoke from a chimney, hearing the German language." Thus, we can see how the experience of near death in which one was the powerless victim of the Nazis might set the stage for an inner life of repeated fear and terror—a reliving so as somehow to come to grips with it.

Death Guilt

The second manifestation of disruption in life symbols is "death guilt" or the guilt over survival. In the face of severe trauma, the ability to anticipate, and thus to think of a way to act, is cut off. In extraordinary amoral circumstances such as the Nazi death damps where there is a massive immersion in death, the potential for both physical and psychic action is virtually eliminated (Lifton, 1979). This immobilization of energy and action sets a stage in which the individual disengages from part of the self, and in so doing, numbs the affective and action parts.

In this numbing pattern, the individual feels responsible for his or her inaction and for the inability to feel. Most of all, he or she senses the difference between the active self that was and the inactive self that is. This moment of transition in the self is the moment associated with the trauma. The person is tortured by the knowledge of the inaction and thus retrospectively replays the traumatic scenario over and over in order to create a more acceptable enactment of the image (Lifton, 1979). Shame and guilt go hand in hand with death guilt. Recovery and relief from shame depend a great deal on the individual's ability to understand and accept the inevitability of inaction in such circumstances.

Lifton (1979) speculates that death guilt leaves the survivor with the fundamental question: "Why did I survive while he, she, or they died?" In the internal shifting of images, the simple next step in dealing with the guilt of inaction is to shift to the feeling state of: "If I had died instead, he, she, or they would have lived." Death guilt is a powerful antecedent to the carrying of images into the next generation. The presence of a child, especially one named for a deceased Holocaust family member, can force the issue of life and how one copes. The resemblance of the child to past generations can trigger an association of guilt. In Fern's family, she was named for her father's mother, and strongly resembled the sister whom he had left behind. She often spoke of her confusion over the warmly affectionate, yet sad, look with which he would greet her. Thus, within the survivor's child lies the seed of death and life, of inaction and mastery, of allegiance to the past and to the present. Shelley (1983) states that 77 percent of her respondents agreed with the statement: "It is our sacred duty to raise families to assure that the death of the six million was not in vain."

Psychic Numbing

I liken psychic numbing to blowing a fuse—the circuits go on overload and the energy for certain functioning goes dead. The individual is left vulnerable, as certain parts of the self are disengaged and unable to respond to stimuli. Shelley (1983) captures the essence of this issue in a statement agreed upon by 41.3 percent of her sample: "The Jews went to the gas chambers like sheep to the slaughter house." And in the following statement, we have a suggestion as to how a blaming-the-victim attitude allows society at large to come to terms with its own death guilt. Slightly more than two-fifths (42.5 percent) of the survivors concurred with the statement, "Without the collaboration of their victims, the Nazis could not have murdered so many Jews" (p. 250).

When taken at face value, we recoil at the thought that society deals with the guilt of inaction by holding the victims responsible for their fates. Shelley (1983) points to Eichman's own testimony during his trial, in which he stated that without Jewish cooperation, the extermination would have encountered serious difficulties. It is my contention that the Nazis instinctively understood and used the effects of trauma to control the minds of their victims. What appeared to the observer as behavioral "cooperation" was, in fact, the outward shell of human beings in the throes of psychic numbness. In this phase, cut off from any semblance of normality and organized by the Nazi military to obey and cooperate, one can only imagine the internal struggle of hope that, through muting of affect and dampening of energy and initiative, one might live. In this adaptive phase, any capacity for feeling was diminished and what appeared, instead, was apathy, withdrawal, and depression (Lifton & Olson, 1976).

We need to appreciate the psychic price paid in this form of adaptation. Mastery, initiative, hope, and a sense of control are suspended and the individual is in a state in which coping imagery is absent. As if in a trance, he or she moves through a process that is too painful and moving too fast to comprehend. Shelley (1983) quotes a survivor who believed that heroes of today would have behaved the same way as the Jews of the Holocaust had they been in that place at that time: "The brain was paralyzed and the Germans knew it" (p. 254).

Nurturance and Contagion (Unfocused Rage)

One can only imagine what it must have been like for the survivors to wake up one morning and realize that the reality of Nazi captivity was over and that suddenly one was permitted to move, to talk, to feel, to plan, and to hope. How does the individual who has been immersed in death guilt and psychic numbing go about the business of living and reconnecting? Lifton (1979) notes that the struggle around nurturance and contagion is directly related to an insufficiently appreciated survivor emotion, that of perpetual anger and frequent rage. Contagion is a simple term for a complex psychological phenomenon in which the individual protects himself or herself and others from the lessons of vulnerability in human relationships. It is as if the survivor has been tainted by the experience and is keenly sensitive to the fact that: "Associations to his experience can activate latent anxieties in others concerning death and death equivalents" (Lifton, 1979, p. 176). Feeling damaged and worthless, the survivor expects that if he or she were to get close and share more of himself or herself, the experience would be difficult, and perhaps intolerable, for others.

Without the option directly to express the range of human emotions that death and violence trigger, the individual is left with feeling angry and, often, rageful. Lifton (1979) states that:

> The survivor seems, in fact, to require his anger and rage—and all, too often, his violence—as an alternative to living in the realm of the annihilated. Many have noted that anger is relatively more comfortable than guilt or other forms of severe anxiety; it can also be a way of holding onto a psychic lifeline when surrounded by images of death. (p. 176)

Aaron, a 38-year-old eldest son of a survivor of Auschwitz, described his father's dilemma to me:

> Recently, my father had to go to the hospital for tests. I dreaded it. I knew what would happen. He can't stand anyone telling him what to do, never mind staying in bed. It was awful. He yelled. He couldn't stay quiet. His anger was out of control. As usual, they called me and I had to go to try to calm him down so they could help him. He understands, but he doesn't. It almost isn't worth it for him to get the care. It's so frustrating.

Thus, the son captures the essence: in the fear of captivity or any reminder of that which was lost; the rage may impede the very connectedness and support the individual requires for coping in the present. Lifton and Olson (1976) describe this state as it related to the Buffalo Creek disaster:

Thirty months after the disaster, survivors are left with diffuse anger they themselves disapprove of, rage they cannot express, and an overall sense that everything (and everyone) is suspect and that life itself has been rendered counterfeit. (p. 7)

Struggle for Meaning or Significance

Survivors of trauma do continue in their lives and somehow come to terms, each in his or her own way, with the experience and its meaning. The essence of the overall task of the survivor is that of finding a way to integrate the trauma so as to find meaning or significance in the effort of living. A leader in this search for meaning is a recent Nobel Peace Prize recipient, Elie Wiesel, who has dedicated his life to "bearing witness" to the events, feelings, and meaning of the Holocaust as an antidote to silence and denial. He confronts us with how he has come to terms with his own need for meaning and his experience of the evil of the Holocaust:

Words have never seemed adequate to convey the evil of the past. . . . I decided to devote my life to telling the story because I felt that having survived, I owe something to the dead. That was their obsession to be remembered, and anyone who does not remember betrays them again (Berger, 1986, p. A10)

Writers can help us face the imagery and those parts of the self that struggle to defy the reality. Aaron Appelfeld (in Alter, 1986), whose mother was killed in the Holocaust, writes metaphorically:

It's just impossible to deal directly with the nakedness of the deaths. It's like looking at the naked sun on a clear summer day. You couldn't stand the temperature. You can never understand the meaning of the Holocaust. You can just come to the edges of it. If you wrote about it directly, you'd end up trivializing it.

The possibility of trivialization is a fear that runs through the literature. The answer for many survivors was in finding a way to carry on or to begin again. Thus, marriage and progeny became an essential way to revitalize and transcend the trauma. Family therapists need to be acutely aware of the special meaning of children and their relevance to mastery of life and its meaning for survivors. Both Epstein (1979) and Kestenberg and Kestenberg (1980) report on the importance of children in finding a way to regain some trust in humanity. What more meaningful way to fight systematic genocide than through the quest for progeny? Moreover, it represents control over biological continuity and the ultimate reconnection of family ties. Epstein (1979) speaks of her own father:

Children were life. Children were the future, he told my mother. They had both survived the war for reasons that were beyond his understanding, but surely their purpose was in part, to build a family. (p. 91)

THE INTERFACE OF TWO SYSTEMS:
THE SURVIVORS AND POSTWAR AMERICA

The Numbing of America: 1942

There is much information about the presence of death anxiety, denial, and psychic numbing in America in the late 1930s and 1940s. In the literature, the term "conspiracy of silence" is used to describe the lack of response of the world at large to the plight of the Jews. Many books and articles have been written about the effect of this silence and its contribution to the murder of six million Jews. Wyman (1984) in *The Abandonment of the Jews* describes the American climate in August 1942, when the first flow of information about Hitler's plan is blocked, not believed, and diverted. He graphically describes the response of the American consulate in Geneva, having received the critical information from a man named Reigner who had informed them that Hitler was planning to exterminate all Jews from German controlled areas once they had been removed to one place (presumably Poland). Three and a half to four million Jews would be exterminated in the process. The American legation found this plan to settle the Jewish question in Europe unbelievable, describing it as "having the earmarks of war rumor inspired by fear" (p. 43). Here we see an outright dismissal and denial with no apparent effort to research or confirm the information.

Described as a "fantastic" report, we can sense the fictionalization of the event. As if in an Asimov novel, the policy makers soothe their vulnerable psyches by negating the possibility of such evil. Thus, by denying the possibility, one need not get involved. Ultimately, as we all know, the United States and the Allies had to become involved. Even then, however, there was never a decision to blow up the train tracks leading into the death camps, in spite of the fact that British and American bombers continuously flew over them. The presence of this silence, both in word and deed, is startling. How much was attributable to the paralysis of the mind in the face of such evil, to antisemitic feelings, or to the politics of war is for history to decide. Recently, I had the occasion to discuss this question with Lewis Weinstein, the chief of liaison section of European Theatre of Operations of the United States Army (personal communication, May 10, 1987). He shed some light on the thinking of the military at that time:

> We were in the war room in Paris. It was February 1945. Eisenhower came in with Chief of Staff Walter Bedell Smith. There was a map on the wall. I saw the details of Auschwitz and noticed that there was a single track leading from a body of tracks into the camp. I said to the general: 'I didn't know that Auschwitz was so big. I've heard that many Jews have been killed there.' I noted the single track and asked if there was any possibility of the bombers targeting it, since they fly in that area. Eisenhower's response was swift and specific: 'Don't tell me how to win the war. We're not spending a man or a plane unless we know it's advancing our aims in the the war.'

Weinstein further stated that groups of officers had previously come to Eisenhower with the same question and received a similar answer. Thus, at the moment that the information about mass extermination is revealed, we note that the response is denial and justification. It is not to be acknowledged; and second, it is processed in terms of the meaning to self—that is, "let's not change, respond, or get involved unless we have to." Clearly, the priority was efficient strategizing to end the war, rather than to sidetrack so as to stop or slow down the exterminations in the concentration camps. This pattern of inaction and silence set the stage for the "conspiracy of silence" that blocked the survivors' ability to process their experiences after the war.

Survivor as Symbol of Devastation

It is difficult to imagine the startling difference in reality experienced by the survivors of the death camps and those who were on U.S. soil during the war. In six years, the United States had emerged from a period of provincial isolationism to a world power that created the most destructive weapon in the history of humankind—the atomic bomb. Although the average citizen yearned for the "good old days" when life was simple, the event of the bombing of Hiroshima and its implications for the future presented the culture with death images and anxiety. Newspapers and magazines carried picture after picture of the massive destructive power of the bomb. U.S. and world citizens could no longer easily deny the possibility of massive vulnerability to instant death. The implication of the introduction of annihilation weaponry is profound and explicitly tied to the event of the Holocaust.

The book *Time Bomb* (MacPherson, 1986) tells the story of how the seeds of the atomic bomb were sown in the soil of the fear of Hitler's potential for further evil. Physicists from the United States and Germany competed to be first in the challenge to create this ultimate weapon. In fact, the fear of the boundarylessness of Hitler's evil and the absence of any U.S. policy about nuclear energy research led Einstein to write to Roosevelt at least twice to try to stir some action:

> Interest in uranium has intensified in Germany. I have now learned that research is being carried out in great secrecy and that it has been extended to another of the Wilhelm Institutes of Physics. (Macpherson, 1986, p. 142)

Ernest Becker (1973) gives us an anthropological perspective as he comments on the paradoxical nature of the human survival dilemma. Human beings are the only creatures who are self-conscious in that they are aware that they are going to die. My dog or cat does not know it is going to die. Furthermore, we also recognize, by virtue of our capacity to think abstractly, that we can die at any minute for reasons that are uncontrollable, and even arbitrary (Solomon, 1986). This dialectic, between the ability for abstraction and the vulnerability of the body, has led humans to the development of culture and the introduction of implements and rituals to reduce death anxiety. With the bombing of Hiroshima, human beings created an unbearable paradox: Out of defense, they produced weaponry that raised the awareness of death vulnerability to unbearable and intolerable levels. The psychic atmosphere of the United States in 1945 and thereafter was permeated by fear, guilt, and shame in the realization that this weapon had actually been used to destroy instantly thousands of civilian innocents. We could now identify with the Japanese citizens of Hiroshima who had no awareness of their impending death:

> Leaflets were dropped on Hiroshima from American planes on July 27, threatening Hiroshima (and other major cities on which they were dropped) with total destruction if Japan did not surrender immediately, but they made no mention of the atomic bomb or of any other special weapon. Nor did the leaflets appear to have reached many people—only a single person among those I interviewed, then a child, remembered picking one of them up, and when he brought it back to his elders, they scoffed at it, whether out of genuine disbelief or, more likely, a sense of how one was supposed to react to such a threat. In any case, the people of Hiroshima received no warning about the atomic bomb: American policy makers, for various strategic reasons, had decided against any prior notice. (Lifton, 1968, p. 17)

In the background of these events, the survivors of the Nazi Holocaust were greeted by a country that was struggling with its own denial, shame, and guilt. Whereas the survivors needed empathy, openness, and caring so as to heal, the U.S. citizenry could not allow themselves to feel, for to do so would mean facing the implications of the change in our cultural symbolism and our responsibility for it. To deal with the trauma of being in the atomic age meant coping with acute death anxiety.

At the end of his life, Becker was asked what it would take for us to survive in the world. Becker said it will take courage, imagination, and dedication: courage to accept ourselves as we are without putting our social construction on others, imagination to conceive of the world other than it is, and, finally, dedication to make that dream a reality (Solomon, 1986). Above all else, the survivors understood this need for a new vision, one that could bring meaning to their lives. They needed the safety of an environment in which their past could be tolerated and dealt with. Trauma theory teaches us that the victim needs to be known, heard, understood, and, above all, believed. Without the ability to be believed, a state called "rigid fixity" (Danieli, 1985) or stuckness in adaptation sets in. Given the emotional and social climate of the mid-40s, we can see how dealing with the imagery of the Holocaust was fraught with facing one's own complicity in the death of others, as well as the possibility of one's own imminent death. No longer could we say, "This cannot happen here." To listen to survivors would mean facing: "It did happen in Germany. It did happen in Hiroshima. It could happen here."

THE SYSTEMIC TRANSMISSION OF PSYCHIC SYMBOLS IN THE SECOND GENERATION

The Atmosphere for Psychic Osmosis

The roots of psychic osmosis are nurtured in an atmosphere of disconnection and fear where silence and foreboding impede openess of affect, information, and the expression of experience. Holocaust survivors, coming to a new land, faced the dilemma of adapting to a new culture, while mourning and integrating the loss of their former world. Children of these survivors speak with puzzlement of this process as they struggle with the pain of the disconnection. In the words of Aaron:

> All across Europe, my father wore big, heavy brown boots. He hid out for most of the war; and everywhere he traveled, his boots carried him through the muck and the terror and the pain. When he saw Ellis Island and the Statue of Liberty, he was overcome by the vision of a new beginning. He took off the boots and threw them overboard. He told me he wanted to start anew, with nothing dragging him down. I understood, but why couldn't he have saved something to help me know, to understand?

What the father understood that the son could not was that no one wanted the dirt and mud tracked into the United States. For this family, as well as for countless others, the ugliness worn as a symbol of pride and survival, got washed away, and the new culture offered no replacement. Survivor families experienced enormous rejection and isolation, thus reinforcing the rupture of the past and setting the stage for great difficulty in finding supports for a bridge to the future.

In systemic terms, we can hypothesize that the Holocaust survivors became the symbolic scapegoats for the shame and guilt over our own complicity in the Holocaust of Hiroshima and Nagasaki. Thus, there was no welcoming of these new immigrants. Instead, there were silence and alienation, a pattern which, to this day, needs addressing by both the first and second generation. Shelley (1983) cites Rappaport, a Holocaust survivor, who found that survivors of the camp were treated as unwelcome disturbers of a lulled world conscience in that their persistent mental anguish after liberation was shrugged off as their resistance against adjustment.

Survivors coped with the cultural wall of silence by building a safety net around themselves. If outsiders could not let them in, they would not let outsiders in, and they would stay bonded unto themselves. Moreover, given their experience, who could be trusted and who could not be trusted? According to Danieli (1985),

> The only option left for the survivors, other than sharing their Holocaust experiences with each other, was to withdraw completely into their newly established families. Children of such families, although remembering their parents' and lost families' war histories only in bits and pieces, attested to the constant psychological presence of the Holocaust at home, verbally and nonverbally or, in some cases, reported having absorbed the omnipresent experience of the Holocaust through "osmosis." (p. 299)

Coming to Terms with the Imagery

I can vividly recall the first time I became aware of the historical transmission process of the symbols of the Holocaust trauma. It was during a therapy session with a woman whose parents were survivors. As we talked one day, she glanced up at the picture on the wall directly behind me: four poignant faces of Indian women in a line, their quiet pain in evidence. She said: "Every time I come here, I see that picture, and I hate it." I was stunned by her intensity and did not totally comprehend its meaning. Other images began to emerge: the Picasso print in the office bathroom that depicted sketches of lean and esthetic faces triggered images of faces from the camps; the image of a train in a children's book was a painful reminder of her uncle's last train ride to the death camps. It was only upon my seeing the film Shoah[1] that I came to understand the symbolism of her emotional experience and its profound connection to the losses in her family.

For those of us who were fortunate enough to be in another place during the Nazi onslaught, the ability to comprehend and respond to the death imagery requires a leap into the unknown. To respond to the underlying symbols and pictures, one must confront one's own anticipatory trauma anxiety. I have found that facing Holocaust imagery means facing my own sense of vulnerability and helplessness. Furthermore, to enable a client to describe and face the acute pain and terror and the fear of victimization in the present requires the therapist to set a tone which is open, safe, and empathic. It is only in the context of openess and empathy that the images can freely occur. We have to deal with our own denial of death and cowardice, which leads to emotional responses such as guilt, anxiety, or disgust (Krystal, 1968).

Danieli (1981), in her study of 61 psychotherapists, reports that therapists' internal reactions reinforce the conspiracy of silence in the therapeutic process. She reports that the most common affective reaction in both therapists and researchers is bystander's guilt or feeling an immense sense of guilt for leading a happy and protected childhood while these people suffered so terribly. Danieli found that therapists who felt guilty were much more fearful of hurting the client, and, therefore, avoided asking some important questions. These questions, according to Danieli, would mean triggering vulnerability and fragility not only in the client, but also in the therapist.

If the client's information is ignored or overreacted to, it has an effect on how the client comes to terms with the experience. To engage at the level of symbolic imagery, the therapist needs to become aware of his or her own[2] unconscious emotional reactivity with its concomitant defensive reactions. In my own case, I found myself wandering through the Holocaust literature. I felt that, to understand, I needed to "know it" through the eyes and experiences of others. I grew up in Portland, Maine, the daughter of parents who did not discuss world events at the dinner table. We were parochial Jews—leading our lives as if the wider community outside of Portland did not exist. For me, the Holocaust was an event of the mind, not of the spirit.

Several of my second-generation clients' abilities to verbalize their imagery triggered my curiosity and need for more information. I consumed literature of the Holocaust. I can only give a partial listing, all of which were highly personal: Epstein (1980); Wiesel (1969, 1970, 1978); Wouk (1973); Appelfeld (1981); Roth-

---

[1] The film Shoah is a documentary in which the producer, Claude Lanzman, returned to the site of the Nazi death machine to interview survivors, bystanders, and perpetrators.

[2] There is no single word in the English language to connote the idea of his/her. For future reference, I shall use the singular "her."

child (1981); Epstein (1979); and Levi (1985). Looking back, I now realize that I was coming to terms with my own psychic numbing and that of my family. Danieli (1981) reports on the "ethical blow"—the shattering of our naive belief that the world we live in is a just place where human life is of value to be protected and respected. Thus, to listen means to open up the necessity of facing the massive and merciless presence of human evil, both in the past and in the present.

NOTING AND DEALING WITH THE TRANSMISSION PROCESS IN THERAPY

As I came to know and tolerate my own emotional responses to the imagery, I came to value the importance of stimulating an environment in which the client could project what she carried inside. The opportunity to process meant the possibility of understanding and dealing with the meaning of the images. Once again, I would like to turn to the therapy of Fern, my 32-year-old client whose father had must managed to escape the camps, leaving his beloved sister and nephews behind. She interpreted as bizarre and crazy her graphic imagery of open graves, in which she saw the bodies of her aunt and cousins writhing with the pain of recent wounds. I encouraged her to keep a journal. Often, in a semiwaking state in the middle of the night, she would write:

> I need to make myself a person separate from those people I've carried with me my whole life. I hate the silence. I hate their screams—or are the screams mine? The silence never allowed them to have the right to their own lives and their own deaths—they've lived on through others—that can be healthy and positive. But when what lives on inside others is anger and fear and a sense of impending danger—then it becomes a burden.

A recent opportunity to travel to Israel gave Fern the chance to work out her feeling that her imagery was "crazy." At the Museum of the Diaspora, she found herself fascinated by the Memorial Column, "a towering sculpture which hung high from the ceiling, traversing multilevels of space, its body imbedded with barbed wire, and an endless light which flowed throughout. I wanted to climb inside, to wrap myself in it, to experience it." Of her experience in seeing the endless pictures from the death camps at the museum and at Yad Vashem, she said: "It was then that I fully realized I was not crazy . . . that the pictures inside me were real for many others. I felt normal at last."

Kestenberg and Kestenberg (1980) report that shared dreams among survivors and children frequently occur. They explain that dreams of persecution resulted when the Nazies assaulted their victims without allowing them the use of defenses. From a systemic viewpoint, the shared dreams allowed a very special connection between survivor and child as the process of sharing connected the generations and reassured the parents that he or she had not been abandoned and alone (Winnik, 1965).

Many other clients, all of whom had family histories of direct involvement with the effects of the Nazi holocaust, reported similar imagery with concomitant intense emotional reactivity. Rebecca, age 34, and married with two sons, reported that she could not stand in line without experiencing intense anxiety and the need to run. She complained, at times, of feeling dissociated and cut off from herself. On and off, a bout of depression haunted her. In one session, she appeared tense and unable to hold her thoughts and concentrate. I noted her difficulty and asked her how she accounted for it. She described an incident immediately before coming to therapy:

> I don't know if you heard it or not—the fire engines that came down the street. I was just coming into the office when they came by. I heard the horns and the sirens. I got so upset inside . . . so frightened and nervous. I noticed the people around me. They didn't seem to notice, or even to care. What bothered me was the one woman nearby. She was laughing loudly. How could she be laughing like that when something terrible was happening to someone somewhere?

Rebecca and I processed the event in terms of her history and the pattern of her family. What was clear was that she had been taught to be hypervigilant and careful at all times. The trigger of the sirens, a sound of foreboding from the concentration camps, stimulates confusion and dissociation. She is aware of the present, but feels as if she were in the past. It is not uncommon for clients to describe this phenomenon as standing between two time zones and behaving as if the past were the present. When she had the opportunity to process and understood this mechanism for survival and its effect on her ability to focus in our session, she became oriented to her current reality.

These clients needed the experience of attaching their "crazy" reactions to some basis in reality. When there is no understanding of this reality, the client can feel disoriented and confused by the insistence and suddenness of feelings and images. Danieli (1987) states that the children of survivors "seem to have consciously and unconsciously absorbed their parents' Holocaust experiences into their lives almost in toto. Holocaust parents, in the attempt to give their best, taught them how to survive, and in the process transmitted to them the life conditions under which they had survived the war" (p. 305).

Recently, Rebecca became aware of a push/pull struggle within herself. She could not figure out how it was that she would make plans to begin an important career change, get right up to it, then back away, only to begin the process again. After several of these "almost" starts, she called her process into question. In the therapy, I traced her feelings: "I spend my time gathering information, trying to make certain that the risk is a good one and that it will be a *safe* move. When I get to the contract stage, the anxiety comes: How do I know that what seems *right* is right? Can I trust the landlord?" When I focused on the trust issue, she agreed that she could not understand her anxiety. "It doesn't make sense, but I can't move forward. The only way out is to back out and look again. Maybe another location will be a better one." When I asked her what "better" was, she could not explain. At the end of the session, I handed her a copy of Danieli's (1981) article on adaptational styles of Holocaust families.

At the next session, she reported that she had read the article. She integrated the connection between her parent's hypervigilant survival pattern and her own, realizing more fully that her parents had spent the entire war wandering throughout eastern Europe in search of a safe location. She then informed me she was about to sign a rental contract that had arrived that day in the mail.

Case Profiles of Second-Generation Clients

Each client has a similar history. The client is part or totally Jewish, age 30 or over, and comes to therapy as an individual or as a member of a couple. The complaints range from symptoms of intense anxiety and somatization to unexplained depression which appears somewhat relevant but not specific to the current reality. The client's genogram reveals a parental history of living in Europe prior to the Nazi persecution. These losses include the deaths of relatives by firing squad, death camps, or merciless attack, as well as the takeover of home or homestead and all their possessions, triggering a pattern of immediate flight, running, or hiding. Experience with dissociative states are common—that is, a sense of numbing, of being out of touch with one's feelings. The client often report behaviors (avoidance of situations, mistrust of a person or situation) with no apparent reason for the sense of foreboding. They also report anxiety states that occur at random, strong issues of separation struggles with their family of origin, dreams with Holocaust imagery, and an enormous fear of abuse or victimization in any form. A sense of belonging is a tantamount goal, while there is an enormous fear of its meaning. There is conflict at every level—between the self that is and the self that wants to be.

Fern speaks to the process of psychic numbing in the following journal report:

> I feel very detached from what I am writing. I'm writing about others—not about me. I feel that burden. I hate it. I have to find some meaning for all this or else their lives—my father's silent pain, and my "burden" of depression and nightmares, will have been for nothing.

Identifying and Restoring the Lost Images

The family therapist has available a wide range of literature about the systemic implications of context and pattern. Hoffman (1981), Keeney (1983), Wynne (1984), and Watzlawick (1978) offer models of thinking and conceptualizing that can enable the therapist to formulate a workable model of intervention. More specifically, theorists and practitioners such as Danieli (1985, 1986), Paul and Grosser (1965), and van der Kolk (1987) address the impact of silence as a rupturing process in communication. They heighten our awareness of the necessity of finding models and methods that will enable us to lead clients safely through a healing process. "Rupturing silence" seals the past in an unmarked tomb, forever blocking the rich memories of those who cannot be recalled, and thus marking the progeny with a sense of hollowness, searching, and rootlessness. The effect of the rupture is addressed by Fern, as she comments about her response to the Holocaust Memorial at Yad-Vashem in Israel: "I felt my father there. For the first time, I could feel how angry I was at him. Silence is destructive. It doesn't allow you to feel proud."

I have previously described the "boot phenomenon"—that is, when the past is so painful and burdensome, it gets the boot and miles and miles of emotions and their contexts are set adrift and buried. Where there is a rupture in the information and images in the past, there can be no pride in what was. Bergman (1982) speaks to the process of unresolved mourning in stating that children of survivors often do not get to live their own lives and adapt either by feeling obliged to undo the trauma or by rebelling vigorously against it. He further states that the therapist must assist the client to work through the mourning process that was cut short when one loss succeeded the other with unbearable rapidity, and when one's daily need to cope made mourning impossible.

The therapist as witness is in a position to enable the second generation to fill in the blank tableau with shapes, forms, and feelings so as to build an affective bridge to the past. A particularly useful tool is that of the genogram (McGoldrick & Gerson, 1985; Danieli, 1986). An objectifying, yet connecting, process, it offers a safe structure in which the second generation can begin to identify the lost family members and some of the attached feelings. What is very useful is that this can be done with or without the first generation. As the search for the people, their lives, and their values begins to take shape, there is a connection of meaning that can bond the two generations. Although the genogram is a very important tool in identifying the lost history, and sense of persona, family patterns, and values, one must be aware that a cognitive frame is not enough. It is essential to uncover and focus on the clients' internalized images and feelings of the lost members. In working with imagery, the therapist needs to guide the process so as to provide this access.

Therapeutic Methods

Many methods can specifically guide and activate the lost images. A word of caution is necessary here, however, in that techniques without grounding in a deeply safe and trustful therapeutic relationship can trigger responses in the client that can feel threatening and abusive. Contextually, it is essential that the client–therapist relationship be as horizontal as possible so as to enable feedback, a sense of control, and safety for the client. Methods such as journal keeping, the introduction of Holocaust literature, guided imagery, story telling, use of images, and hypnosis are useful in this process. Danieli (1985, 1986), in her work with the Group Project for Holocaust Survivors and Their Children, highly recommends the group process. The Group I most often refer to in the Boston area is "One Generation After." The goal for therapy is to search for a context that will explain the floating behaviors and feelings which recur with no apparent trigger in the present.

Journal keeping is a method in which I instruct the client to select a notebook in which she can write down the events and feelings that cause anxiety and worry. I further instruct the client to keep the journal with her, and whenever she feels overwhelmed or puzzled, to make a note or to sit and write. I further state that what is important is that the client break her own internal silencing pattern and share with the self that which she has difficulty expressing or stating.

I then recommend she make selections which she wants to share and bring them into sessions to process. In the session, I will encourage the client to read the material aloud so as to integrate it. If the client is not ready to so this, I read the material out loud and then we discuss it. Witnessing in this way makes the information real and present.

The introduction of Holocaust literature which lends itself to imagery and response is a way to offer a common language and experience between the therapist and client. Appelfeld (1984), Rothchild (1981), Trunk (1979), Ettinger (1970), Sichrovsky (1987), and Wiesel (1969) are but a few of the many descriptive and compelling authors whose imagery can enable the bridging of affect. The children of Holocaust families are seen as having a very different cultural experience; and, thus, the parent cannot imagine how the images or feelings could be so pressing when the child has not lived it. The child, in return, has integrated this difference and wonders how it is that she feels so strongly when she "should not" as it is her parents' experience. The therapist and client join as mutual witnesses who are affected as human beings. From there, the therapist is able to help the client move to her own ancestry and the meaning of this loss.

The use of photographs and guided imagery (picturing) enables the client to get at a more specific and concrete level of imagery by "seeing" what the lost family members were like. The therapist, as witness to the lost members, comes to know and appreciate these people and their meaning to the client. Hanna, age 30, was beset with a sense of "invisibility" about herself and her ability to let people know about her vulnerability. A highly successful professional, she was beset by anxiety over maintaining her poise and calmness, and bewildered by high reactivity to change and the fear of loss of control. When I introduced guided imagery and asked her to imagine who else in her family might have experienced the need for "invisibility" while maintaining a sense of absolute control, she pictured her mother and her maternal grandparents, who were forced to leave their apartment in the middle of the night, act like non-Jews, and present an impeccable image that would give no cause to notice any possible relationship to Jewishness. All through the war, they wandered, masquerading for survival. She also spoke of an image of her mother, at age six, crouching on the roof of a school bus going through the German lines, absolutely still and invisible so as not to be seen. Her job was to be the courier who daily brought food back for the family's survival. At the end of her guided journey, she saw their return to the apartment in France. "It was absolutely barren. The Nazis had removed everything." In that process, she came to appreciate how the pattern of invisibility and control in 1943 was life saving, and how in 1987 it was debilitating and limiting.

Another integrative technique is that of the story-telling method in which I match stories of other second-generation survivors with similar issues with those of my client. This method is Ericksonian (Rosen, 1982; Gordon, 1982). By telling a story with which the client can identify, it shifts the pattern from silence and disconnectedness to one of sharing and connecting.

Finally, hypnosis and the use of dream states is a highly useful tool in enabling the client to gain access to images, to practice ways of shifting them, as well as to access affect. Information from the literature on hypnotherapy and the post-traumatic stress syndrome is especially useful. Brown and Fromm (1986) speak to the importance of using hypnotherapy and imagery techniques gradually to reveal the traumatic images of dreams and the unconscious with the goal of ultimately tying them to affect and context. Emphasis is on integration of the past into the present, with the therapist enacting the role of respectful and supportive guide who is witness to the uncovering and its meaning in the present.

Case Example: Fern

Fern's therapy demonstrates the essentialness of moving to the unconscious, imagistic level that provides access to the affect and its sources. I have selected parts of the treatment process which specifically focus on her identification with the losses experienced by her father so as to demonstrate the therapeutic goal of individuation with this population. Fern's family fits Danieli's (1981) description of the numb, silent family in which children rarely learned the specific details of their parents' life histories, yet they had the sense that their parents were stuck in the past. Fern grew up experiencing confusion between behaviors and affect, facts and feeling. The area in which there was the greatest confusion were some of the lessons her father taught her about curiosity. She learned that whenever she asked questions about nonfamily issues, he would respond affirmatively and with interesting information. When she made the mistake of asking about his past or that of his family, he would become rageful and frightening, often leaving the room to calm down. Fern was always left with the feeling that she had done something bad, and gradually could not trust herself easily to ask any question of him. Early in the therapy, I assigned journal writing. The following entry describes her childhood confusion:

> When I was nine or ten years old, I remember I went to get the mail and there was a postcard from the synagogue we attended notifying my father of the Yahrzeit of his mother's death. The card read something like, "Reminding you that the anniversary of the death of Fern Z., this year will be on . . ." I remember reading the card, feeling frightened, and running in to show my mother—I know she probably explained the whole thing, but couldn't acknowledge my feelings. I remember trying to explain to myself that I had not died—but who was this other Fern Z.? No one could tell me about her—or no one would tell me—especially my father.

Children of silent families need to identify resources that will enable an identification and enlargement of their life context. In Fern's case, there was an aunt, her father's remaining sister, who had willingly shared the family album with Fern and then came to therapy to tell the stories of the past. In the session, she claimed that the opportunity for witnessing gave her presence value and meaning. In the process, Fern struggled with both the relief of knowing and the pain of exposing her aunt's suffering, even though her aunt experienced relief from the opportunity to witness and share information. Fern writes:

> I think that what my aunt was able to do last week was to make the people in my images, nightmares, and fears into real people . . . with their own lives and values. They became, on some level, people who lived and died and for whom I

cannot be responsible. . . . I think that the part of me that feels like it has died is the depressed, frightened victim who was a victim in this life and who relived, in my mind, . . . in the images of another generation. Until they had their own lives and deaths, they weren't buried . . . it feels very strange but it feels like, in the mourning for those people my aunt talked about, especially my grandmother and the two children, my cousins, I have allowed myself to feel fully alive.

Fern's statement again exemplifies Daniele's (1987) perspective that survivors taught their children how to survive; and in so doing, transmitted the extreme conditions under which they had lived. For years, Fern struggled with a life-threatening depression. Only after she had dealt with some of her numbness and had better control over her dissociated states could she identify what was happening to her. In one session, she stated: "Did I ever tell you that when I wanted to kill myself? It was to stop the screams—I needed to put them to rest. . . . But not myself. It was a terrible struggle." In many of her journal writings, she would come back to: "What is he trying to say to me? He was always saying something in his silence. It's that screaming silence. How I hate it. It makes my whole body shake."

The death of her father and its finality broke through Fern's wall of emotional silence. Two weeks after his death, Fern came to my office. She looked a little pale, but strong and clear eyed. Her father had been dead for only two weeks, and her headaches had disappeared. She likened it to a miracle, as they had haunted her for years. When I asked her when it was that she noticed the pain was gone, she talked of the funeral: "I stood at the grave and watched them put his casket in the ground. Was he in the casket?" she asked, not really wanting a reply. She went on, "I wonder if he is with them now." I replied: "Who do you mean? His family?" She replied, "Yes . . . you know what I mean. I saw them at the funeral. While I was standing at the grave . . . All of a sudden . . . they were there . . . for an instant . . . I felt crazy . . . I watched them all file into the grave with him . . . and then I felt at peace."

The therapeutic process is repetitive and compelling. Fern's headaches returned as she struggled with the meaning of his silent look. Again, it was through a dream that she finally came to integrate the meaning of this look: "I guess what I never realized was . . . that I saw the pain in his eyes every time he looked at me . . . it wasn't fair . . . How do I know all about them?" Over time, Fern has come to understand how it is she carried the lost images; and, with time, she has found ways to integrate and mourn and, ultimately, to find meaning in the resolve. In Israel after her experience at Yad Vashem, she decided to create a living memorial for her father and his lost family. She went to a section near Jerusalem where the land was being restored and bought two seedlings: one young tree to commemorate her father and another for his lost family. I have an image of her on her knees, hands in the earth, carefully smoothing and covering and mounding the soil. As she told of her experience, she cried. I shared those tears of sadness in the knowledge that, at long last, she had found a place for "them."

CONCLUSION

Wiesel has heightened the awareness of the need to bear witness and deal with one's own pain as a means of integrating the past with the present. A survivor of Auschwitz, he speaks of despair: "We have to go into the despair and go beyond it, by working and doing for somebody else, by using it for something else" (in Berger, 1986, p. A10). After he received his Nobel Peace Prize, he stated:

> It's normal to forget what hurts us. But those are the things we should not forget. When you suppress pain, it comes back with terrifying violence to haunt you. To supress memories is to provoke inner turmoil. It's good to open yourself up to your own pain. Once you confront your pain, you can cope with it. (in Christy, 1987, p. 87)

In the context of therapy, the therapist becomes the lost witness to the person(s) whose images and feelings could not be heard or acknowledged by the outside world. In this chapter, I have selected cases primarily from silent families where despair was present, but never directly expressed. Other literature deals with the adaptation of children whose families were more open, and thus were more easily able to integrate the past into the present (Danieli, 1981, 1985). Through case examples of Fern and others whose silent past was a main factor in the search for therapeutic witnessing, I have tried to show the debilitating aspects of organizing one's life through two sets of lenses: the past and the present, or those of the parents and those of the self. The child grows up with conflictual messages: to prove to the world that we/you are normal; and to remember the silent message that she must not forget the past in which there was betrayal, evil, and despair. This creates a conflict between following the family's coping patterns and adapting one's own which are flexible and appropriate for the present. Psychic numbing, anxiety, obsessive behaviors, night terrors, and other defenses are symptomatic of this conflict and create distance in present day relationships. The silenced Holocaust child needs the understanding of the past and its effects in order to integrate her day-to-day reality in a meaningful context.

Danieli (1985) speaks to the danger of fixity, the tendency for psychotherapists to dwell on certain periods in the survivors' lives at the expense of others, in that it hinders survivors and their offspring from meaningfully dealing with the flexible, mastery aspects of their lives. She further states that getting better involves a continuous and consistent unraveling and working through of the individual's or the family's particular victim-survivor pattern that has become rigidified and inappropriate in the present context. Survivor families have confused fixity with stability and operate from the fear that change will stir up the feelings that surround the trauma. Therapy, then, becomes a safe and resourceful environment in which old images and feelings are released so that new images and feelings can be formed and practiced.

The search to explain the psychic osmosis phenomenon in the second generation of Holocaust survivors has taken me to paths of information, images, and feelings that have both stretched my sense of being and heightened my awareness of the meaning and dangers of anticipatory trauma anxiety and denial. To deny means not to attend to what is present and to condemn that which is present to invisibility. Invisibility is the most dangerous outcome in dealing with the event of trauma. The legacy of the Nazi Holocaust is the legacy of the meaning of rupture: fixity, unpreparedness, and the inability to adapt to the meanings of events and experiences around us. The antidote is engagement at the level of facing the images and the feelings of fear, suffering, and despair so as to reengage all parts of the self and restore energy for adaptation, integration, and meaning in the present.

I would like to thank my clients, both past and present, through whose honesty and openess I have begun to appreciate the meaning of victimization and its dangers for humankind.

REFERENCES

Alter, R. (1986, Nov. 2). Mother and son lost in a continent [review of *To the land of the cattails* by A. Appelfeld]. *New York Times, 7,* 34.
Appelfeld, A. (1981). *The age of wonders.* Boston: David R. Godine.
Appelfeld, A. (1984). *The retreat.* London: Penguin Books.
Appelfeld, A. (1984). *Tzili.* London: Penguin Books.
Becker, E. (1973). *The denial of death.* New York: Free Press.
Berger, J. (1986, Nov. 15). Witness to evil: Eliezer Wiesel. *New York Times,* A10.
Bergman, M., & Jucoy, M. E. (1982). *Generations of the Holocaust.* New York: Basic Books.
Brown, D., & Fromm, E. (1986). *Hypnotherapy and hypnoanalysis.* Hillsdale, N.J.: Lawrence Erlbaum.
Christy, M. (1987, Feb. 1). A survivor remembers: Conversations with Elie Wiesel. *The Boston Sunday Globe,* 87, 90.
Danieli, Y. (1981). Differing adaptational styles in families of survivors of the Nazi Holocaust. *Children Today,* Sept.-Oct.
Danieli, Y. (1981). Therapist' difficulties in treating survivors of the Nazi Holocaust and their children (doctoral dissertation, New York University). *University Microfilms International.*
Danieli, Y. (9185). *The treatment and prevention of long-term effects and intergenerational transmission of victimization: A lesson from Holocaust survivors and their children.* In C. Figley (Ed.), *Trauma and its wake* (pp. 295–313). New York: Brunner/Mazel
Danieli, Y. (1988). Treating survivors and children of survivors of the Nazi Holocaust. In F. M. Ochberg (Ed.), *Victims of violence and post traumatic therapy.* New York: Brunner/Mazel
Epstein, H. (1970). *Children of the Holocaust.* New York: G. P. Putnam's Sons.
Epstein, L. (1979). *King of the Jews.* New York: Coward, McCann, & Geoghogan.
Ettinger, E. (1970). *Kindergarten.* Boston: Houghton-Mifflin.
Gordon, D. (1982). Ericksonian anecdotal therapy. In J. Zeig (Ed.), *Ericksonian approaches to hypnosis and psychotherapy.* New York: Brunner/Mazel.
Hoffman, L. (1981). *Foundations of family therapy: A conceptual framework for systems change.* New York: Basic Books.
Keeney, B. (1983). *Aesthetics of change.* New York: Guilford Press.
Kerstenberg, J., & Kerstenberg, M. (1980). Psycho-analysis of children of survivors from the Nazi persecution: The continuing struggle of survivor parents. *Victimology: An International Journal,* 5, 368–373.

Krystal, H., & Niederland, W. G. (1968). Clinical observations on the survivor syndrome. In H. Kyrstal (Ed.), *Massive psychic trauma (pp. 368–373). New York: International University Press.*

Levi, P. (1985). If not now, when?. New York: Penguin Books.

Lifton, R. J. (1968). *Death in life, survivors of Hiroshima.* New York: Random House.

Lifton, R. J. (1973). *Home from the war.* New York: Simon & Schuster.

Lifton, R. J. (1979). *The broken connection.* New York: Simon & Schuster.

Lifton, R. J., & Olson, E. (1976). The human meaning of total disaster, the Buffalo Creek experience. *Psychiatry, 39,* 1–18.

MacPherson, M. (1986). *Time bomb.* New York: Dutton.

McGoldrick, M., & Gerson, R. (1985). *Genograms in family assessment.* New York: W. W. Norton.

Paul, N., & Grosser, G. H. (1965). Operational mourning and its role in conjoint family therapy. *Community Mental Health Journal 1,* 339–345.

Rosen, S. (1982). *My voice will go with you: The teaching tales of Milton Erickson.* New York: W. W. Norton.

Rothchild, S. (1981). *Voices from the Holocaust.* New York: New American Library.

Shelley, L. (1987). Jewish Holocaust survivors' attitudes toward contemporary beliefs about themselves. (doctoral dissertation, The Fielding Institute, 1983). *University Microfilms International.*

Sichrovsky, P. (1987). *Strangers in their land.* New York: Penguin Books.

Solomon, S. (1986). The terror in being human. *Skidmore Voices.*

Van der Kolk, B. A. (1987). Psychological trauma. Washington, D.C.: American Psychiatric Press.

Watzlawick, P. (1978). *The language of change.* New York: Basic Books.

Wiesel, E. (1969). *Night.* New York: Avon Books.

Wiesel, E. (1970). *The accident.* New York: Avon Books.

Wiesel, E. (1978). *One generation after.* New York: Pocket Books.

Winnik, H. (1965). Further comments concerning problems of late psychopathological effects of Nazi persecution and their therapy. *Israel Annals of Psychiatry, 5,* 1–16

Work Group to revise DSM-III of the American Psychological Association (1985). *Traumatic stress points1,* 1.6.

Wouk, H. (1973). *The winds of war.* New York: Little, Brown

Wyman, D. (1984). *Abandonment of the Jews.* New York: Pantheon Books.

Wynn, L. (1984). The epigenesis of relational systems: A model for understanding family development. *Family Process, 23,* 297–318.

17

FAMILY THERAPY WITH SOUTHEAST ASIAN FAMILIES

Evelyn Lee, Ed.D.

Family therapy with Southeast Asian refugee families is both challenging and rewarding. Unlike many American families, they bring a unique set of political, cultural, social, and linguistic factors to the therapeutic encounter. To treat Southeast Asian families successfully, the therapist needs to understand their unique life experiences and world view and to develop culturally attuned interventions at various phases of the treatment process. The purpose of this chapter is to identify some of the special cultural and environmental issues relevant to the experiences of Southeast Asian families. A model for diagnostic assessment and treatment is recommended.

This chapter is divided into two parts. The first part explores the impact of war, family interactional patterns, and the effects of cultural transition on the Southeast Asian family system. Four questions will be addressed:

1. What are the psychological effects of war trauma on the Southeast Asian refugees?
2. What are the effects of migration and acculturation stresses on the family system?
3. What are the traditional and transitional cultural characteristics of Southeast Asian families?
4. What are the clinical manifestations of mental health problems of this population?

The second part of this chapter attempts to translate our understanding of the refugee experiences into effective clinical strategies. A family assessment model that takes into account the political-social-cultural variables will be presented. Practical guidelines for effective treatment will also be discussed. The suggestions are meant to be a general framework within which to approach families in a clinical situation. Southeast Asian individuals vary as to their country of origin, migration pattern, degree of trauma, and socioeconomic level. Effective therapy requires the therapist to see the refugees as individuals rather than in terms of ethnocentric stereotypes.

THE TRAUMA OF MASS VIOLENCE AND TORTURE

Background

The United States is accepting the largest number of displaced persons since World War II. Over 70% are Southeast Asians (Mollica et al, 1987). The total Southeast Asian refugee population in the United States was 711,001 as of September 1984. Half of the five major ethnic groups of Vietnamese, Chinese Vietnamese, Cambodians, Hmong and Lao have settled in the Western States and a third have become residents of California (Office of Refugee Resettlement, 1985).

There have been two major groups of Southeast Asian refugee settlement in the United States: from 1975 to 1977 and from 1978 to the present. Major economic, and sociocultural political, differences exist between these two waves of refugees. The first group admitted to the United States was almost all Vietnamese. They were generally well-educated, young, urban dwellers and in the company of family (Montero, 1979). The second wave of refugees included much greater numbers of Hmong, Lao, Khmer, and Chinese-Vietnamese ethnic groups. They were generally less well educated, less literate, of rural origin, and much more traumatized during their escape.

Many Southeast Asian refugees have suffered serious war traumas. A significant number of them are survivors of hunger, rape, incarceration, forced migration, and torture. Between 1977 and 1980, an estimated half million "boat people" left Vietnam, and 200,000 of them died at sea. More than 80 percent of the boats were boarded by pirates who robbed, raped, assaulted, and killed the refugees (Knoll, 1982). The survivors who reached the shores stayed for years in overcrowded and unsanitary refugee camps awaiting an uncertain future. Since 1975, an estimated 300,000 refugees have left Laos. The Pathet Lao tried to halt these refugee flights by exterminating the Hmong with napalm and nerve gas. Entire villages were destroyed. Some estimate that one-half the people who fled died on route to Thailand. Many died from starvation (Knoll, 1982). The most seriously traumatized Southeast Asian refugee group is the Cambodians. Between one and three million of Cambodia's population of seven million died under the Pol Pot regime. Hundreds of thousands were executed. The horror is described as one of the most violent blood baths in the twentieth century (Kinzie et al., 1984).

Psychological Consequences of Trauma

The human response to sudden and overwhelming life experiences is increasingly recognized as a stable psychological entity (Horowitz, 1986; Figley, 1985, Van der Kolk, 1987). Two recent studies of Kinzie, Fredrickson, Ben, Fleck, and Kares (1984) and Mollica, Wyshak, and Lavekle (1986) have suggested that many Southeast Asian patients suffer from both depression and the post-traumatic stress disorder (to be discussed later).

There are no specific studies on the impact of trauma on Southeast Asian family systems. Contemporary studies of trauma in other groups have largely emphasized individual and intrapsychic responses, with little attention to the effect of trauma on the family. One of the very few studies conducted on the family is the work of Danieli (1985) with Nazi holocaust survivors and offspring. She formulated four major categories of survivor families: victim families, fighter families, numb families, and families of "those who made it." Like families of survivors of the Nazi holocaust, many Southeast Asian families suffered from tremendous trauma and losses. The management of rage, aggression, despair, guilt, grief, and hopelessness was an enormous problem for them. Life during the war and the escape process did not afford the survivors adequate opportunities for expression of these feelings. Denial and repression of negative feelings were also encouraged by the Asian culture. During the postmigration period, many expressed such repressed emotions in the form of somatization, nightmares, compulsive work, drug abuse, and physical abuse of family members. Parental fighting sometimes took the form of uncontrollable rage, usually followed by outbursts of tears and self-pity. Adolescent children often feel an intense obligation to compensate for the parents' helplessness and sorrow (Lee, 1988).

EFFECTS OF MIGRATION AND ACCULTURATION STRESSES ON SOUTHEAST ASIAN FAMILIES

Refugee status presumably is more stressful than voluntary emigration as it involves unwilling separations, disenfranchisement, and exposure to trauma, both in the home country and in the search for sanctuary. Caught in varying degrees of unpreparedness, many suffered personal losses in many aspects of their lives. Five types of losses are associated with refugee status: (1) material losses, such as properties, business, career, and investments; (2) physical losses, such as disfigurement, physical injuries, hunger, malnutrition; (3) spiritual losses, such as freedom to practice religion, support from religious community; (4) loss of community support and cultural milieu; and (5) loss of family members, other relatives, and friends. Such losses are particularly traumatic for the Southeast Asian refugees to whom the family, community, and religion are exceedingly important.

While still actively mourning for the losses, refugees must also cope with the oppressive load imposed by the sheer need to survive while reconstructing a new life during the postimmigration period. They need to learn a new language, find a new job, locate housing, and deal with the culture shock in a multiracial racist society.

In recent years, several studies have been conducted to evaluate adjustment problems as perceived by Southeast Asian refugees. Not unexpectedly, the lack of English-language skills ranked as the most serious problem. Family separation was another problem frequently cited by refugees. Other areas of concern are related to more general issues of employment and economic self-sufficiency, difficulties with American agencies, and understanding American life (Strand & Jones, 1985).

What are the effects of stresses on the family system? Migration produces a transitional crisis in the family in predictable stages (Sluzki, 1979). Not only must individual family members adapt to the cultural transplantation, but also the family unit itself must often be reconstructed. New patterns of interaction emerge as a result of changes in family composition. Separation and reunions of family members during the migratory process require structural functional reorganization (Falicov, 1982). A majority of Southeast Asian families have gone through several major changes of family composition. For example, some families sent their "chosen sons or daughters" to the United States during the first refugee exodus in 1975. Their children reunited with another set of family members who fled their home countries by boat in the early 1980s and, for some fortunate families, reunited again with another set of family members who arrived recently by plane. Separation and reunion require constant changes of the family boundaries and structure.

In addition to the changes in the internal family organization, the external stresses caused by the extreme cultural and value differences between Southeast Asians and the host country can be also stressful for family members. Many Southeast Asian refugees came from agricultural societies with no experiences in dealing with life stresses caused by urbanization and industrialization. Many families face a sudden lack of extended family and community support at a time when these are most needed. Where the external stresses are extreme and the internal support systems are not sufficient, family pathologies may develop. Families may become isolated, enmeshed, or disengaged (Landau, 1982).

While family members try to recover from migration stresses, further imbalances may occur during the process of acculturation. Family members usually experience different acculturation rates, and this inevitably leads to transitional conflict. For example, a refugee wife may stay at home with the children and become increasingly isolated and loyal to the original culture, while her husband is learning the new language and values. An adolescent girl may speak better English and become the "cultural broker" or intermediary between the parents and American society, weakening the authority of the parents and aggravating intergenerational conflicts.

McGoldrick (1982) provided an excellent insight regarding the effects of migration on different stages of family life cycles. The readjustment to a new culture is a prolonged developmental process of adjustment, which will affect family members differently, depending on the individual and the family life cycle phase the person is in at the time of transition. For example, families that migrate with young children are perhaps strengthened by having each other, but they are vulnerable to the parental reversal of hierarchies. Families migrating when their children are adolescents may have more difficulty because they will have less time together as a unit before the children move out on their own. Thus, the family must struggle with multiple transitions and generational conflicts at once. In addition, the distance from the grandparental generation in the old country may be particularly distressing as grandparents become ill, dependent, or die. The parents may experience severe stress in not being able to fulfill their obligations to their parents in the country of origin. It is not uncommon for symptoms to develop in adolescents in reaction to their unexpressed distress.

CULTURAL CHARACTERISTICS OF SOUTHEAST ASIAN FAMILIES

Traditional Values

Asian family values are very different from Western family values. The agricultural background and the teachings of Confucius and Buddha have had a profound influence on Asian values and family interactional patterns. In traditional Southeast Asian families, interpersonal interactions are determined more by prescribed roles, obligations, and duties than by a person-oriented process. The individual is seen as the product of all the generations of his or her family from the beginning of time. Family members learn to respect elders, authority, status, and clear expectations from other members. Interdependence and obedience are valued. Independence and self-determination are discouraged. Shame and loss of face are frequently used to reinforce adherence to prescribed sets of role and obligations. Family members are obliged to make all kinds of self-sacrifices for other family members.

Marital subsystem

In the extended Southeast Asian families, the dominant relationship is more likely to be placed in an intergenerational dyad than in a husband–wife dyad. Leadership and authority are also vested in the intergenerational tie. The husband assumes the instrumental role of the provider, decision maker, and protector of the family and the wife assumes the expressive role of homemaker. Marriage is arranged to ensure the family prosperity and continue the man's family line rather than on a basis of romantic love. In marital relationships, it is considered a sign of maturity not to express love overtly, especially not in front of the children and elders. When things go wrong in a marriage, the difficulties may be repaired by other adult mediators or confidants. Divorce is not a common practice. However, emotional divorce is not uncommon. In such cases, the mother transfers her love to the children, and the father compensates by working compulsively and spending his leisure time with other men. A woman is usually dominated by the authority of her father, husband, son, and mother-in-law. She achieves status only when she becomes an elder. Because of the closeness of the mother and the son, the working out of the mother-in-law and daughter-in-law relationship is crucial to the success of the marriage.

Parent/Child subsystem

The traditional role of the father is to discipline and control, and the role of the mother is to provide nurturance and support. The Father's and mother's functions tend to be complementary rather than symmetrical. As the relationship between parents and children is considered to be more important than the marital relationship, the strongest emotional attachment for a woman is usually not to her husband, but to her children, especially the sons. Hierarchies in most Southeast Asian families are clearly defined, and most parents demand filial piety, respect, and obedience from their children.

Affective ties for children are not focused solely on their parents, but are spread over a wide range of adult figures. Generally speaking, children are not believed to be capable of acting independently until they reach "maturity." Maturity is defined according to the cultural rules regardless of physical and emotional development of the child. Traditionally, parents are expected to be taken care of in their old age and have strong connections with their adult children. A daughter does not move out until she marries. A son is expected to live in the parental household with his bride. Thus, Southeast Asian parents may never experience an empty nest.

Sibling subsystem

Siblings play important roles for each other throughout life. The ties among siblings are very strong in the Southeast Asian family tradition. Sibling bonding is especially strong for those who suffered together during the war. Because of the large number of siblings, parents usually delegate some supervisory functions to the older siblings and encourage children to have their own siblings and cousins as playmates. Cooperation, sharing, and even sacrifice for other siblings are stressed. However, quarrels and resentment among siblings are common. Within the traditional agricultural Asian cultures, sons are more valued. The executive power rests with the father, and eventually passes to the son. The oldest daughter is still seen primarily as the caretaker of the household and the nurturant parent for the younger siblings in the absence of the mother.

Families in Transition

Repeated contact with the new values over a prolonged period of time changes the family's outlook on such issues as sex role, child rearing, educational achievement, and philosophy of life. The values, norms, and role behaviors learned in the home country become a source of stress when the family comes into contact with the new culture. Many Southeast Asian families are in transition from an extended family to a nuclear unit through the inevitable changes induced by migration, urbanization, and modernization. Refugee families are forced to move from settings where there was stability of values and ideas based on tradition, generational continuity, and authority to American society where the family is based on the centrality of the marital dyad and the cultural codes and norms of the Western industrial world. Family members are usually struggling to hold on to the old ways while trying to develop new rules congruent with the new environment. Some families eventually accomplish this task, but some develop symptoms when attempting to force a blend between two contradictoy sets of rules.

Generally speaking, Southeast Asian families in the United states can be divided into three major types: traditional families, transitional families, and bicultural families (Lee, in press).

Traditional families

These include families from agricultural backgrounds, families who are recent arrivals, refugees who are older at the time of immigration, and families who live in an ethnic neighborhood. Family members speak in their native language and make little attempt to be "Americanized."

Transitional families

Such families usually arrived a decade ago when their children were young, or are families with American-born children. The family system usually experiences a great degree of cultural conflict between the acculturated children and the traditional parents. Individual goals of the individual member are in conflict with family goals. Intergerational conflicts, marital difficulties, and cultural identity confusion are common problems.

Bicultural families

Such families usually came from the urban cities of Southeast Asian and are familiar with Western culture. Family members are very well acculturated, bilingual, and bicultural. They want to be able eventually to integrate the two cultures, to make sense out of the apparent cultural confusion and contradiction.

These families all have different help-seeking patterns. The traditional families generally come to agencies with many environmental problems that require concrete assistance and language interpretation; the transitional families usually need help in resolving generational conflicts, role confusion, and communication problems. The bicultural families require little help from outside agencies and appear to be quite adaptable in the new country. (Lee, in press).

CLINICAL MANIFESTATIONS OF MENTAL HEALTH PROBLEMS OF SOUTHEAST ASIAN REFUGEES

Anxiety and depression are the most frequent nonpsychotic conditions for which Southeast Asian patients will seek help from their doctors or mental health professionals. The typical symptomatology includes a rich variety of com-plaints: headaches, dizziness, poor appetite, fatigue, aches and pains in the limbs, feeling of constant chill, poor concentration, sleep disorder, and suicidal thoughts (Kinzie & Manson, 1983; Nguyen, 1982; Tung, 1985; Lee, 1985; Lee & Chan, 1985).

The post-traumatic stress disorder (PTSD) is exprienced as occurrences of repetitive nightmares of catastrophic events, intrusive thinking, restlessness, irritability, recurrent explosive anger, hyperalertness, poor concentration, and "survivor guilt." Patients who experience somatization present a description of "weak heart" (palpitation, fatigue), "weak kidney" (sexual dysfunctions, lower back pain, headache, decreased intellectual function), and "weak nervous sys-tems" (inability to concentrate, irritability, poor memory) (Tung, 1980). Many patients hide their depressive illness behind somatic complaints.

Schizophrenia accounts for 20 percent of the diagnoses in Southeast Asians in an inpatient hospital (Lee, 1985). One type of psychotic reaction that is of particular interest involves a systematized paranoid delusion that affects an individual who has had no symptoms until sometime after he or she arrives in the United States (Tung, 1985).

Alcoholism, substance abuse, and gambling are more common among the single male adults and late teens. Finaly, clients present with family problems includeing (1) parital conflicts resulting in physical violence and or threat of divorce; (2) parent/child conflicts resulting in child abuse, runaways, teenage pregnancy, and so on; (3) in-law conflicts; and (4) sibling rivalry.

SUGGESTED GUIDELINES FOR FAMILY ASSESSMENT

Because of the refugee experiences and their unique cultural background, the evaluation and assessment of Southeast Asian refugee families must include information beyond traditional intake data. The following section provides an assessment model, which includes (1) assessment of major family stressors, (2) assessment of family strengths, and (3) assessment of culturally specific re-sponses to mental health problems. (Lee, in press.)

Assessment of Family Stressors

Migration stress caused by war and relocation

When taking a thorough case history, the clinician should not concentrate solely on recent symptoms and traumatic events. A chronological approach focusing on three major aspects of the family's migration history is needed (Lee & Lu, 1989).

1. Premigration experience (life in the homeland)
●Socioeconomic status of the family before the war
●Type of community where the family lived
●Major caretaker(s) before the escape

●Educational, medical, and recreational systems in the home country
●Traumatic events in the family: death of family members, loss of significant relatives, loss of family properties, and so on
●Significant physical injury and/or emotional difficulties
●Traumatic events encountered: degree of exposure to death and dying, degree of torture, degree of assault

2. Migration experiences (the escape process and life in a refugee camp)
●Decision to leave: why, when, and who
●Degree and type of trauma during escape: e.g., attacks by pirates, rape, hunger, exposure to death
●The refugee camp experience: physical safety, psychological support
●Separation and losses of significant others
●Stress induced by legal immigration process: uncertainty of sponsorship, duration of waiting

3. Postmigration experiences (life immediately after the arrival in United States):
●Problems encountered caused by language difficulties
●School adjustment and academic demands
●Financial worries
●Culture shock
●Changes in living environment and neighborhood
●Significant changes in family composition and relationship
●The reception experience in the host environment.

Acculturation stress

As indicated earlier, there are major differences between the traditional Southeast Asian values and the contemporary urban industrial values. After the refugees have settled in the new country for awhile, they usually do not fall into the two extremes of the opposite cultural forces. The degree of acculturation of each individual refugee depends on the age at immigration, past and present exposure to Western culture, and degree of interaction with other ethnic groups. The therapist needs to assess the acculturation rate of each family member and the family changes associated with cultural transition.

Family stress caused by role changes

There are role changes in these families that are very stressful. First, Intergenerational conflicts may be caused by the disparity between the children's and the parents' values. Asian parents expect their children to be quiet, obedient, polite, humble, hard working, and respectful to them and other extended-family members. Good sons and daughters are expected to take care of younger siblings, take care of their aged parents, and bring honor to the family. However, many acculturated children identify more with American values that have strong emphasis on independence, self-reliance, assertiveness, "open communication," and competition. As many adolescents live with their grandparents, many families face not only gaps between two generations, but triple generational gaps.

Second, conflicts may be caused by role reversal between parents and children. Many monolingual parents depend on their English-speaking children in negotiations with the outside world. Such dependence can evoke anger and resentment on both parts. The need to supplement family income has forced refugee women, who did not work in Southeast Asia, to seek employment. Though this new freedom and economic power are generally valued by the women, it undermines traditional patriarchal authority and causes marital conflict.

Third, family stress may be caused by the fact that many refugees did not receive their parenting from their biololgical parents, because of the extended-family system and multiple losses and separation from family members during the war. Family reunion in the United States after years of separation may trigger many unresolved family conflicts and resentments.

Finally, there are conflicts that arise with the sponsor. With no other alternatives, many refugees have to be quite dependent on the sponsor's financial, legal, and emotional support, especially when they first arrive in this country. The legal sponsor is often given a great deal of power in many family decisions, including where to live, which school to go to, which agency to receive help from, or even which family members should be sponsored to come to the United States. The role of the sponsor (usually assumed by the adult children or other siblings who migrated earlier than their parents) is at times in conflict with the traditional role in refugee families.

Work and financial stresses

Hope of improving the family's economic status is one of the major reasons for migration. However, because of language barriers and lack of job opportunities, many refugees suffer from unemployment or underemployment. "Status inconsistency" or "downward mobility" leads to low self-esteem, insecurity of the individuals, and role reversal in the family system. The upwardly mobile segments of the refugee population also face hidden stress. Upward mobility often requires long working hours and dissociation with their ethnic groups. Family members may feel compelled to make a choice between moving ahead and loyalty to other family members who stay behind. This, in itself, can be a source of severe identity conflict for family members (Lee, 1982).

Stress caused by legal problems

Many refugees place their hopes and dreams on sponsoring other family members to come to the United States. Because of language difficulties, unfamiliarity with the legal procedure, financial costs (legal fee, transportation, etc.), many families are under tremendous stress. In addition, which family member should be sponsored also cause family disagreements and arouse many unresolved family conficts in the past.

Stress caused by the living environment and community attitude

Many refugees live in poor neighborhoods where they encounter problems of inadequate housing, racism, crimes, drugs, prostitution, and the like. Within the refugee communities, family members also have to cope with the issues of shame or losing face because of the stigma of emotional problems. Therapists need to assess carefully the degree of support or vulnerability felt by the refugee family with regard to the outside American society and the refugee community.

Physical problems caused by war and refugee experiences

Because of physical injuries, malnutrition, and lack of adequate medical treatment during the war, many refugees need medical attention. For psychiatric patients, their psychiatric symptoms may have an organic etiology that requires careful clinical observations and medical examinations. It is very important routinely to request information on the patients' physical condition and family medical history. Close consultation with physicians or indigenous healers and working together as a team wherever possible are highly recommended. In addition, the therapist needs to take a detailed history of medicines (including herbal medicine) used by patients and other family members. (It is quite common for refugees' family members to share medication and send medication to their relatives and friends back home.) Attention paid by the therapist regarding physical health and medication can enhance the credibility of the therapist because Southeast Asians are more likely to believe that emotional problems are caused by organic factors.

Assessment of Family Strengths

In addition to the assessment of stress, careful assessment is necessary with respect to individual and family strengths in past adaptation, coping, and problem solving. The Southeast Asian families arrive in the United states with many problems associated with their refuge experiences. They also bring along thousands of years of Asian culture and culturally specific coping strategies in response to stress. In addition to their cultural strengths, many refugees draw support from many sources in their immediate environmemt, such as family, school, friends, relatives, sponsors, teachers, peers at home, the refugee community, and service providers.

Culturally Specific Responses to Mental Health Problems

In coming to understand the causes of mental illness or emotional problems, many traditional Southeast Asians rarely invoke psychological explanations. A mental problem is conceptualized as a manifestation of organic disorders, hereditary weakness, imbalance between yin and yang elements, supernatural intervention, or emotional exhaustion caused by external situation factors (Lee, 1982). They usually seek help in a state of crisis with the expectation of an immediate "cure." In the assessment process, it is essential for the therapist to encourage the patient and his or her family members to discuss openly their cultural viewpoints on the causes of the problem, their past efforts in coping with the problem, and their treatment expectations. The discussion can be based on the following questions: (Lee, in press).

- What are the symptoms and problems as perceived by family members?
- What do family members think of as the causes of the problem?
- Are the presenting problems related to the refugee and war experiences?
- Where did the family go to get help?
- What are the family's treatment expectations?

Summary of Assessment

In summary, the assessment of special family stressors, strengths, and cultural responses to the presenting problem provides a practical guideline in the diagnostic inquiry of Southeast Asian refugee families. In the process of evaluation, there are several potential problems that can create difficulties:

First, many refugees do not understand the significance and procedures of evaluation. They are either not used to detailed history taking or do not understand the relationship between the question and the presenting symptoms. Some may even suspect that such information will be put to political use, thus jeopardizing their immigration status.

Second, refugees tend to be very discreet about family problems. Family members feel loyal and protective of each other and of the clan and will readily censor any public inquiries that could cast a bad light upon the family group or ethnic group (Tung, 1985). Such protection may lead to an understatment of the family pathology.

Third, there is a lack of bilingual, bicultural assessment tools. Many psychological testing and mental status examination questions are irrelevant to the refugees' experiences and may lead to misdiagnosis. It is important for the therapist to be sensitive to such issues and search for culturally relevant materials for psychological evaluation.

SUGGESTED APPROACHES FOR SUCCESSFUL TREATMENT

The strong family orientation of Southeast Asian refugees would indicate that family therapy is the ideal treatment modality to deal with this population. However, Southeast Asians generally do not seek family treatment or they only seek treatment when all other alternatives have failed. Besides underutilization of services, there are also problems of premature termination of services and poor therapeutic outcomes. The following reasons highlight some of the possible difficulties.

First, mental health concepts as they exist in current practice are foreign to the majority of the Southeast Asian groups. For example, clinical psychology and psychiatric social work as professions are almost unheard of in Southeast

Asian countries. For Southeast Asians, mental health is viewed in terms of "being crazy" and "not being crazy." Therefore, going to see mental health counselors is highly stigmatized by other relatives and friends and avoided at all costs.

Second, mental health techniques as practiced by American therapists are not compatible with Southeast Asian cultural values. The training of American therapists has been usually permeated by the U.S. middle-class values of individualism, egalitarianism, change and future orientation, self-determination, and self-fulfillment. The therapist usually expects the family to work things out together, to talk things over, to keep appointments weekly and be on time, to take responsibility for their own actions, to gain insight into the causes for the problems, and to plan for change. In contrast, traditional Southeast Asian values stress family interdependence and loyalty, age and sex hierarchies, collectivism and cooperation, and protection of family boundaries and secrets.

Third, family members usually do not see individual problems as family related (Tung, 1980). Southeast Asians are rarely agreeable to the suggestion that the problem is the group's instead of the identified patient's. They usually do not understand the need for family therapy as a way to improve the individual's pathological symptoms. In addition, owing to the family communication style and the family hierarchy, parents will abstain from disclosing their feelings in front of the children. Children will refrain from saying anything negative about their parents. And all resent a therapist who wants to suggest that the problem is caused by the family.

Fourth, there is a reluctance to deal with the emotional pain caused by the trauma of war. Almost all refugees have faced terrible personal encounters of brutality and cruelty. In the process of resettlement in a new country, many of them want to put aside the horror stories and go on with their lives. Many of them may not have even shared their horror stories with other family members. Therefore, family therapy can be very threatening to the refugees who try to repress these painful memories. In addition, countertransference issues on the part of the therapist in dealing with traumatized clients can also lead to inappropriate treatment and premature terminations. The majority of American therapists did not experience war themselves. Clinical contact with refugee clients may stir up feelings of helplessness, rage, anger, and self-doubt of the own capacity to endure similar traumatic conditions.

Fifth, there are language and communication difficulties. As a result of different linguistic patterns and cultural assumptions, interpretation poses many barriers. Using interpreters to work with patients and families is considered to be particularly problematic because of the difficulties in translating both words and emotions. In addition, most likely the refugee interpreters are trauma survivors themselves. Their countertransference issues also present special problems in the therapeutic encounters.

Finally, other barriers are present, such as accessibility of the agency, office hours, service fee, and so on.

TREATMENT RECOMMENDATIONS: STRUCTURE AND STRATEGIES

Structural Aspects

Membership

The therapist should encourage all family members to come to the first session so that the interaction among family members can be observed. However, in many instances, the "Let's get together and talk openly" approach would not be possible or appropriate. Family therapy does not always require all-encompassing family involvement. Therapists should pay special attention to the readiness of family members to communicate as a group, and the natural groupings within thew family.

A flexible subfamily system approach in the establishment of therapeutic relationships with family members at times can be very helpful. For example, an effective method is for a therapist to interview the parents first, then the subgroup, and then bring the whole family together for a feedback session with the therapist. The parents can discuss their adult concerns or express their emotion in the absence of the children. The children, usually more acculturated and more fluent in English, can negotiate issues they might not bring up with their parents present. Parents will tend to respect the feelings that the children have for each other as a sign of sibling solidarity.

Goal setting

A problem-focused, goal-oriented, and symptom-relieving approach is highly recommended. Rather than defining goals in abstract, emotional terms, goals may be best stated in terms of external resolution or symptom reduction. Long-term goals may best be broken down into a series of easy-to-understand, achievable, measurable, short-term goals. Once the family is engaged in the therapeutic relationship, the therapist can gradually introduce other, more insight-oriented goals and renegotiate with the family members.

Timing and number of sessions

The first session is usually the most crucial one, which may determine whether or not the family will stay in treatment. Therapists should take advantage of the family energy mobilized by the presenting family crisis to conduct an extensive evaluation and offer immediate help if possible. Allowance of an extended period of time for the first session is often necessary. The ending of the session should not be based on the clock, but on clinical observations. In the beginning phases of therapy, the traditional 55-minute, once-a-week session may be inappropriate. To capitalize on the heightened energy induced by crisis, the family should be seen more frequently during the beginning phases of therapy and gradually move to once a week or once a month if clinically indicated.

Office interviews versus home visits

For the family members who are motivated to engage in treatment, office interviews can be very therapeutic and cost-effective. Although travel to the home increases the expense of therapy, family therapy in the home offers many unique benefits. Patients and families are more relaxed in their own homes. During the home visits, family members can reenact family disputes and rehearse more effective communication and problem solving in the natural setting. Furthermore, the home visits may enhance the therapeutic alliance. Family members may see such visits as symbols of the therapist's caring and commitment to help.

Treatment Strategies

Forming a social and cultural relationship
with family during the initial phase of treatment

During the first session, the therapist should pronounce the family name correctly and address the Southeast Asian family in a polite and formal manner, using last names to introduce himself or herself and when speaking to the adults. Given the culture's emphasis on interpersonal relationships, a social phase that transmits the therapist's interest in the persons involved rather than focusing on procedures (such as referral sheets or billing forms) is helpful. Asking non-threatening personal pquestions at the beginning phase of conversation can put the family at ease. "Have you had lunch yet?," "Is today your day off?," Unstructured formal questions such as, "What brought you here?," "Can you tell me more about the family problems?," and "How do you feel?" may arouse discomfort and distrust (Lee, in press).

As influenced by the Asian culture, Southeast Asian refugees in general are very interested in the personal background of the therapist. During the initial stage of relationship, the family may expect the therapist to do a certain amount of self-disclosure concerning his or her family, cultural, academic, and professional background. Self-dislosure allows the family to assess the therapist as a person and enables the development of a necessary level of trust and confidence. It is helpful for the therapist to share some of his or her own cultural background, and familiarity with the refugee culture (such as philosophy, migration history, food, music, humor) to establish credibility. If the therapist has had similar migration experiences in his or her family, sharing them may facilitate positive cultural alliance.

With respect to the traditional age/sex hierarchies, it is advisable to address questions to the father first, then to the mother, then to other adults, and finally to the older and then younger children. Directing the opening to the parents helps establish culturally consonant generational boundaries. It is also important at the beginning of the relationship to avoid direct confrontation, to demand greater emotional disclosure, or to discuss culturally taboo subjects. (Lee, in press)

Defining the problem

Since cultural norms emphasize the importance of the parent–child dyad

over the marital dyad, during the initial stage, a focus on parent–child interactions is more readily accepted than a focus on marital issues. In fact, it is
almost unheard of for Southeast Asian couples to ask for marital counseling. In
most instances, family members ask for professional help because of the difficulties they encounter with one particular family member (the identified parent).
Parents are either unaware of their roles in contributing to the problem, or are
unwilling to discuss it openly in front of their children.

In order to engage the family in therapy, it is important for the therapist to
(1) acknowledge the identified patient as the problem, (2) assist the family to
shift from person-focused to problem-focused attitudes, (3) focus on the effect
of the problem on each family member, (4) verbalize the family pain caused by
the difficulties, and (5) reinforce the sense of family obligation and the significant
role of the family members in solving the problem together. At times, it may
be helpful to encourage family members to elaborate their previous attempts in
dealing with the problem. The realization of their coping failures and the unpleasant consequences if the problem is uncorrected may motivate the family
to continue in treatment. The therapist should take on a nonblaming attitude
toward the family and the identified patient. In some situations, the therapist
may use the family sense of guilt and obligation to participate in treatment for
the sake of the family name. (Lee, in press)

*Educating the family about the procedures, the illness, and how the family
members can be of help.*

In order to motivate the family to come back, it is important to help the
family to understand how talking about problems to a third party can result in
the alleviation of emotional, physical, or behavioral distress. It is also very
important for the therapist to explore the family's perception of the causes of
problems and their treatment expectations. A general verbal agreement about
what problems would be addressed and an estimate of the number of sessions
should be made. (An explicit formal contract may be too task oriented.) Treatment objectives should be phrased simply and focused on either specific symptoms or on emotional/environmental problems with which to work.

Education is highly valued in Southeast Asian cultures. The psychoeducational approach (McGill & Lee, 1986) based on social learning principles may be
compatible with many Southeast Asian values and beliefs. Such intervention
focuses on four major areas: (1) education about the illness (or problem), (2)
communication training, (3) problem-solving training, and (4) behavioral management strategies. (It is beyond the scope of this chapter to discuss each technique in detail.)

Establishing power, credibility, and authority.

The therapist should convey expertise and use caution in establishing an
initial egalitarian therapeutic relationship. Because Southeast Asian families view
family relationships in terms of a vertical hierarchy, extreme caution is advised
against adopting a democratic attitude in the therapeutic relationship. The therapist will need to take a much more authoritative attitude than may be customary, as Southeast Asian family members view the therapist as the problem solver

and expect him or her to behave in an authoritative or parental manner. They will feel very uncomfortable if put on a peer level with the therapist. Credibility refers to the client's perception of the therapist as an effective and trustworthy helper (Sue & Zane, 1987). An air of confidence, empathic understanding, warmth, maturity, and professional mannerism are all important ingredients in developing credibility.

If the therapist does not know a cultural norm or wishes to find out what a particular norm means to the family, he or she can ask such questions as, "How old do you think your daughter should be to be allowed to go to the school dance?" This approach has the advantage of acknowledging the parents' authority and of avoiding making cultural misinterpretations. If the therapist works with a knowledgeable interpreter from the same cultural background as the family, he or she should use the interpreter as the cultural expert. If possible, the therapist should not make an issue of his or her ignorance as this would tend to decrease the therapist's authority and credibility.

Talk therapy is not common in most of the Asian countries. Many come to see an "expert" with the cultural expectation of receiving directives. Nonjudgmental listening and neutrality in the therapist's responses may be viewed as a lack of interest or incompetence. As verbal expression of feelings is not encouraged in Southeast Asian cultures, the client's dissatisfaction may not be made known to the clinician.

The ways of acquiring therapeutic power include (l) obtaining sufficient information about the patient and the family before seeing the family, (2) offering some possible explanations for the cause of the problem, (3) showing familiarity with the family's cultural background and making necessary "cultural connection," (4) providing a set of cues that help the family to judge the therapists's expertise (i.e., "according to my experience working with Southeast Asian refugees the past ten years," and (5) utilizing the crisis intervention approach of offering the client some immediate solutions to the problems. (Lee, in press)

Building alliance with members with power.

Treatment will not be effective without the permission of the leader(s) in the vertical, hierarchical structure. Therefore the therapists should acknowledge their power in decision making and engage them in therapy with all possible means. Generally speaking, there are two types of power in the family system: role-prescribed power (usually given to the grandfather, father, oldest son, or the sponsor), and psychological power (usually maintained by the grandmother or the mother). Until the therapist has gained the necessary respect and authority in the eyes of the decision makers, it is important to support the existing power structure. (Lee, in press)

Assuming multiple helping roles

Because of the lack of understanding of the role of mental health professional, flexibility and willingness to assume multiple helping roles enhance the therapeutic relationship. Many refugee families expect the therapist not only to be a "talking" doctor, but also to play the role of teacher, advocate, family advisor, consultant, cultural intermediary, interpreter, and so on. Actions such as tele-phoning the client's physician, talking to the teacher, or getting the client a job can be very therapeutic. However, the therapist should be aware of which roles are therapeutic for the client. The use of paraprofessionals in a team can be effective in allowing for a diversity of therapeutic roles, although it is important to have one primary therapist.

Showing empathy and caring

Southeast Asian clients usually do not view their therapist as merely a profes-sional. They expect the therapist to care about them as people and to guide them as friends. Among refugee patients with a history of long years of sepa-ration from their loved ones, there is a yearning for an actively empathic parental figure. A giving therapist who exhibits warmth is more able to gain the trust of his or her clients. This requires not only careful listening to the clients, but also trying to do something that will be helpful in relieving symptoms. Because of the strong sense of obligation in the culture, clients may view keeping appoint-ments or taking medication as doing something for the therapist in return for the therapist's concern.

Mobilizing the family's cultural strength

Creative use of the client's cultural strengths is encouraged. Strengths such as support from extended-family members and siblings, the strong sense of obligation, the strong focus on educational achievement, the work ethic, the spiritual beliefs, and their survival spirit should be respected and used creatively in the therapeutic process.

Overcoming language barriers

The majority of the refugees do not speak English. There are also marked subgroup differences of dialect and communication style among the various Southeast Asian refugee groups. It is important for the therapist to work with interpreters who can provide both correct language and cultural translation. In order to minimize misdiagnoses and inappropriate treatments, both the inter-preter and clinician need to be trained in cross-cultural communication skills. A training videotape recently developed by Lee (1987) on working with inter-preters in mental health can be used for such training. The therapist needs to pay special attention to his or her own nonverbal communication style (Lee, in press).

Other Treatment Approaches

Normalization reers to a process by which the refugee client comes to realize that his or her thoughts, feelings, or experiences are common and that many individuals encounter similar experiences. The purpose is not to deny unique experiences or to trivialize the client's problem. Rather, it is intended to reassure clients who magnify problems and who are unable to place their experiences in a proper context because of a reluctance to share thoughts with others (Sue & Zane, 1987). The client can be further helped by knowing that other persons who have similar difficulties are treated successfully. This approach appears to help many refugees to feel less alone and ashamed of their distress, as well as to promote a sense of hope.

Generalization is an especially helpful approach in the engagement phase of treatment. The therapist makes general statements relevant to the refugee experiences, and helps the client to make personal connection with the universal problem. For example, the therapist may ask, "Most of newly arrived refugees have difficulty in finding jobs. Did you have the same problem?" Or, "Refugees who escaped by boat experienced a great deal of hardships on the way. What were some of your experiences?" Generalizations using familiar philosophical and religious sayings and examples are found to be especially effective.

Therapeutic use can be made of the "trauma story." Almost every refugee has at least one traumatic experience that figures prominently as an essential aspect of his life or her history. The gentle sharing and acceptance of the trauma story, at the client's own pace and direction, can significantly diminish the refugee client's sense of hopelessness, shame, fear, and guilt. Sharing the story with other family members can also strengthen the empathy among family members. However, the *readiness* of the client must be assessed with care. Too much disclosure may lead to serious, and often unremitting, psychotic distress.

CASE EXAMPLE

Presenting Problem

Mei Le, a 21 year-old Chinese woman from Vietnam, was admitted to the psychiatric ward because of a weight loss of roughly 50 percent. The patient reported that she had been active in school and at work until about 18 months prior to presentation, when she began to lose weight following a loss of appetite. She would eat an average of one meal per day at dinnertime, and then would sometimes vomit "because of stomach upset." She became too weak to go to work, too thin to carry books to school, and too sick to go out with friends. Gradually, in the past few months before admission, the patient had become increasingly socially isolated. She was admitted to a medical ward for a medical checkup for her weight loss, diarrhea, vomiting, and sleeping difficulty. At admission, she weighed only 55 pounds. The initial psychiatric impression was that the patient probably had anorexia nervosa and bulimia.

Because of Mei Le's refugee experiences and her unique cultural background, the evaluation and assessment of her case must include information beyond traditional intake data. Based on the suggested assessment guidelines as outlines in this chapter, the following vital information on the patient and her family was obtained.

Major Stressors

Migration stress caused by war and relocation

Mei Le was born in a rural fishing village in Vietnam, the youngest of seven children in a Chinese, Cantonese-speaking family. The first two siblings died from childhood diseases and another two children died during the war. Life in the fishing village before the war was peaceful and relatively pleasant. Her father worked as a fisherman while her mother took care of the household responsibilities. Mei Le spent most of her time with her siblings and her grandmother.

At the age of 14, Mei Le escaped with her family from Vietnam by boat. Her grandmother stayed behind. Although the patient reported no major incidents on the way to the refugee camp in Malaysia, the escape process was very stressful owing to the many horror stories of robbery and rape she had heard from other refugees. Mei Le spent one year in the refugee camp and then immigrated to the United States with her parents. Unfortunately, her brother and his family were sent to New Zealand and her sister was sent to France. The "forced" separation from her brother and sister was very painful for Mei Le, as she felt she was much closer to her siblings than to her parents.

The postmigration experiences immediately after arrival in the United States were quite difficult for Mei Le and her family. In the fishing village back in Vietnam, Mei Le did not attend any school. At the age of 16, she had to enter junior high as soon as she arrived here. The problems she encountered caused by language difficulties, school adjustment, racism, and academic demands were overwhelming. Her elderly parents (in their late 60s) were not able to obtain employment. To supplement welfare assistance, Mei Le had to go out to work part-time after school in a restaurant. The family also had difficulties in finding suitable housing. All three lived in a small one-bedroom apartment.

Acculturation stresses

While Mei Le tried to recover from migration strresses, she had to learn to adapt to the contemporary urban industrial values, which are almost opposite to the traditional Asian values with which she was brought up in Vietnam. As an adolescent, she was confused by the comparative freedom of American life-style and the definition of her responsibilities to her aging and lonely parents.

Family stress caused by role change

After a few years in the United States, value differences gradually caused conflicts between Mei Le and her parents. As do most traditional Chinese parents, they expected their daughter to be hard working, obedient, dependent, polite, and respectful to elders. Mei Le was expected to take care of her aging parents and to bring honor to the family. However, like many acculturated adolescents, Mei Le also identified with American values with their strong emphasis on independence, self-reliance, and assertiveness. When Mei Le was 17, her parents tried to arrange a marriage for her to a Chinese man from Vietnam. Mei Le refused. Her conflict with her parents was also intensified by role reversal. Her monolingual parents depended on her as the cultural broker and interpreter in negotiations with the outside world. Her economic power as the sole breadwinner also undermined traditional parental authority. In addition to the adolescent and cultural identity crisis, Mei Le also had to struggle with her sexual identity. With her older brothers absent, she had to play the role of the "good son" to support and comfort her parents. She refused to date, and eventually refused to eat.

Our Western understanding was that Mei Le's eating disorder reflected an attempt to become childlike and unattractive to men so that she could stay home and care for her parents. This would resolve in favor of her Vietnamese heritage the powerful conflict she experienced between her old culture's prescription for loyalty and obedience and her new culture's focus on autonomy and independence.

Work and financial stresses

Mei Le was enrolled full-time in public school, attended English classes to improve her English, and worked part-time in a restaurant, sometimes staying as late as 1:00 a.m. During the summer, she worked for a government agency as a clerk. Like many refugees, she buried herself at work in order to bring in extra money and also so that she would not have time to think about her worries.

Other stressors

Other stressors included legal problems (Mei Le's mother wanted to migrate to New Zealand to join her son) and health problems (both parents claimed to have severe heart problems, her mother had been recently hospitalized); and stress caused by the living environment (the family lived in a high-crime neighborhood, and Mei Le had witnessed at least three deaths on the streets).

Assessment of Strengths

Mei Le was a very intelligent, attractive young woman who did very well in school. She worked hard, was very dedicated to her job, and had a very clear career goal for herself. She was well liked by her peers and her co-workers. In spite of the trauma of war and relocation, the family members demonstrated a great deal of love and caring with each other and a strong sense of commitment and obligation to take care of each other. They also received a considerable amount of emotional support from other family members, relatives, teachers, and counselors from the refugee community.

Assessment of Culturally Specific Responses to Mental Health Problems

At the beginning of the admission, all family members denied that the problems of weight loss, vomiting, and sleep difficulty were mental health-related problems. The parents attributed the causes of all symptoms to physiological explanations. They were extremely angry with the inpatient hospitalization. The mother cried for hours in front of the ward before visiting hours, declaring that her daughter was "not crazy." Both parents even threatened to have a "heart attack" after the hospital put their daughter on involuntary admission. In the meantime, the patient denied any emotional difficulty and was initially very upset about being hospitalized.

The family's belief in the physical cause of the patient's problems was not openly challenged by the therapist. Instead, the parents were encouraged to talk about traditional Chinese medicine and the cultural belief in the causes of eating disorder. When they were asked during one interview whether they believed in ghost possession, they were very relieved and revealed a family secret—their daughter was possessed by a male ghost who haunted her at the new apartment (near a funeral home). The patient acknowledged that hypnagognic visions of this ghost beckoning to her for several months. The family first prayed for the patient's release from this ghost, and then began consulting spiritual healers from the refugee community. One day, the spiritual healer came to the house with a "paper boat" and chanted for hours in order to free the patient from the "spell" of this ghost. The parents also consulted a local fortune teller in the community to find out the fate of their daughter. After their failure, the patient and her parents sought help from several herbalists and several Western-trained Chinese physicians located in Chinatown. The patient was hospitalized in a community-based hospital before finally turning to an "American" hospital for an answer. Getting help from mental health professionals was considered as the last resort, and they entered treatment with extreme anger, resentment, and a sense of hopelessness. However, their fortune teller prescribed that Mei Le would meet a man in July who could save her. In July, a male resident arrived who took primary responsibility for Mei Le's treatment. The strength of the relationship and his ability to help Mei Le were in large part based on the family's belief that the arrival of this "rescuer" was predetermined and his power indisputable.

Treatment

It is beyond the scope of this chapter to discuss the treatment approaches of this case in detail. the patient stayed in the hospital for eight weeks with successful treatment outcome. The patient's weight increased to 90 pounds at discharge and she was referred to a local outpatient clinic in Chinatown with a bilingual, bicultural therapist for individual psychotherapy and family therapy. Several important treatment strategies contributed to success in this case.

1. Forming a social and cultural relationship with the patient and her parents during the initial phase of treatment. The patient's and her parents' anger and denial of problems and feelings of shame were acknowledged with understanding.

2. Encouraging the patient and her parents to discuss openly their cultural viewpoints on the causes of the problem, their past efforts in coping with the problem, and their treatment expectations.

3. Educating the family about the Western concept of eating disorders, including the diagnostic procedures and treatment process. In this case, the patient was referred to a medical clinic for extensive workups to rule out organic causes.

4. Demonstrating care by assuming multiple helping roles. The therapist helped the patient and her parents with financial, medical, dental, legal, and employment problems and school placement.

5. Providing the patient and her parents with empathy and caring by a multidisciplinary team. This case was assigned to a team of psychiatrist, social worker, nurses, occupational therapist, and a dietician. The treatment plan was developed with inputs from all disciplines.

6. Providing the patient with a supportive milieu in the ward. The patient had the chance to attend small therapy groups and community meetings and participate in other group activities. She improved her self-esteem dramatically by demonstrating her leadership skill in the ward.

7. Establishing credibility and authority by being the "problem solver" for the family. After the establishment of trust, the patient was put on a behavioral modification program to help her gain weight. The parents were advised to find a bigger apartment as a condition for discharge so that the patient could have some privacy and distance from her parents.

8. Mobilizing the patient's and the parents' strengths. The patient's strong desire to return to school and work were highly valued in the discharge plan. Continued family support was encouraged. Community resources available for the refugee community were utilized extensively during hospitalization and after discharge.

CONCLUSION

This chapter offers practical guidelines for family assessment and treatment that take into account the political, social, and cultural background of Southeast Asian refugees. Effective family therapy requires knowledge, skills, respect, and empathy. A therapist needs to know about the specific cultural and family strengths and pathologies of the Southeast Asian family and the unique effects of war, trauma, and cultural transition on the family system.

The therapist must also exhibit an understanding of his or her own cultural identity, communication style, treatment orientation, and countertransference issues. In addition, professional skills are required to translate this knowledge into effective, culturally appropriate treatment strategies. The establishment of a therapeutic alliance with a Southeast Asian family is based on trust through mutual respect and the therapist's ability to empathize with compassion. The goal is to help the refugee family members overcome their sense of loss, find meaning in their traumatic past, develop confidence in the present, foster new hopes for the future, and find peace and family harmony in their new homeland.

REFERENCES

Danieli, Y. (1875). The treatment and prevention of long-term effects and intergenerational transmission of victimization: A lesson from holocaust survivors and their children. In C. R. Figley (Ed.), *Trauma and its wake: The study and treatment of post-traumatic stress disorder* (pp. 295–313). New York: Brunner/Mazel.

Falicov, C. J. (1982). Mexican family. In M. McGoldrick, J. Pearce, & J. Giordana (Eds.), *Ethnicity and family therapy* (pp. 134–161). New York: Guilford Press.

Figley, C. R. (Ed.), (1985). *Trauma and its wake: The study and treatment of post-traumatic stress disorder.* New York: Brunner/Mazel.

Horowitz, M. J. (1986). *Stress response syndromes.* New York: Jason Aronson.

Kinzie, J. D., Frederickson, R. H., Ben, R., Fleck J., & Karls, W. (1984). Post-traumatic stress disorder among survivors of Cambodian concentration camps. *American Journal of Psychiatry. 141,* 645–650.

Kinzie, J. D., & Manson, S. (1983). Five-year experience with Indochinese refugee psychiatric patients. *Journal of Operational Psychiatry. 14*(2), 105–111.

Knoll, T. (1982). *Becoming Americans.* Portland: Coast to Coast Books.

Landau, J. (1982). Therapy with families in cultural transition. In M. McGoldrick, J. Pearce, & J. Giordana (Eds.), *Ethnicity and family therapy* (pp. 552–572). New York: Guilford Press.

Lee, E. (1985). Inpatient psychiatric services for Southeast Asian refugees. In T. C. Owen (Ed.), *Southeast Asian mental health: Treatment, prevention, services, training, and research* (pp. 307–328). (DHHS Publication No. ADM85-1399) Washington D.C.: U.S. Government Printing Office.

Lee, E. (1982). A social systems approach to assessment and treatment for Chinese American families. In M. McGoldrick, J. Pearce, & J. Giordana (Eds.), *Ethnicity and family therapy* (pp. 527–551). New York: Guilford Press.

Lee, E. (1988). Cultural factors in working with Southeast Asian refugee adolescents. *Journal of Adolescence. 11, 167–179.*

Lee, E. (in press). Assessment and treatment of Chinese/American immigrant families. *Psychotherapy and the Family.*

Lee, E., & Chan, F. (1986). The use of diagnostic interview schedule with Vietnamese refugees. *Asian American Psychological Association Journal, 1, 36–39.*

Lee, E., & Lu, F. (1989). Assessment and treatment of Asian American survivors of Mass Traumatic Stress. *Journal of Psychotherapy and the Family.*

McGoldrick, M. (1982). Ethnicity and family therapy: An overview. In M. McGoldrick, J. Pearce, & J. Giordana. (Eds.), *Ethnicity and family therapy* (pp. 3–30). New York: Guilford Press.

Mollica, R. F., Wyshak, G., & Lavelle, J. (1986). *the psychosocial impact of war trauma and torture on the Southeast Asian refugee.* Unpublished manuscript.

Mollica, R. F.; Wyshak, G.; de Marneffe, D.; Khum, F.; and Lavelle, J. (1982). Indochinese versions of the Hopkins Symptom Checklist-25: A screening instrument for the psychiatric care of refugees. *American Journal of Psychiatry. 144*(4), 497–500.

Montero, D. (1979). *Vietnamese Americans: Patterns of resettlement and socioeconomic adaptation in the United States.* Boulder, Col.: Westview Press.

Nguyen, S. D. (1982). The psychosocial admustment and the mental health needs of Southeast Asian refugees. *The Psychiatric Journal of the University of Ottawa, 7*(1), 26–33.

Office of Refugee Resettlement (1985). *Refugee resettlement program: Report to the Congress.* Washington, D.C.: U.S. Government Printing Office.

Sluzki, C. F (1979). Migration and family conflict. *Family Process. 18,* 379–390.

Strand, P. J., & Jones, W. (1985). *Indochinese refugees in America.* Durham, N.C.: Duke University Press.

Sue, S., & Zane, N. (1987). The role of culture and cultural techniques in psychotherapy. *American Psychologist. 42*(1), 37–44.

Tung, T. M. (1980). *Indochinese patients: Cultural aspects of the medical and psychiatric care of Indochinese refugees.* Washington, D.C.: Action for Southeast Asians.

Tung, T. M. (1985). Psychiatric care for Southeast Asians: How different is different? In T. C. Owen (Ed.), *Southeast Asian mental health: Treatment, prevention, services, training and research* (pp. 5–40). (DHHS Publication no. HDM85-1399.) Washington D.C.: U. S. Government Printing Office.

Van der Kolk, B. (1987). *Psychological trauma.* Washington D.C.: American Psychiatric Press.

Part V
The Threat of Nuclear Holocaust

18

SOME IMPLICATIONS OF THE THREAT OF NUCLEAR WAR FOR FAMILIES AND FAMILY THERAPISTS

Donna Hilleboe DeMuth, M.S.W., L.C.S.W.

> At present, most of us do nothing. We look away. We remain calm. We are silent. We take refuge in the hope that the holocaust won't happen, and turn back to our individual concerns. We deny the truth that is all around us. Indifferent to the future of our kind, we grow indifferent to one another. We drift apart. We grow cold. We drowse our way toward the end of the world. But if once we shook off our lethargy and fatigue and began to act, the climate would change. Just as inertia produces despair—a despair often so deep that it does not even know itself as despair—arousal and action would give us access to hope, and life would start to mend: not just life in its entirety but daily life, every individual life. (Schell, 1982, p. 230)

As I let myself experience the impact of Schell's statement and the threat of nuclear holocaust, my role as family therapist does not make me any different from the rest of the human race as we all face the possibilities of our own extinction. I am, in fact, consoled by feeling that connection, even though it strips me of the hierarchical status that sometimes gives me the illusion of having power to create change in the therapy room. I begin to realize that even without status, my skills as a family therapist may offer some opportunities for understanding and action outside of the therapy room. I am finding an antidote to personal despair. There are even times when I dare to hope that what I know from my work with troubled families may have some impact on the larger world, particularly by releasing some of the individual and collective problem solving energy now locked into that "lethargy and fatigue."

As I deal with being a therapist in the nuclear age, I struggle with the pull between objectivity and subjectivity, knowing I am not an effective therapist when I separate my personal responses from "objective reality." Such a person/object split replicates a dangerous pattern in society, which Caldicott (1984), among others, has identified as a central psychological factor in the escalation of the nuclear arms race. So my work must be both personal and empirical; I hope to have the wisdom both to differentiate and to integrate.

I also struggle between objectivity and taking a moral stance. With regard to nuclear issues, I want my work to be intellectually rigorous; the field is new, and most of us who work in it need to be very honest so that we can be credible. But the ethical imperative for me is very strong. I cannot pretend that this work is unbiased. I do want therapists to define their functional arena more broadly, using their expertise to help families cope more effectively with the impact of the nuclear threat. I want to persuade others to work, in their own way, toward understanding and solving the basic moral dilemma of our times.

I come to my work with the stance of a child protective worker, where the preservation of life itself is always the first order of business. Only after a child is physically safe can one begin to sort out what is going on in the family and how to make change. My first priority now is that the world's children should be protected from destruction; therefore, full understanding may have to come later.

I also come to this work with humility. I have only recently begun to face the nuclear threat, both personally and professionally. I am also deeply aware of the psychological and cultural barriers to this kind of exploration. I hope to persuade but not to preach. And I am supported in this stance by the work of Robert Coles (1986) and Robert Jay Lifton (1967, 1979, 1986, 1987), who have spoken eloquently for the therapeutic community about dealing with the social and political dilemmas of our time. They remind me that all of our explorations are approximations of the truth, no matter how rigorous our thinking may be. We are looking at enormous moral issues. We cannot be blinded into believing that our work can come close to knowing a reality which, as Schell (1982) points out, is beyond our ability to know, or even to imagine—that everything should end. Coles (1986) wisely reminds us that conventional research interviews, particularly of children, may not be enough to tap the depths of their complex feelings about the larger world. We need to remember this as we explore how family members interact with one another on nuclear age topics.

In this chapter, I present some empirical data about how the threat of nuclear war affects children, adults, and families, and some of the coping strategies used by individuals and families in response to this threat. I will develop some ideas about what is normative and what is pathological in family coping strategies, and then propose a model for effective family functioning vis-à-vis nuclear issues.

Finally, I develop some ideas about how family therapists can empower themselves to become more involved in the psychology of the nuclear world, using my own personal journey into social activism as a metaphor.

NUCLEAR ISSUES RESEARCH

Scarcity of Information about Families

The startling fact, as I present research data on how families deal with nuclear issues, is that so little work has yet been done by family therapists. At this writing, no papers have been published in either *Family Process* or *The Journal of the Association on Marriage and Family Therapy*, and very few have been presented at family therapy conferences. As of April 1987, there were no recorded doctoral theses. A recent book entitled *Families and The Prospect of Nuclear Attack/Holocaust* (Marciano & Sussman, 1986) contains only one chapter dealing directly with nuclear anxiety and the family (Perlmutter & Ringler, 1986). Greenwald and Zeitlin (1987) outline the issues for families brilliantly in their book *No reason to talk about it: Families Confront the Nuclear Taboo*, but their work is a pilot study based on extensive family interviews with no control group.

I know of only five current research projects being undertaken by family therapists, one of which is my own. There may be other studies to be found in journals of social psychology and sociology, but they have not yet cross-fertilized into the work of family therapists.

The research questions are infinite. For example, we can assume that there is an effect on family functioning because of the existence of the potential for nuclear destruction, but is that assumption true? If so, how is the impact manifested? Is there any connection between response to the threat and clinical symptomatology? What kinds of families are most affected? What kinds of family structure and/or family coping devices are most effective? What, indeed, are normal family functions in a world that could blow up?

Lacking answers, and having questions that lead to more questions, we must look at studies of individual responses of families to other catastrophic events for illumination.

Historical Context of Research in the Psychology of Nuclear Issues

The first major research project of nuclear age psychology was conducted by Lifton (1967), who studied the psychological effects upon survivors of the first atomic bomb dropped on Hiroshima in 1945. He found evidence to support the existence of powerful, long-lasting damage from the bomb on the psychological health of the population. He developed the concept of psychic numbing to describe the coping strategies that allowed survivors to carry on their daily lives in the presence of previously unimaginable horrors. Escalona (1962) and Schwebel (1965) followed with studies of the impact of knowledge of the existence of nuclear weapons on American children, and were the first to point out that the majority of children had serious worries about the possibility of nuclear war and feared that they would not survive it.

Then, for many years, direct investigations into the psychology of the nuclear age stopped. Foundations were being laid through research into the effect of other large-scale disasters. Crisis theory (Parad, 1965) had come of age with significant studies to document the ways in which the psychological functioning of individuals and families was affected by traumatic external events. But it was not until 1977 that the American Psychiatric Association published Beardslee and Mack's study of 1,100 American high school children that documented the widespread extent of children's fears of nuclear annihilation.

Following some critical world events of the early 1960s (the signing of the

Nuclear Test Ban Treaty, the Cuban missile crisis, the assassination of John Kennedy), the psychological community was silent about nuclear issues. Interestingly, this silence was replicated with regard to the other major devastation of modern history, the Holocaust for Jews under Nazi domination in the 1930s and 1940s. The first psychological studies of Holocaust survivors and their families also emerged in the late 1970s (Epstein, 1979). The psychological effects of other large-scale disasters have also been followed by silence; for example, posttraumatic stress disorders (PTSD) following Vietnam (Figley & Sprenkle, 1978) and the Three Mile Island reactor accident (Cunningham, 1982).

Significantly, in the past ten years, the mandate for silence about intrafamily devastation caused by alcoholism and physical or sexual abuse has also begun to be lifted. Researchers are presenting substantive information on the extent of these formerly secret horrors, and therapists are engaged in designing remedial interventions now that the secrets are beginning to be exposed.

I suspect that the development of nuclear psychology, holocaust studies, and other related phenomena needed to be based on a rethinking of death from a contemporary perspective. The works of Becker (1974), later reinforced by Lifton (1979), lamented the inability of many people in Western civilization to face the issues of death directly, which leads them to create defensive structures that weaken their ability to deal fully with their lives. Kubler-Ross (1969), focusing primarily on children, illuminated the price paid by both children and parents by their inability to share the experience of dying together. Her early work with medical personnel brings to mind parallels with the experiences of those of us who have recently begun to call for more open discussion of nuclear concerns. She experienced similar criticism for opening up issues too painful to be borne, and was cautioned that parents and children needed to be protected from the impact of dealing directly with issues of death.

We seem to be at the very beginning of a period of significant change in our ability and willingness to look at the psychology of deep and universal tragedy. Perhaps we are just beginning to redefine the American dream of infinite peace and prosperity even as the culture of materialism, addictions, and easy answers seems to be running rampant. Are we at last willing to push beyond the denial of death? We may have learned something from other social phenomena of the 1960s and 1970s; from the human potential movement that fostered openness of expression; from the women's movement, which validated the existence of vulnerability; from the civil rights movement, which demonstrated the possibilities of major change in social structures; from the influence of Eastern philosophy, which counters the increasing technologization of Western civilization.

We know that all systems flow through an ongoing process of development, changing over time in cycles of homeostasis and growth. Growth requires openness to new information and the release of barriers to that information. It may be that silence can last only so long in a developing open system.

Another interesting aspect of this opening to the psychology of horror is that much of the impetus of exploration has come from second-generation survivors (Holocaust, ACOA groups, incest victims, children of PTSD victims) who have banded together to aknowledge their common realities, for mutual support, and for empowerment. We now have the first generation of adults who have grown up with awareness of The Bomb. If we accept Lifton's view (1967) that we are *all* survivors of Hiroshima Nagasaki, then we may now be in the generation that allows us to face with our "peers" the effects of our "parents' " disfunctions upon us, and to support each other in the process.

Therefore, I will now examine what we do know—from research on individual nuclear psychology, on social stress, and on family coping strategies.

Research Data on the Psychology of Nuclear Issues

Reactions of children and adolescents

As previously mentioned, Escolona (1962) and Schwebel (1965) were the first scholars to document the potential deleterious affect of the nuclear situation on children. In a cross-cultural group of 311 students aged ten to 17, Escalona (1962) found that 70 percent spontaneously mentioned issues relating to nuclear war in responding to an open-ended question about their concerns for the future. Following the Cuban missile crisis, using a written questionnaire, Schwebel (1965) reported that of 300 high school students, 42 percent expected nuclear war in their lifetime.

More recently, Berger-Gould (1986), following the shooting down of an American plane by Russians over Korea, used the Schwebel questionnaire on a sample of ninth-graders, and found that 64 percent anticipated that a nuclear war would occur. Other large-scale studies based on written surveys (Goldenring & Doctor, 1986; Diamond & Bachman, 1986) show that 32 to 45 percent of teenagers believe that a nuclear war will take place, and most believe that they will not survive it. Seventy percent of students in Beardslee and Mack's (1982) study felt the country would not survive a nuclear war.

Even when nuclear concerns were embedded in questions that ranked many kinds of adolescent worries, they were rated very high. Goldenring and Doctor (1986), for example, found that this issue ranked third, behind worry about parental death and failing grades. These studies did not link nuclear anxiety to critical nuclear events in the world. (This information is adopted from Eisenbud et al [1985].)

Few developmental studies have been done, but there are indications that children's concerns exist as early as the age of four (Friedman, 1984). Young elementary school children in a nuclear education program spoke eloquently and easily of their awareness and fears. Yet, by adolescence, many of them seem to have developed a more cynical or apathetic position (Roberta Snow, personal communication, 1982).

Even more compelling are the verbatim statements that children gave to researchers (Beardslee & Mack, 1982; Berger-Gould et al., 1986). Children report vivid and concrete imagery, speak movingly of not wanting to die, of wanting to grow up. Younger children, in particular, speak of the terror of loss of and separation from family as they face the possibility of nuclear war.

For other excellent reviews of the research data see Berger-Gould et al. (1986), Schwebel (1986), and Children's Fears of War, U.S. Government Document (1983).

Looking more closely at the studies of adolescents previously cited, we find some very significant data for use in our understanding of family dynamics. Young people who have concerns do not talk much about them, and almost none talk to their parents. Young people who do think about nuclear issues more often rank higher on indexes of normal adolescent functioning and have fewer fears for the future than do teenagers who rarely think about nuclear war. The concerned youngsters have more of a sense of personal power, feel more hopeful, and are much more apt to be engaged in activities that express social concern of varying kinds. Diamond and Bachman (1986) emphasize that the presence of concern is not paralyzing; indeed, it serves as a mobilizing force.

Young people who think about nuclear war seem to function better than their counterparts. We do not know exactly how this process works. It seems reasonable that a more functional child can better tolerate painful challenges. It is equally conceivable, especially when we look at studies of children who have survived major catastrophes (Sheehy, 1986; Rutter, 1987), that grappling with touch issues can lead to a sense of strength and to higher functioning.

In summary, research on children indicates that they are indeed concerned about nuclear war, and that actively concerned adolescents are well adjusted and not immobilized by this worry.

Adults and the nuclear threat

Interestingly, there are relatively few studies of adults' concerns about nuclear war. We dare to ask children questions we have not been willing to ask ourselves (a fact that, we will soon see, fits into Zeitlin's [1984] theory of displaced parent/child boundaries around nuclear issues). A very large number of adults who spoke to me while attending educational programs about children and the nuclear threat consistently reported being very worried, trying not to think about the future, not talking about their worries. They felt helpless in relation to their children's concerns and so said nothing. My experience is replicated over and over again by family therapist colleagues, as well as in the family interviews conducted by my research team and others.

All of the important explorations of adult nuclear psychology seem to reveal the coexistence of strong feelings of worry about nuclear war and very little focus on or discussion of these concerns.

Lifton's (1967) post-Hiroshima study is the major base for our understanding of this phenomenon. At Hiroshima, life events took place in which the most intense intrapsychic terrors of total annihilation became real. Even after substantial time had elapsed, the scars remained. Ultimately, for emotional survival, a kind of psychic numbing took place. In order to maintain daily life, survivors created an interior world in which the images of the bombing were sealed off from their ordinary consciousness. Lifton called this phenomenon double life. These images were retrievable at early stages, but gradually faded. However, the impact of the terror and loss from the bomb was not erased; survivors suffered symptoms normally associated with grief reactions, but did not attribute them to memories of the bombing.

Lifton found that survivors who were geographically distant from the event felt its impact over time. Concentric rings of psychological reaction spread from the epicenter, as did the radioactive effects—so that, in a sense, according to

Lifton, we are all survivors of the bomb. (See Locatelli and Holt [1986] for a sensitive critique and expansion of the psychic numbing concept.)

Lifton's research and thoughts have been central to conceptualizations of nuclear psychology. But his recommendation for further studies of Japanese survivors were not followed up. By his own statements, his work was not completed.

In addition, Frank (1986), Schell (1982), Schwebel (1986) and Macy (1981, 1983) all speak of the psychic effort that it takes *not* to be aware of the awful possibilities of nuclear devestation; of the potential deleterious effects of seperating out such a large area of consciousness, of the terror and despair lying underneath the apparent apathy of many people. These notions make total sense to me, but are not as yet supported by substantial research data.

Two small studies reported in Schwebel (1986) have some relevance to my thinking about adult functioning and family coping efforts. Van Hoorn, (1986) looked at the effects of viewing a television film *The Day After*, a fictional account of the aftermath of the nuclear bombing of a large midwest city. She found that people exposed to this highly charged visual material reported substantial immediate affective impact, but that they showed little change in political attitudes or in their willingness to engage in social activism. The author speculates (and cites evidence from studies in other areas to support her contention) that strong feelings will diminish without an orderly process leading people in sequential steps to a change of consciousness. Arousing fears without offering hope of a method of risk reduction does not result in attitudinal or behavioral change. Therefore, I would propose that adults may not be able to face the existence of the nuclear threat without some sense of appropriate action that they could take to deal with it in some way.

Another study of adults also replicates the findings about adolescent concerns about nuclear issues. Locatelli & Holt (1986) contrasted the attitudes of adult peace activists with others who believe in nonviolent political solutions but do not act on them. The former report more strong feelings and experience more concrete images of war, but also maintain more feelings of personal competence and hope.

Being concerned and being active are factors correlated with positive mental attitudes toward the world situation (see Macy [1983] for an in-depth discussion of this notion). Contrary to popular wisdom, moderate anxiety levels may be necessary, and even helpful, in coping successfully with nuclear stress. As Schell (1982, p. 230) has pointed out, "arousal and action . . . give us access to hope."

Data about family coping strategies

Research informs us that children are concerned about nuclear war and that adults have often learned to cope by remaining frozen and numb in relation to the danger. What role does the family play in resolving this dilemma? What do we know about how parents and children interact around nuclear concerns? My own working assumption is that the existence of the nuclear threat has a substantial effect on family life in ways yet to be fully documented, and that, ultimately, family therapists will need to find a role in assisting families to deal with that stress.

At this writing, I know of research, based on direct interviews with families, that has been started by Steve Zeitlin and Jon Reusser, by David Greenwald and Wendy Forman, by Robert Garfield (Peace Research Associates), by Jules Riskin of the Mental Research Institute, and by the Family Interviewing Project, a research collaborative of which I am the founder. To date, results have been published only by Greenwald and Zeitlin (1987).

Our work presents some interesting and fairly consistent hypotheses. Zeitlin (1984) has defined the problem as one of dysfunctional generational boundaries, in which parents feel helpless to protect their children from an unimaginable horror and thereby abdicate their function as guides and guardians. They become paralyzed. They respond with hollow optimism, mechanical reassurance, lectures, and defensive postures that barely hide guilt; they change the subject, do not hear what kids say, use dogmatic religious or philosophical statements rather than responding empathetically. Children protect parents primarily by silence, by down-playing their concerns, or even by reassuring their parents that the world will be alright. Parents also abdicate responsibility by openly giving children the mandate that they, the younger generation, must take responsibility for political/social change.

Greenwald and Zeitlin (1987) state that this behavior serves as a protective mechanism in which either avoidance or minimization is used to defuse potentially strong affective responses to nuclear issues. They also note that families frequently use blame as a coping device, venting anger against political figures or social forces as a way of discharging frustration.

There is some indication, also, of structural factors that could underly dysfunctional communication. I have observed that when otherwise well-functioning families attempt to discuss this highly charged subject, weaknesses in family structure (i.e., marital disagreement, an overinvolved parent–child dyad, a distancing member) may be revealed that, under other circumstances, might not surface so easily. The consequences may be to discourage families from facing issues of nuclear concern (or, indeed, of other subjects of potential serious emotional impact).

According to Greenwald Zeitlin (1987), families can use positive affirmation to help deal with the stress of facing nuclear issues. Some families do share grief and fear openly; family members support each other with words and physical gestures and attempt to reassure each other in more meaningful ways. We do not yet know what circumstances lead to these more positive exchanges, or in what kinds of families members find it possible to support each other more effectively. We do have consistent anecdotal reports from families in all the current research projects that indicate that family discussions about nuclear issues, even those that showed dysfunctional patterns, were viewed positively by the families themselves. Almost all families have indicated relief of tension after the interviews, greater closeness, and, in some cases, a greater sense of empowerment regarding social activism.

My own research group is currently studying the impact of a structured family interview about nuclear issues on family cohesiveness and on individual members' feelings of hopelessness and/or despair. We will compare families in which the parents have had a short preparation for the interview and those in which there has been no parental preparation. We postulate from Zeitlin's work

(1984) that in families where the parents have had more support, family cohesiveness will be greater and the sense of hopelessness decreased.

The studies previously cited are based on family members' reactions to the possibilities of nuclear war. We also have some information about families that have already faced the adverse effect of a nuclear explosion Ellis, Greenburg, and Murphy (1987) have interviewed families of American servicemen who were directly exposed to radiation from nuclear explosions during above-ground testing in the early post-World War II era. Like the other research subjects, these families had not previously discussed together their concerns over the impact of this exposure, even though both the survivor and the children were known to be more vulnerable to cancer and to genetic defects. Again, these families expressed gratitude for an opportunity to talk together with the researcher.

In summary, preliminary research studies of families facing nuclear issues have focused on family coping strategies, primarily those of family discussion. They indicate that famijlies rarely discuss the threat of nuclear war, and that when they do, many have considerable difficulty in supporting each other directly. Parents, feeling a loss of appropriate role, have particular difficulty in supporting their children's concerns.

FAMILIES FACING NUCLEAR STRESS—WHAT IS NORMAL FUNCTIONING?

Risk of Silence and Suppression

As there are so few data from direct observation of families dealing with nuclear stress, and as our conceptualizations are so new, it is difficult to have a clear sense of what is normal. How can we define healthy family functioning in an area in which there is so much silence? One must ask whether it is truly maladaptive for families to remain silent about nuclear concerns. Conventional psychologial wisdom tells us that expressing feelings of anxiety, sadness, anger, and so on to a sympathetic listener is conducive to healing and growth; the practice of individual psychotherapy is built on this foundation.

Family therapists are not united in believing that expressing feelings is valuable for families coping with stressful situations. A strong case for the value of open communication as the basis for effective family functioning comes from the work of Satir (1983). Satir, who with her colleagues has interviewed thousands of families over a period of 25 years, has demonstrated experientially that when families members can talk with each other in an open and congruent way, individual symptoms can be relieved and a sense of family well-being enhanced. In addition, several major indices of family functioning, from the research of Epstein et al. (1983), Beavers (1981), and Olson et al. (1979) stress that direct communication about affective matters is a positive factor in family well-being.

However, many other schools of thought in family therapy seem to deemphasize the value of open affective exchanges between family members in favor of other approaches; for example, the use of problem solving (Haley, 1976), tasks (Minuchin, 1974), and strategic interventions (Madanes, 1981) that effect system change without exploring feelings. Indeed, there is little evidence from the original family therapy research that communication about difficult topics promotes healthy functioning. (Donald Bloch, personal communication, 1986)

Researchers studying families of PTSD victims also disagree in their findings. For example, Rosenheck and Thompson (1986) found the family discussions about the traumatic events need to be deferred until the survivor's emotional reactiveness has decreased. However, the weight of evidence seems to demonstrate that family discussions can be very helpful in the recovery process. Figley and Sprenkle (1978) found, for example, that the survivor's reactive symptoms decreased after discussing his painful memories with family members. Ritterman, in Chapter 14 supports Figley and Sprenkle's findings from her work with families that have survived serious political oppression.

Perhaps the most solid evidence for the value of family communication in coping with PTSD comes from the work of Solomon et al. (1987). This study of Israeli combat survivors shows a high positive correlation between their recovery rates and the ability of their families to express feelings openly and with appropriate affect. However, other family therapists do not encourage whole family communication as a coping strategy for dealing with catastrophic events. Sgroi (1982), for example, advises delaying family discussions around incest issues until the victim has had sufficient time to recover self-esteem through individual and group therapy. Others discourage family communication around catastrophic illness (Baider, 1977; Barbarin & Chesler, 1984; Johnson et al., 1985). Even the stance of the researcher can imply that it is not wise for families to talk to one another about matters of life and death. In three major journals, *Family Process, The Journal of the American Association of Marriage and Family Therapy*, and *Family Systems Medicine*, studies of families coping with illness are almost entirely based on individual rather than family interviews.

Insights from Social Stress Literature

In the work of social psychology, we find further information on the complex question of suppression as normative for families coping with severe stress. Here, we learn that the essential nature of the nuclear threat, described by Schwebel (1986) as insidious because of its ongoing nature and lack of resolution, fits into Boss and Greenberg's (1984) definition of ambiguity, seen as among the most debilitating aspects of stress for families.

Furthermore, McCubbin and Patterson (1983) show us that the impact of a stressor on family functioning is determined not only by the nature of the stressor itself, but by the community's definition of the stressor, and by the family's definition of the stressor based on its values and its shared paradigm (an implicit set of assumptions about the nature of reality). Stress becomes *distress* only when it is subjectively defined as unpleasant or undesirable by the family and/or communitiy. One could assume, for example, that the family that believes that the evil of the world will lead inevitably to nuclear disaster and that its faith will bring eternal life, may not experience stress from the nuclear situation. Mojtabai (1986) writes movingly of the prevalence of Armageddon thinking in Amarillo, Texas, where all manufactured components for nuclear missils are assembled. Families develop constructs that minimize the nature of the threat, and thus could be described as having normal coping strategies, because their shared definition allows them relief from anxiety.

Oliveri and Reiss (1982) find the following internal factors to be significant in effective family coping with external stress:

1. The extent to which the family believes problems in the environment can be solved (regardless of the family's coping skills per se).
2. The way in which the family believes the stressors can be understood and dealt with from its own past experiences.
3. The extent to which the family can deal with the stressor(s) as a unit rather than as separate beings.

Using this schema, we could assume that the nuclear threat poses extraordinary demands on family coping devices. The threat of nuclear catastrophe is overwhelming, and does not seem solvable to many families. There is no easy way to understand it or or any equivalent disaster in previous experience from which the family can learn. We know from studies previously cited (Greenwald & Zeitlin, 1987; Goldenring & Doctor, 1986) that teenagers do not discuss nuclear issues with their families and choose to deal with their concerns separately. According to all Oliveri-Reiss indices, families would not do well in coping with nuclear stress. Lack of cohesiveness is exemplified by the many teenagers who feel isolated from their families in relation to nuclear issues.

Given that the coping strategies for families are seriously stressed by the nature of the threat of nuclear destruction, it is no wonder that they may seek relief by suppression and minimization in order to maintain daily life. Normal human beings learn to adapt to anything, partly by selective attention that involves suppression of painful affect, particularly if there seems to be no focus on which to direct that affect (Locatelli & Holt, 1986). This suppression may not be ultimately functional for families, but it is certainly understandable. Ironically, the suppression of affect may lead to a decreasing sense of family cohesiveness, which according to the study of Israeli PTSD victims already cited (Solomon et al., 1987), is another major factor in effective recovery. It appears that what may be normal for immediate daily survival, is not sufficient for long-term recovery.

Further evidence for this notion comes from the work of Levine et al. (1987) which found that coronary attack victims who did not discuss the serious nature of their condition made more rapid recovery while in the hospital but did not fare as well over the long haul. It may be that long-term survival for these patients, and perhaps for the world at large, does require facing and discussing painful matters as the first in a series of necessary steps toward a lasting "cure."

Possible Pathology Resulting from Family Coping Devices

It is important to remind ourselves again that we have as yet no definitive research linking reactions to the nuclear situation with any kind of individual or family psychopathology. There have been, however, suggestions as to what those links might be. Mack (1986) believes, for example, that the high incidence of substance abuse among American teenagers may well be related to nuclear age despair, and that widespread rebellion against adult authority may be rein-forced by the inability to trust adults who have created such an unsafe world. Wetzel and Winnawer (1986) believe that the presence of such a powerful family secret could lead to developmental stagnation over the generations, and cor-ruption of values and mutual insensitivity in the present.

A further indictment against silence is demonstrated in studies of female learning patterns. Social expectations that pressure women to curtail speaking out in school, at home, and in other social situations may lead to lower feelings of self-esteem, cognitive blocking, and possibly depression and learned help-lessness (Belenky et al., 1986)

My own experience is that there is potential for serious dysfunction when family members are not able to talk to one another about serious concerns. I believe that the ability to communicate painful feelings appropriately, according to the family's ethnic and typal style (Kantor & Lehr 1975; McGoldrick et al., 1982), is crucial to the development of a sense of family cohesiveness and to the self-esteem of its individual members. I believe that children do gain when they are encouraged to share their deep concerns with parents and interested adults, and there is potential for dysfunction when this talking function is shut off. I know the price paid by children growing up in families where talking is not encouraged. Children of the Holocaust survivors, for example, have stressed this pain (Epstein, 1979; Bergmann & Jucovy, 1982). Goleman (1986) cites ex-tensive research to prove that silence and self-deception about the nature of painful realities takes a heavy psychic toll.

I agree that there is potential for dysfunction in otherwise normal families as a result of the erosion of trust in parental competence when parents are silent in response to children's concerns (Zeitlin, 1984). I also have seen other poten-tially dysfunctional interactions related to the rule of silence around nuclear issues.

I watched the depressive affect increase in one father as an interview pro-gressed. He was the only member of the family expressing deep concern about a possible nuclear war. Other family members deflected from his expressions of concern, minimized them, and showed in many ways their lack of tolerance for his intensity. His isolation from the family increased, until, finally, other members were able to engage him with another topic. He became included in the family again only by putting aside his powerful feelings about nuclear war and being left to handle them in other ways.

I have seen couples show tension around their different needs to discuss nuclear issues, and become at least temporarily isolated from each other rather than joining in mutual support. I have also seen a couple disagree as to the degree of protection from discussing nuclear issues they would try to provide their children, and then witnessed a parent–child coalition develop that sepa-rated the parents further.

I have seen the whole affect of a family become flat and dull in response to queries about nuclear issues. My probes seemed to reveal that there are other issues of strong concern within this family that have been silenced, and the inability to face nuclear issues directly is part of a more generalized posture with regard to the basic struggles of life itself.

These examples suggest to me that repeated interactions of this nature might have the potential for developing into more serious forms of family difficulties.

I believe that families that are not able to discuss the nuclear threat can be seen as dysfunctional, even though they may not show some of these structural difficulties, and even though, as previously seen, their silence may seem to help them face more easily the realities of daily living. Rutter's (1987) work on the mechanisms of psychosocial resilience to high risk makes it clear that children who survive well in response to serious life stressors profit from gradual exposure to stressors, and thereby develop a better sense of their own abilities to cope with the risks. From this work, it follows that family silence on matters as serious as the nuclear threat truly deprives children of an important opportunity to feel more competent in response to a dangerous world by gradually becoming familiar with its essential nature while they are still in a nurturing environment.

For me, the real significance of this issue lies in the fact that coping strategies that work when you look only within the boundaries of day-to-day family functioning become dysfunctional when you look at the global system. The reality is that our whole world is in serious danger of nuclear destruction. Silence suppresses alertness to the danger and cuts off possibilities for individuals to develop truly functional skills that would lead to solving the external problem (Goleman, 1985). We have already seen (Locatelli & Holt, 1986) that greater awareness of war isues in adults is correlated with activism and that awareness is correlated with both activism and positive mental attitudes in adolescents (Goldenring & Doctor, 1986). Intragroup cohesiveness (Oliveri & Reiss, 1982) and connectedness to the larger global system (Macy, 1983) are extremely important for coping with nuclear issues and, potentially, for empowerment toward action for change. I believe that the most serious evidence of pathology in families who do not discuss nuclear issues is the loss of this potential for a sense of mastery and the loss of a matrix that would support children in a conviction that solutions to global tension can indeed be found.

A Theory of External Boundary Dysfunction

In trying to assess what is normal and what is pathological for families as they deal with nuclear stress, it has been helpful to me to expand Zeitlin's (1984) ideas on boundaries. He focused on internal boundary dysfunctions, noting that parents became like children in their responses to the nuclear threat. In addition, I see serious external boundary dysfunction: I believe that most modern families have drawn a rigid boundary in their *affective* response to the outside world, whereas boundaries with regard to *information* are very loosely drawn. For example, studies of the effects of television on children indicate that information about world events is often indiscrimately available to young children (Liebert et al., 1982). Indeed, watching the news may be even more evocative of depression and antisocial behavior in certain vulnerable children than watching fictional shows depicting violence. Yet, we suspect that families rarely share affective responses to this material.

There can be many consequences when a boundary is too rigid with regard to affect, too permeable with regard to information. I have indicated that Caldicott (1984) sees depersonalization of affective response to the bomb and its impact as a major factor in the political ideology of deterrence by massive arms buildup. To me, chilling evidence of this split is found in the "normalization" of the atomic bomb's effects by citizens who live near and work in the Hanford nuclear reactor plant in Washington. Cheerleaders in this high school wear a yellow exploding bomb on their sweaters as they root for the Hanford Bombers. They have daily cognitive reminders of the serious nature of nuclear weapons, but they split off and dismiss their affective reactions to it. There exists extensive apathy, masked depression, and high use of addictive chemicals by teenagers and adults in this community. (Loeb, 1983).

We do know of the potentially serious psychological consequences for individuals who have a serious internal split between their affective responses and the intellectual constructs they build around them. This depersonalization is found in patients suffering from obsessive-compulsive neurosis, from substance disorders, and, in its most extreme form, from schizophrenia.

I see the problem of the boundary definition and affective/information split not only in the individual and social pathology it may encourage, but also in the opportunities that may be cut off. I agree with Macy (1983) that Western concepts of individualism lead to rigid boundaries that prevent individuals (and families) from utilizing the healthy natural connections with the sense of the planet as a whole. If one sees the ecological system as potentially self-healing, cutting off the sense of one's connections to that world also cuts off vast opportunities for growth. We know that families recover from trauma more readily when they have strong connections to the community; we know that death rates soar and indices of mental and physical health are lower for people who live alone (Lynch, 1977). Families with rigid boundaries are more apt to reverberate with the intensity that magnifies and perpetuates personal stress. The cutting off of opportunities for growth and enrichment operates not only in the sense of global connections, but internally, depriving families of opportunities to develop a sense of competence and mastery. I have been influenced by Kegan (1982) and Gilligan (1982) in whose developmental schema compassion and a sense of social responsibility are seen as the highest levels of adult functioning. We deprive ourselves and our children when we do not allow ourselves to be affectively connected to the whole world, in both its good and its evil aspects. We may, as Lifton suggests (1979), be depriving ourselves of the essential meaning of life, and limiting ourselves to a duller, shallower form of existence.

We have interesting anecdotal reports from children who grew up in the 1930s as "red diaper babies," whose parents were dedicated Communists, committing their lives to political and social change (Chernin, 1983; Kaplan & Shapiro, 1985). There were, of course, some adverse psychological effects for these families whose lives were focused on their connections with the suffering of the world. But primarily the memories of those now-adult children are very rich. They were energized from the sense of mission and of connection with the community that they experienced.

In a recent *New Yorker* article, Schell (1986) sums it up.

> The lines which connect the individual citizens to the body politic and beyond that to the world at large appear to have become attenuated. . . . Events themselves have failed to make deep and lasting impressions. Nor has television filled the breach: on television, it seems, the world draws closer but matters less. (p. 84)

A Model for Effective Family Functioning in Response to the Threat

In daring to develop a model with so few data to work from, I turn to the work of Dennis Jaffe (1985). He studied cancer patients who survived despite a terminal prognosis. This strikes me as a most appropriate metaphor for the nuclear dilemma. Jaffe found the following personal characteristics in the cancer survivors: a belief system that makes some kind of sense out of the occurrence of the disease; a sense of power to affect positively the course of one's illness; and a strong, active support network (i.e., family, friends, medical team, community). I propose that these factors may also be central to effective family functioning in a world that may have been given a terminal prognosis.

First, using Jaffe's schema, families would attempt to understand the nuclear situation and its meaning in relation to their own unique life goals and values. The rule of silence would have to be broken in order to achieve this end. A clearer philosophical or spiritual dimension would emerge as family members talked about their concerns for the world, and could then reinforce the family as it dealt with painful feelings.

Second, Jaffe reminds us again that talking about nuclear issues is not enough and that the survivor must have a sense of mastery. We have seen that anxiety is more effectively channeled into action if discussion of fearful topics is followed by sequential steps leading to action; for example, discussing feelings, evidencing mutual support, evoking problem-solving alternatives, modeling action possibilities (Macy, 1983). Children feel safer and more validated when parents themselves take appropriate action around their concerns (Goldenring & Doctor, 1986; Solantus & Rimpela, 1986.)

In our "model" family, there would not only be discussions, but some active involvement in world affairs, with parents leading the way. Fortunately, a great many possibilities are available for families that wish to take action for world peace—some directly political, some spiritually based. There are peaceful conflict resolution techniques for parents to teach children, citizen diplomacy efforts in which to engage, and much more.

Third, the feeling of connectedness to one another and to all of life on this planet would be part of our model for families. I have already cited other evidence to support this belief. Several of our research families have spontaneously asked to talk to other families about nuclear concerns after being interviewed. As a consequence, we plan to offer multiple-family group experience to all participants after our research interviews have been completed. Our own research "family" has found that the most important base for continuing our work is a sense of a supportive connection to one another and to others who share their concerns.

Furthermore, in this proposed family model, we would recognize that children's needs differ according to developmental stages. Children need different kinds of parental support and guidance at different ages. Preschool- and early-school-age children need protection from exposure to more graphic depictions of the consequences of nuclear war, and more physical contact and reassurance when the topic comes up. School-age children need help in sorting out facts as well as feelings and much guidance in taking some action steps. Adolescents need the opportunity to debate, develop their own opinions, and bond with peers to develop their own peace-making activities.

Families in different developmental stages would have appropriate differences in their boundaries to the external world. For example, in early stages of family formation (newly married couples and families with young children), it is appropriate that their energies be primarily directed inward. As families mature, however, there would be a healthy broadening of boundaries to include a more active concern for the larger world as children and career building require less time involvement. Senior citizens would perhaps be most active of all. Indeed, the largest and most enthusiastic audience I have ever addressed on the topic of families and the nuclear threat was one made up primarily of retired persons in a coastal Maine community.

Finally, our model would include recognition of and respect for variations in style based on ethnic values and family typology. Talking together does not necessarily mean in the nonheirarchial style of the open system (Kantor & Lehr, 1975). For example, dissenting political opinions in the healthy versions of a more hierarchial family type might be dealt with indirectly. However, regardless of style and tradition, I would consider it normative for there to be a set of agreed-upon processes in which nuclear concerns could be shared and dissent monitored, so that family members could support one another both by words and by actions.

It would be normative for families facing the nuclear threat to call upon outside resources, appropriate to the family style, for assistance. Even families that function extremely well without assistance in other areas, or whose members' style do not normally lead them to seek outside help, may flounder in trying to operate in total autonomy as its members deal with nuclear issues.

In summary, I propose that a normal family coping well with nuclear stress might call upon Jaffe's survivor principles by developing a set of meanings that have value to them about the nuclear threat, taking an active stance leading to a feeling of greater mastery, and joining with each other and and with others in a support system. In addition, a healthy family would respond to the nuclear threat in ways appropriate to its developmental stage and would learn to use coping measures that would fit its ethnic and typal preferences.

HOW FAMILY THERAPISTS ARE DEALING WITH NUCLEAR ISSUES

Value of Systems Thinking in Approaching the Nuclear Dilemma

Capra (1982) pointed out that Western civilization may be at the beginning of a cultural and intellectual revolution equivalent to that of the age of enlightenment in the 18th century. He believes that systems thinking is the core concept of this new revolution, and that we are moving from intellectual constructs that see the individual as primary to ones in which individuals are seen as part of a network of interlocking units that operate with predictable rules as part of a total ecological system.

In family therapy, we see directly the change in treatment approaches when pathology is viewed as residing solely within the individual and when it is viewed as a function of dysfunctional relationships within the entire family. Family therapists now assume that most individual disturbance can be treated best when the whole family is involved in therapy in some way.

At first glance, it might appear that thinking systemically about nuclear issues would be overwhelming. If the family dysfunction we have seen occurring in response to nuclear stress can best be treated by making changes in the larger world system, our job as effective charge agents can seem impossible. I believe that family therapists may sometimes avoid looking at nuclear issues because of this very issue. We are action-oriented problem solvers, and it is not at all clear how we can gain access to that larger system.

However, systems thinking has been more helpful to me than it has been overwhelming. It has allowed me to conceptualize from data on small systems in a way that illuminates the whole. For example, in our research group, we have polarized around affective versus cognitive approaches to problems, and the polarization was eased when we moved to a deeper level of sharing our mutual concerns and common purpose. It is likely that change on a global level can take place in similar ways.

Furthermore, systems thinking can help address the problem of apathy and despair in facing the nuclear dilemma. Linear approaches to problem solving tend to reinforce despair, because too many sequential steps seem necessary before one reaches a solution. Systems thinkers know that transformation can take place in a large system by an effective intervention in one of its subsystems, if the whole system dysfunction is clearly understood. Not every individual in a family needs to change, one at a time, in order for dysfunctional patterns to be interrupted.

Family therapists do have experience and expertise in working with larger systems as a way of intervening in the life of specific families. Often these families, like families experiencing nuclear stress, do not see the link between their symptoms and the chronic social stress (i.e., poverty, disenfranchisement, exploitation) that supports the existence of those symptoms. Here the wise family therapist, rather than dealing only with symptoms, serves as an advocate for the family in dealing with the agencies and institutions whose dysfunction contributes to family dysfunction. She also can sometimes find ways to offer consultation to warring agencies in whose conflict the family is caught, even if she does not have enough power personally to effect major changes in agency policy. Her systems thinking reframes the immediate problem to a larger scale that offers greater challenges for intervention but also greater hope for solutions.

The hopeful aspect of most systems thinking has been particularly useful to me in thinking about the nuclear threat. Systems thinking is relatively blame-free; it looks primarily at how and not why things work. In many ways, it offers models for successful conflict resolution that could as well be utilized by varying nations as by warring social agencies or family members. Because the systems thinker does not see issues in terms of polarities, she is freer to reframe conflictual issues and develop a more broadly based plan for solution.

This kind of thinking may seem grandiose. Indeed, it is dangerous to make quick assumptions that expertise can be transformed directly from one context to another. Yet this approach offers a very new direction for family therapists (see Chapter 20).

Current Interventions by Family Therapists

In this section, I will report some of the efforts that family therapists have made to ease nuclear-based tension and to create change in families and small groups. It is important to remember that all of these efforts have begun very recently. Therapists are at the familiar stage of joining. In this intance, joining with families around nuclear concerns is extremely difficult because of the previously noted existence of suppression as a coping mechanism. Therapists literally have to buck the system to gain access. As we have seen, there are firm boundaries around families that serve to protect them from affective response to external events and to maintain the privacy of the family as a sanctuary (Lasch, 1975).

Group educational projects

To date, most of the efforts to affect family responses to the nuclear threat have been through educational and/or experiential groups. The focus has been on repairing dysfunctional generational boundaries by empowering parents, teachers, and therapists to deal more effectively with children's needs. Most of these projects have been offered under community auspices, such as churches, schools, and social action groups.

The examples that follow offer a combination of information sharing, group discussion, and experiential exercises that allow adults access to their own deep concerns about nuclear war. They rely heavily on developing a supportive and nurturing group environment as an aid to personal empowerment (Van Ornum & Van Ornum, 1984; Macy, 1983; McVeigh, 1982).

Wendy Forman (personal communication, 1984) has gathered parents together at Peace Breakfasts to share informally their concerns about raising children in the nuclear age. Berger-Gould (personal communication, 1983) is particularly impressed with the results of multifamily groups that allow adults and children to empower each other within their own generations, as an aid to increasing competence and empathy.

In my role as family therapy consultant I have offered over 25 workshops to community groups, ranging in size from six to 60 participants and from one and a half to nine hours in length. I am impressed with the effectiveness of role playing. Participants take turns playing the roles of child and adult, as they talk about nuclear war. Speaking as children, adults seem to find it easier to articulate their own deep feelings. Then, speaking as parents, they can try out ways of responding more appropriately to children's concerns, having allowed themselves to experience more directly the part of themselves that becomes childlike in response to nuclear terror.

My efforts to educate and support parents, I believe, will be even more effective when our research is completed. We believe our data will support both the beneficial nature of family discussions and the effectiveness of parent preparation. We hope, in collaboration with other researchers, to develop training films from tapes of family interviews that can aid in the preparation process.

Public acceptance of the value of training for enhancing family functioning around nuclear issues has been slow to come. However, the consistently positive responses from adults who have participated in such training leads me to feel hopeful that we will be able to expand these programs.

Research as intervention

Research into family nuclear issues can be seen as a direct intervention into family life, as well as a necessary step in broadening our cognitive understanding. I have already mentioned the positive responses we have had from research families. In addition, under the auspices of a research project, it is easier to gain access to families. It also becomes easier to engage professional audiences when speaking from a research perspective.

A single-parent family interviewed as part of our pilot studies had never discussed nuclear war, although all members showed a very high degree of social and political concern. The children talked easily and the parent responded with empathy. At the end of the interview, one child confronted the parent directly with her wish to see the parent become actively involved in the peace movement. The family asked for a return interview, and, in the two months that elapsed, the parent had actually taken a step toward involvement. The children expressed pride in her, and immense relief. We had made an intervention, both into the family and into the external world, by simply opening the door to communication within a healthy family system.

Clinical interventions

Clinical interventions by therapists are at an embryonic stage, awaiting not only evidence of a clearer correlation between nuclear stress and clinical symptoms, but also the development of therapeutic skill in appropriately reframing pathology into larger systems terms, and the development of the links between immediate family experiences and global issues.

EMPOWERING FAMILY THERAPISTS TO DEAL WITH NUCLEAR CONCERNS

Problems of Role Definition for the Therapist

When dealing with the nuclear threat, being inside the system so totally affects the therapist/researcher that her view of therapeutic distance is necessarily revised. Since, in the event of nuclear war, we are as much at risk as our clients, we are truly part of the systems we are attempting to affect. Therefore, we need different conceptualizations of our role and our process.

On our research team, we have gone through cycles of apathy and hope-lessness, grandiosity (a form of denial we think!) and polarization between affect and thinking. We replicate what we find in families, and in the social structure as a whole. I forget to tell my husband of our appointment to be interviewed by the team. I am teased (and supported) by my colleagues about contaminating the research because I am brought to tears as parents and children speak about their worries. All of us, experienced clinicians, try to intervene so as to make things better. We reassure and interrupt process too soon when we feel parents are not supportive or children not clear in their expressions. For example, I found myself directly colluding with a parent to cut off the first personal com-ment her quiet daughter had made about her concerns.

We all have a great deal to learn. But as families experience relief, a sense of competence, and greater cohesiveness after making contact around uclear issues, so do we. All of us need to reframe our dilemmas, connecting the symp-toms with larger systems issues—and this requires transformation of the first order, a new epistomology, and literally, a new world view.

My Own Story—Development of a Nuclear Consciousness

Although it can be deceptive to extrapolate from one person's experience alone, I would like to discuss my own evolution as a family therapist interested in nuclear issues. In talking with others, I have found that our similarities are more apparent than are the idiosyncratic variations.

I began with a family mandate toward social activism. From my early child-hood, my parents had assumed that my intelligence was to be used for the benefit of the world. In my adolescence, this injunction conflicted with the world of my peers, which instructed me to be pretty and compliant. I followed both mandates. I went to a college that also stressed intellect as a tool for service and entered a graduate school of social work, but primarily I presented my social self to the world. I rejoiced in Times Square when the bomb dropped. I married young and "gave up" my career to be a wife and to raise children. My social concerns were primarily private; my husband was to do the work of changing the world and I would be his helpmate.

The assassinations and the political excitement of the 1960s coincided with my increasing freedom from child care, my restlessness as a homemaker, and the fledgling women's movement, which encouraged my reemergence into the public arena. With my husband, I worked hard in the civil rights movement, seemingly with no effect on our affluent suburban community. Only later did I see how our small efforts were part of the changing nature of society.

I burned out! and again I devoted myself to private pursuits, this time to building a professional career. I fell in love with family therapy. The children left home, and I became successful. My husband and I, alone together, started a new family. We built our dream house. I tried not to read about or listen to international news. I felt guilty *all the time*, and I stuffed it down, consciously. It was like the years when I smoked, and knew it would kill me, and I also knew I had no power to stop.

Like the impetus to quit smoking, the opening to a possibility of political awareness came from the voice of someone who cared about me. One of my daughters sent me Joanna Macy's article "Despair Work" (1981). The door opened.

Macy pointed out that I already had a skill that could be useful in developing a more peaceful world. That excited me. I had lost interest in the usual kinds of political efforts. But Macy used group process to reach people below the surface of their seeming apathy, and, from their sense of community and connection, to help them regain hope. "Just like working with families," I thought—a naive, but useful, concept to start with. I began the process of making connections with Macy and with others who could help me learn how to relate this new work to my profession.

My first public move was to offer a nuclear issues interest group at the American Family Therapy Association annual meeting in June 1982. Ten people came. I showed tapes of Brookline third-graders talking about nuclear war. None of us knew what to do except to cry. It was a beginning of awareness. I had gathered a group in order to begin talking to other family therapists about matters that none of us knew anything about as yet. I took leadership not because I had knowledge or experience, but because I had to start somewhere.

Next, I offered a variation on Macy's despair and empowerment work to other therapists. To my surprise, I learned that their primary interest in the psychology of nuclear issues was not for their clients but for themselves, in their role as parents. Out of this, I developed an educational/experiental process called "Helping Children Grow Up in a Nuclear World," which I began to present to community groups.

The groups were well received but I burned out again. This time my body gave way. I had no local support system, I worked alone, above and beyond my normal professional and personal activities. The intensity of the experiences as group leader was overwhelming.

So I stopped, and healed—and began to gather a group to work with in my own community. First, I joined with a small group of women peace activists to share both the personal and global concerns in our work. Then I moved from education/healing to research. I had felt on thin ice making recommendations to parents on the basis of so little direct experience. Work on a research project would lend credibility to community inverventions, and, I thought, would give me some more distance from the emotional involvement of the work.

That, too, was a mirage. As our all volunteer research group began to work, our original excitement and energy began to give way to the all-too-familiar apathy and discouragement. We had been clear from the beginning that maintaining ourselves through mutual support was of the highest priority. We addressed our slump in the following ways:

1. We did our own despair work, sharing together both our fears and our hesitancy to express these.

2. We interviewed each other's families, to break through our own concerns about breaking the taboos of silence around the nuclear threat.

3. We had a chance to present our work to an interested community group and were validated for it. Here we were assisted by an increase in public aware-

ness coming from the possibility of a nuclear waste dump being located in southern Maine.

The energy returned. A year later, we now have a fine research design, the beginnings of a plan for implementing it, and a hard working core group of ten members. We still have no funding, and the possibility of a despair cycle starting again is always present.

In this process, another major shift in my own thinking was taking place. I was stimulated by work with Sarah Conn and Sarah Pirtle of Interhelp, a national group working to support the raising of nuclear consciousness. My unspoken frame of reference had been to spare children the terrible damage that might result from their parents' inability to help them cope with nuclear anxiety and to heal families from the illness of repression and denial. The reframing came with my awareness that opening family boundaries to the world was not just for the healing of pathology but for the developing of new opportunities. I began to believe that supporting children and adults to connect with the whole human condition was a gift, a growth-inducing experience we need not deny ourselves because of the dangerousness of the world.

I subsequently have been re-energized by the preparations for writing this article, by the growth of my own work, through colleagues at AFTA, Interhelp, and Ortho, and by making concrete plans to cut down on other professional responsibilities. I am not a martyr. There are times when I need to shut down. I take a lot of breaks, many more than other peace activists do, it seems. I work in my garden, read mysteries, swim, ski, play with my grandchildren, travel with my husband, make quilts. These activities, which produce immediate and concrete results, compensate somewhat for the slow process of developing awareness of the implications for families living in a nuclear age.

I am more prepared now for the recurrent despair. Systems thinking has given me a better way of understanding and getting beyond it. I have given up the American dream which views progress as a line starting from the beginning of a problem and moving to an ultimate solution. I understand now that all movement, my own, my family's, the world's, is in cycles of activity and in-activity, hope and despair.

The Despair and Empowerment Cycle

Macy's (1983) despair/empowerment cycle has given me a new world view (see Table 18-1).

Of course, there are idiosyncratic variations in this cycle, based on personality variables, ethnic considerations, the availability of community support, and the stage of the life cycle one is in. Some people move quickly through the feeling stage to activism. Many move into the feeling stage as a result of activism, without going through extensive paralysis. In this cycle, the apathy/paralysis phase is a time of rest that is necessary before renewal can take place. It is not at all pathological, given time and the existence of support. I look now to my previous periods of seeming political inactivity as times when I was gathering necessary skills, experiences, ideas, support, and energy for the next movement back into the world. As the socially conscious therapist develops, she must

Table 18-1
The Despair/Empowerment Cycle

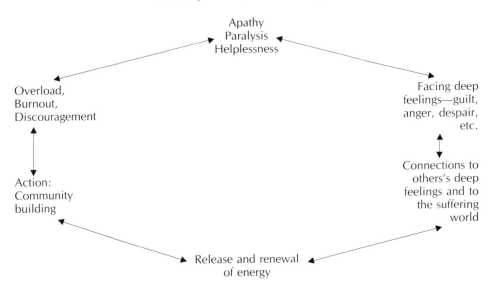

recognize and validate all aspects of the cycle, especially when she is at a point where the outcome of the immediate phase may not be clear.

Jaffe's (1985) three characteristics of cancer survivors are also relevant to my own life as an an activist. I do have some influence on the course of the nuclear "disease." I have a project or two, which may be useful in freeing up some of the forces that prevent people from putting their full energies into solving the nuclear dilemma. My sense of power increases as I see myself connected with thousands of others working in the same direction.

I have developed a sense of the meaning and ultimate purpose of the nuclear illness. I fully believe that the enormity and imminence of the threat of nuclear annihilation have the power to lead people to suppress affect, to close off their boundaries, and to resist activism. This threat also has the power to force a crisis in society that can drastically revise outmoded and ineffective ways of dealing with political and social conflict, create a new consciousness, and lead to increased connections between people. I feel energized by the drama of being at a crossroads in history.

Finally, I have a powerful support system. I know for sure that the exacting and demanding work of facing the terror can only take place in community. The people with whom I live and work care not only about the world, but about me. We will be present for each other during the hard times, even if our work should lead us nowhere.

The following are some of those people:
From my research group: Joe Melnick, Kathleen Sullivan, Carol Lohman, Bonnie Lazar, Mary McCann, Ben Chandler, Denis Noonan, Macy Whitehead, Paulette Gosselin, Cheryl Ebenstein, Mary Jean Mork, Bruce St. Thomas, Cindy Lambert, M.J. Ferrier.

From The Day Before Project: Sharon Hayes-Whitney, Priscilla Kelly, Marge Hodgton, Wendy Roberts, Don Hodgson, Susie Schweppe.

From the Smiling Moose Family Therapist Alliance: Ron Zorn, Jim Smith, Jim Maier, Peter Allen.

From my affinty group: Sr. Claire DeRoche, Marby Payson, Denise Ewell

From All the "Kids and Nukes" Groups: Especially the organizers, Diana Wyatt, Jim McCullough Smith, Renee Lebrun, Judy Roman, Tony Scucci, Donna Bailey Miller, and many others.

From Interhelp: Joanna Macy, Kevin McVeigh, Sarah Pirtle, Sarah Conn, Suzie Pearce, Tova Green, Mona Barbera, Berne Weiss, Harris Peck, Mara Pavel, Rosa Lane, Barbara Hazard, Malachy Shaw-Jones, Nancy Moorehead, Sue Schwartz, Erwin and Sylvia Straub, Sylvia Blanchet, Janine Maland, Bob Housman, Stephanie Merrin, and many more.

From the Avanta Network: Virginia Satir, Bill and Anne Nerin, Joanna Schwab, Margarita Suarez, Jane Gerber, Yetta Bernard, Joan Herrick, Michele Baldwin.

From AFTA: Benina Berger-Gould, Don Bloch, Hinda Winnawer, Erika Waechter, Dick Chasin, Steve Zeitlin, Dave Greenwald, Wendy Forman, Faye Snider, Jules Riskin.

From the American Orthopsychiatric Association: Jon Reusser, Priscilla Ellis, Bianca Cody-Murphy, Peter Rees, Joe Miller

My editor, Marsha Mirkin (and the editiorial assisistance of Carol Burdick, Sarah Pirtle, Mary McCann, Carol Lohman, & Robert Jay Green)

And, most important, my family, especially my grandchildren, Kristofer, Alia, Mischa, Michele, and Caitlin; and my special friend, Eleanor Warner.

REFERENCES

Baider, L. (1977). The silent message—Communications in a family with a dying patient. *Journal of Marriage and Family Counseling, 3,* 23–28.

Barbarin, O. A., & Chesler, M. A. (1984). Coping as interpersonal strategy: Families with childhood cancer. *Family Systems Medicine, 2,* 279–289.

Beardslee, W., & Mack, J. (1982). The impact of nuclear developments on children and adolescents. *Psychological aspects of nuclear developments,* Task Force Report 20. Washington, D.C.: American Psychiatric Association.

Beavers, R. (1981). Healthy families. In G. Berenson & H. White (Eds.), *Annual review of family therapy:* Vol. 1 (pp. 63–91). New York: Human Sciences.

Becker, E. (1974). *The denial of death.* New York: Free Press.

Belenky, M. F., Clinchy, B. M., Goldberger, N. R., & Tarule, J. M. (1986). *Women's ways of knowing: the development of self, voice, and mind.* New York: Basic Books.

Berger-Gould, B., Moon, S., & Van Hoorn, J. (Eds.), (1986). *Growing up scared: The psychological effect of the nuclear threat on children.* Berkeley, Calif.: Open Books.

Bergmann, M. S., & Jucovy, M. E. (Eds.), (1982). *Generations of the Holocaust.* New York: Basic Books.

Boss, P., & Greenberg, J. (1984). Family boundary ambiguity: A new variable in family stress theory. *Family Process, 23,* 534–546.

Caldicott, H. (1984) *Missile envy.* New York: Morrow.

Capra, F. (1982). *The turning point: Science, society and the rising culture.* New York: Simon & Schuster.

Chernin, K. (1983). *In my mother's house.* New York: Harper Colophon.

Children's fears of war: Hearing before the select committee on children, youth, and families. (1984). Washington, D.C.: U.S. Government Printing Office.

Coles, R. (1986). *The moral life of children.* Boston: Atlantic Monthly.

Cunningham, A.M. (1982, Oct.). Is there a seismograph for stress? *Psychology Today,* 46–52.

Diamond, G., & Bachman, J. (1986). High-school seniors and the nuclear threat, 1975-1984: Political and mental health implications of concern and despair. *International Journal of Mental Health, 15,* 210–241.

Eisenbud, M. M., Van Hoorn, J. L., & Gould, B. B. (1985). Children, adolescents and the threat of nuclear war: An international perspective. *Advances in International Maternal and Child Health, 6.*

Ellis, P., Greenburg, S., & Murphy, B. C. (1987, March). The atomic vereran's survivor project. Paper presented at the meeting of the American Orthopsychiatric Association, Washington, D.C.

Ellis et al. (see "Cody Murphy)

Epstein, H. (1979). *Children of the Holocaust.* New York: Bantam.

Epstein, N. B., Baldwin, L. M., & Bishop, D. S. (1983). The McMaster family assessment device. *Journal of Marital and Family Therapy, 9,* 171–182.

Escalona, S. (1962). *Children and the threat of nuclear war.* Child Study Association of America.

Figley, C. R., & Sprenkle, D. H. (1978). Delayed stress response syndrome: Family therapy implications. *Journal of Marriage and Family counseling, 4,* 53–60.

Frank, J. D. (1986). Psychological responses to the threat of nuclear annihilation. *International Journal of Mental Health, 15,* 65–71.

Friedman, B. (1984). Preschoolers' awareness of the nuclear threat. *California Association for the Education of Young Children Newsletter, 12*(2).

Gilligan, C. (1982). *In a different voice: Psychological theory and women's development.* Cambridge, Mass.: Harvard University Press.

Goldenring, J. M., & Doctor, R. (1986), Teen-age worry about nuclear war: North American and European questionnaire studies. *International Journal of Mental Health, 15,* 72–92.

Goleman, D. (1985). *Vital lies, simple truths: the psychology of self-deception.* New York: Simon & Schuster.

Gould, J. (1986). Exploring youth's reaction to the threat of nuclear war. In B. B. Gould, S. Moon, & J. Van Horne (Eds.), *Growing up scared? The psychological effect of the nuclear threat on children* (pp. 49–56). Berkeley, Calif.: Open Books.

Greenwald, D. S., & Zeitlin, S. J. (1987). *No reason to talk about it: Families confront the nuclear taboo.* New York: Norton.

Haley, J. (1976). *Problem solving therapy.* San Francisco: Jossey-Bass.

Jaffe, D. T. (1985). *Self-renewal: Personal transformation following extreme trauma* (Research Rep. IV). Los Angeles: Holmes Center for Research in Holistic Healing.

Johnson, M. C., Muyskens, M. J., Bryce, M., Palmer, J., & Rodnan, J. (1985). A comparison of family adaptations to having a child with cystic fibrosis. *Journal of Marital and Family Therapy, 11,* 305–312.

Kantor, D., & Lehr, W. (1975). *Inside the family: Toward a theory of family process.* New York: Harper Colophon.

Kaplan, J., & Shapiro, L. (Eds.), (1985). *Red diaper babies: Children of the left.* Somerville, Mass.: Red Diaper Productions.

Kegan, R. (1982). *The evolving self.* Cambridge, Mass.: Harvard University Press.

Klein, D. M. (1983). Family problem solving and family stress. *Marriage and Family Review. 6,* 85–112.

Kubler-Ross, E. (1969). *On death and dying.* New York: Macmillan.

Kubler-Ross, E. (1983). *On children and death.* New York: Collier.

Lasch, C. (1975). *Haven in a heartless world.* New York: Basic Books.

Liebert, R. M., Sprafkin, J. N., & Davidson, E. S. (1982). *The early window: Effects of television on children and youth* (2nd ed.). New York: Pergamon.

Levine, J., Warrenburg, S., Kerns, R., Schwartz, G., Delaney, R., Fontana, R., Gradman, A., Smith, S., Allen, S., Cascione, R. (1987) The role of denial in recovery from coronary heart disease. *Psychosomatic Medicine, 49,* 109-117.

Lifton, R. J. (1967). *Death in life: Survivors of Hiroshima.* New York: Simon & Schuster.

Lifton, R. J. (1979). *The broken connection.* New York: Simon & Schuster.

Lifton, R. J. (1986). *The Nazi doctors.* New York: Basic Books.

Lifton, R. J. (1987). *The future of immortality and other essays for a nuclear age.* New York: Basic Books.

Locatelli, M. G., & Holt, R. R. (1986). Antinuclear activism, psychic numbing, and mental health. *International Journal of Mental Health, 15,* 143–161.

Loeb, P. (1983) *Nuclear culture: Living and working in the world's largest atomic complex.* Philadelphia: New Society Publishers.

Lynch, J. J. (1977). *The broken heart: The medical consequences of loneliness.* New York: Basic Books.

Mack, J. E. (1986). Approaching the nuclear threat in clinical work with children and their families. In B. B. Gould, S. Moon, & J. Van Horne (Eds.), *Growing up scared? The psychological effect of the nuclear threat on children* (pp. 25–38). Berkeley, Calif.: Open Books.

Macy, J. (1981). Despair work. *Evolutionary Blues—An Interhelp Quarterly, 1.*

Macy, J. (1983). *Despair and personal power in the nuclear age.* Philadelphia: New Society.

Madanes, C. (1981). *Strategic family therapy.* San Francisco: Jossey-Bass.

Marciano, T. D., & Sussman, M. B. (Eds.), (1986). *Families and the prospect of nuclear attack/holocaust.* New York: Haworth.

McCubbin, H. I., Dahl B. B., Metries, P., Hunter, E., & Plag, J. (Eds.), (1974). Family separation and reunion. Washington, D.C.: U.S. Government Printing Office.

McCubbin, H. I., & Patterson, J. M. (1983). The family stress process: The double ABCX model of adjustment and adaption. *Marriage and Family REview. 6,* 7–37.

McGoldrick, M., Pearce, J. K., & Giordano, J. (Eds.), (1982). *Ethnicity and family therapy.* New York: Guilford Press.

McVeigh, K. (1982). The hunger to be heard: Children and nuclear war. *Humpty Dumpty Reports: An Interhelp Journal.*

Minuchin, S. (1974). *Families and family therapy.* Cambridge, Mass.: Harvard University Press.

Mojtabai, A. G. (1986). *Blessed assurance: at home with the bomb in Amarillo, Texas.* Boston: Houghton-Mifflin.

Oliveri, M. E., & Reiss, D. (1982). Families' schemata of social relationship. *Family Process, 21,* 295–312.

Olson, D. H., Sprenkle, D. H., & Russell, C. (1979). Circumplex model of marital and family systems: I. Cohesion and adaptability dimensions, family types, and clinical applications, *Family Process, 18,* 3–28.

Parad, H. (Ed.), (1965). *Crisis intervention: Selected readings.* New York: Family Service Association of America.

Perlmutter, M.S., & Ringler, D. (1986). Nuclear anxiety: social symptomatology and educational therapy. In T. D. Marciano & M. B. Sussman (Eds.), *Families and the prospect of nuclear attack/holocaust* (pp. 59–84). New York: Haworth.

Rosenheck, R., & Thompson, J. (1986). ''Detoxification'' of Vietnam War trauma: A combined family-individual approach. *Family Process, 25,* 559–570.

Rutter, M. (1987). Psychosocial resilience and protective mechanisms. *American Journal of Orthopsychiatry, 57,* 316–331.

Satir, V. (1983). *Conjoint family therapy* (3rd ed.). Palo Alto, Calif.: Science and Behavior Books.

Schell, J. (1982). *The fate of the earth.* New York: Avon.

Schell, J. (1987 Jan.). History in Sherman Park, part II. *The New Yorker,* 57–87.

Schwebel, M. (1965). Nuclear cold war: Student opinions and professional responsibility. *Behavior science and human survival.* Palo Alto, Calif.: Science and Behavior Books.

Schwebel, M. (Ed.), (1986). Mental health implications of life in the nuclear age. *International Journal of Mental Health, 15.*

Schwebel, M. (1986). The study of stress and coping in the nuclear age: A new specialty. *International Journal of Mental Health, 15,* 5–15.

Sgroi, S. M. (1982). *Handbook of clinical, intervention in child sexual abuse.* Lexington, Mass.: Lexington Books.

Sheehy, G. (1986). *The spirit of survival.* New York: Morrow.

Solantus, T., & Rimpela, M. (1986). Mental health and the threat of nuclear war—A suitable case for treatment? *International Journal of Mental Health, 15,* 261–275.

Solomon, Z., Mikulincer, M., Freid, B., & Wosner, Y.. (1987) Family characteristics and postraumatic stress disorder: a followup of Israeli combat stress reaction casualties. *Family Process, 27,* 383–394.

Van Hoorn, J. (1986). Facing the nuclear threat: Comparisons of adolescents and adults. In B. B. Gould, S. Moon, & J. Van Hoorne (Eds.), *Growing up scared? The psychological effect of the nuclear threat on children* (pp. 57–76). Berkeley, Calif.: Open Books.

Van Ornum, W., & Van Ornum, M. W. (1984). *Talking to children about nuclear war.* New York: Continuum.

Venaki, S. K., Nadler, A., & Gersoni, H. (1985). Sharing the holocaust experience. *Family Process, 24,* 273–280.

Wetzel, N. A., & Winnawer, H. (1986). The psychological consequences of the nuclear threat from a family systems perspective. *International Journal of Mental Health, 15,* 298–313.

Zeitlin, S. (1984). What do we tell mom and dad? *The Family Therapy Networker, 8,* 31, 38–39, 62.

19

DOES DISCUSSION OF NUCLEAR WAR HAVE A PLACE IN FAMILY THERAPY?

Robert Simon, M.D.

Studies of Americans in all age groups have demonstrated the psychological impact of the threat of nuclear war. Fear, anger, despair, and denial form a tangle of affect surrounding this issue, visible once the taboo against discussing it has been removed. These observations have been made with both individuals and families, but from a clinician's point of view, two questions remain: (1) How does nuclear fear relate to dysfunction within the family system? (2) How would that relationship be approached in the specific enterprise called family therapy?

In the abstract, it is hard to see how the nuclear issue would *not* affect every aspect of therapy. First, we know that therapy is a "benevolent ordeal" involving a major commitment of time, effort, and money. Willingness to undergo the ordeal springs not only from the patients' suffering but also, implicitly, from their hope for a better future. This idea may not be stated explicitly, but it is clearly present, and it would be at its most powerful when children are involved. No matter what problems they represent, children are parents' best link to a hoped-for future, ultimately, the future beyond the parents' own lifetimes. Robert J. Lifton (1983) has cited hope for the future as a transcendental issue in human psychology. Even without children, humans will cling to the eternal future of life on earth as antidote to the awareness of death. And yet in this age we confront a world issue that threatens to cancel that future, that negates hope not only for one's family but for all the world family. The reality of the threat cannot be rationally denied, so it must be a silent specter in an undertaking like therapy that pivots on the hope of future happiness. Meaning and the ethical commitments attached to meaning can be preserved, even beyond one's personal death, through the fantasied succession of generations or even the enduring earth itself. But if the earth is not fated to survive, what else has meaning? To use Lifton's terms, nuclearism creates a "broken connection."

Another unique aspect of this problem is that it is inescapable for the therapist as well as for the clients. In most psychotherapy, a major anxiety shared by therapist and client would be considered an important danger signal, and perhaps a contraindication to the therapeutic contract. Training analysis, supervision, and other forms of self-examination are part of the therapist's continuing quest not to allow this to occur. Yet, in nuclear war, we meet an anxiety of severe proportions (were it to be fully conscious) that cannot be neutralized by one's personal analysis, by introspection, or by research into one's family of origin. This death's head sits grinning in the mirror no matter who looks.

The field of family therapy is largely silent on this problem. No therapist of the many I have questioned is willing to bring up nuclear fears in family sessions, although almost all would discuss it if the family brought it up. The 25 families reported by Greenwald and Zeitlin (1987) who did discuss the issue did not do so in the course of therapy sessions, but had been specifically recruited for the study. How can a crucial world issue be so pervasive in modern consciousness and at the same time be so little encountered clinically? The following two stories give some clues.

THE DAY AFTER: **A PERSONAL EXPERIENCE**

It has long been debated whether popular media shape public consciousness or whether they only reflect it. Probably both were true in November 1983, when the American Broadcasting System (ABC) presented its dramatic version of life after a U.S.-Soviet nuclear exchange. The film received poor reviews, and apparently had been clumsily edited from a much longer (and perhaps more coherent) original. It was also not helped by the soporific panel discussion tacked on at the end. Nevertheless, the first hour had a shocking power. This initial segment depicted the inexorable march of events leading up to the firing of the missiles, and then the explosions themselves. These images in the living rooms of America may well have given the *coup de grâce* to an era in which the physical threat of nuclear war was largely denied, and also may have played a part in laying to rest the government's absurd program of civil defense.

Even more striking, however, was the impact of *The Day After* in the month *preceding* its presentation. ABC's well-organized public relations campaign produced leaflets, discussion materials for schools, and a brief trailer for the film. The trailer wisely concentrated on the stunning early sequences rather than on the trite human-interest stories that made up most of the script. Among other organizations, Physicians for Social Responsibility (PSR) became aware of the forthcoming presentation and recognized an opportunity to augment its perennial message to the public: that nuclear war would be devastating. Local chapters of PSR were notified of the telecast and urged to take action in their communities, organizing discussion groups, mobilizing the psychiatric and medical societies, speaking in schools and churches, and so on.

My personal experience began through membership in a district chapter of PSR. Most significant was the opportunity to see ABC's trailer for the film. Its intense emotional impact supported the PSR view that children should not watch

The Day After without their parents, and that perhaps younger children should not watch it at all. (One did not realize at the time that the complete film would be such an anticlimax.) Shortly before the airing date, at a conference of the Ackerman Institute for Family Therapy, I chaired a session on nuclear anxieties and the family. In the course of my remarks, I mentioned the film and its possible impact on children.

The following day, the *New York Times* story about the conference centered on what I had said about the film. There followed the "15 minutes of being a celebrity" that Andy Warhol said everyone will enjoy at some point. Out-of-town newspapers called. I was interviewed on three radio programs and two television news shows. (On one of these, the other panelist was the local civil defense chief. He said that, upon nuclear attack, residents along the Connecticut shore should gas up their cars, take the New England Thruway to New Haven, and turn north on I-91. After several hours of driving, they would arrive in Vermont, where kindly local citizens were sure to give them food and shelter.) Phyllis Schlafly's office called to commend my emphasis on the family and to invite me to speak (I declined). And so on. This bizarre experience perhaps gives the flavor of what was washing through the media at that time. Pushed by all the excitement, not just my own "celebrity," I felt fully justified to ask families I was treating, "What do you intend to do about *The Day After?*"

Their responses were interesting because, naturally, each was tinted by the family's usual colors. One loud and bullying father handled the question with typical bluster. When his son voiced some fears, he became red-faced and lectured the boy on how absurd it was to think that anyone would so deliberately commit suicide. "It can't happen! Nobody could be so crazy!" Later on, without the children present, he revealed a lifetime fear of dying. Another father told how, when his college-age son had given a passionate speech against nuclear war at the Thanksgiving table, he had criticized his son for using an abrasive tone of voice. The response was consistent with this man's insensitivity to the feelings of others. Not all responses were dramatic, of course, but that was not the point. What had happened in the heat of that national moment, and of my personal moment, was that nuclear war seemed to have entered legitimately into the process of therapy. I felt that a new dimension might be opening for theory and practice.

Nothing came of it. In the weeks following the broadcast, I followed up with nearly all my patients about what the effect of the experience had been. The results were diffuse and inconclusive. People seemed to be thinking about the issue more than they previously had, but no one seemed deeply troubled and there were no dramatic conversions to political activism. The usual personal and family problems, like jungle vines, quickly recaptured the territory. *The Day After* resurfaced briefly during the 1987 controversy over a National Broadcasting Company drama, *Amerika*, about a supposed Russian takeover of the United States. Otherwise, it seems to have gone to wherever they bury the vast wasteland's junk. Its once-vivid emotional impact has apparently been sucked into the encompassing vacuum of psychic numbing.

THE STORY OF *HALFLIFE*

In the spring of 1982, a group of faculty members at the Ackerman Institute for Family Therapy began to meet weekly during their lunch hour to discuss their increasing concern over the nuclear threat, on both a political and a clinical level. The central psychological question was whether Lifton's "broken connection" might be playing a silent role in young adults' increasing aversion to personal commitments, in their disinterest in starting families, and in the spreading use of cocaine and other intoxicants. This was not a group of tut-tutting defenders of the status quo; in fact, they were inclined more to empathy and support for the younger generation, and had themselves struggled through many of the same issues. Their concerns had accumulated through repeated experiences in the consulting room, in which baffled parents with severely "turned-off" adolescents and young adults came and went. These patients were afflicted not only with the textbook problems of family life but also with a failure in the transmission of ideals and values from one generation to the next. It was recognized that many factors in contemporary life probably played a part in this phenomenon, but, especially after the publication of Jonathan Schell's *The Fate of the Earth* (1982), one had to face the possibility that the prospect of future nuclear devastation might somehow be rotting the psychological fabric of the family. At the suggestion of the Institute's director, Donald Bloch, the group took the name Halflife; it was simultaneously a reference to atomic physics and to the uncertain human future.

Halflife meetings promoted an atmosphere of support so that participants could share their fears, their sense of powerlessness, and their own tendency toward psychic numbing. It was always understood, however, that the meetings would have to be more than rap sessions if they were to be productive. Plans for action within the family therapy field were discussed and implemented in the meeting format.

Two major achievements resulted: First, the Halflife group proposed to the remainder of the faculty that all large conferences given by the institute, no matter what their themes, include a luncheon session devoted to family aspects of the nuclear threat. The faculty adopted this resolution, and the sessions became a popular feature of the institute's professional meetings (at that time, two or three per year). Second, Halflife members used the group's support and suggestions to develop advocacy in larger forums such as the American Family Therapy Association, the American Orthopsychiatric Association, and the American Association for Marriage and Family Therapy. Each of these organizations still features workshops and plenary sessions on the topic at their annual conferences—not solely an achievement of Halflife, but certainly on its list of contributions.

A more subtle result was the empowerment and stimulation that Halflife offered its members to publish articles about the effect of nuclear anxiety on families and upon the practice of therapy. (Bloch, 1984; Penn, 1984; Simon, 1984; Wetzel & Winawer, 1986). It was also supportive and enriching to its members' participation in other organizations such as Physicians for Social Responsibility, SANE, and Council for a Livable World.

One thing that Halflife could not accomplish, however, was to design a model for incorporating the nuclear issue into the actual practice of family therapy. A short demonstration videotape was developed by Marcia Sheinberg and Peggy Penn,* centering on a family in which a child had actually voiced fears of nuclear holocaust in connection with his chronic anxiety. There was a lot of discussion about developing a library of such clinical vignettes, but nothing came of it because no one else could come up with suitable clinical material. In general, Halflife members reported increasing frustration in attempts to bring nuclearism into the practice of therapy.

After the Reagan landslide in 1984, Halflife turned out to have a "half-life" of its own. Meetings grew dispirited and pessimistic, and fell off in regularity. Members said that they felt they had done all they could within this particular format. The conference luncheon sessions continued, but were frequently organized at the last minute and without a sense that something unique and valuable was being brought to the participants. By the fall of 1986, the group effectively was no longer in existence, although it was never officially terminated.

In preparation for writing this chapter, the author polled nine members of Halflife by questionnaire in order to tap their understanding of what had happened. The questions were as follows.

1. From a systemic point of view, why do you think Halflife has become so inactive?

2. Are you currently involved in a specific antinuclear war group?

3. If the answer is Yes, did this activity or commitment change with the demise of Halflife, and in what way?

4. Do you currently work with the threat of nuclear war in family therapy, and how do you do it?

As might be expected, the first question produced the greatest variety of answers. Halflife's demise was attributed to ennui within the antinuclear movement itself; to characteristic impatience of systemic therapists for long-range solutions; to internal politics of the Institute itself, and so on. No one will ever know the correct answer, but it is likely that Halflife's small, seminar-style format had much less resilience for change in membership and motivation than would a national organization such as PSR with its thousands of members. In reply to question 2, nearly everyone identified himself or herself with some established antiwar group, though the level of commitment and activity varied. Activity in these other organizations was perceived as uninfluenced by the fate of Halflife, but in the author's opinion the availability of other structures for expressions of activism was the greatest reason for Halflife's decline.

Question 4 produced a nearly unanimous response. No one currently makes a practice of introducing nuclear issues into family therapy unless the family itself brings it up, and this happens rarely, if ever. It seems that Halflife's inability to bridge the gap to therapy has remained unresolved despite all of the organizational, political, and theoretical activity it engendered.

*Respectively, senior faculty member and Director of Training, Ackerman Institute for Family Therapy.

TREATMENT IN CONTEXT

Both of these stories remind us that, just as individuals cannot be separated from their relationship context, neither can the process of treatment itself. Therapy of any kind exists in a network of social, ethnic, financial, and political realities. This network is invisible for the most part, but when it is looked for, its presence and power can be felt. A mundane example: the fee usually is paid by mail, "untouched by human hands" as it were, or in a polite zone of silence tacitly agreed to by both sides. If the patient falls behind in payments, however, or if the therapist decides to increase the fee, then the issue may spring to the center stage with intense affect on either side, whether publicly acknowledged or not. So it is with the nuclear issue. Suppose a patient expressed uncertainty about which candidate to vote for in a national election. It is more likely that the therapist would bring up the patient's past experience with divorced parents, or the obsessive need to see all sides of every issue, rather than ask, "What about candidate A's record on the MX missile?" Perhaps such a comment by the therapist would be acceptable in a country where the average citizen thinks about politics as matter-of-factly as about sex or physical fitness. In America, however, political activity is usually on the fringe of personal concerns, a special interest such as music or stamp collecting. It takes a major media event like *The Day After* to provide a context in which a political theme can be introduced in treatment without its seeming to be tacked on and, therefore, suspect as favoring the therapist's personal convictions. The topic could be legitimized if the patient introduced it, because bringing up problems is an implicit privilege of the patient. In practice, however, this almost never occurs.

But "almost never" is not "never," and there are isolated instances in which nuclear fears either surface directly or in thinly disguised anxieties about the future. Despite the rarity of these situations, some consideration of therapeutic response is worthwhile. One never knows when the social context may again stimulate openness about nuclear fears in the way that *The Day After* did. Some family discussions about the issue have been reported. The study of 25 families by Greenwald and Zeitlin (1987) is a valuable resource. These were volunteer families, not in the process of therapy. Nevertheless, the authors illustrate many important themes underlying the family's response to the issue: feelings of vulnerability, the sense of powerlessness, and reactive blaming.

These families illustrate the notion of nuclear war as a special kind of family secret—the "open" type that everyone knows but no one will mention. Its difference from more mundane versions such as mom's drinking or dad's pornography collection lies in its vast scope, its finality, and the lack of well-defined clinical options once it comes into the open—not to mention the fact that it is deeply shared by the therapist. Nevertheless, Greenwald and Zeitlin correctly emphasize that "breaking the taboo" (against talking about it) is a vital first step. Their approach also emphasizes the necessity for further action, especially by the parents, once the topic has surfaced. There is sometimes a sentimental tendency to equate family therapy with "talking it over," but experienced therapists know that talking is only a precursor to a therapeutic plan for change. This is especially true when the family has been touched by such realities as abuse, incest, poverty, unemployment, and political oppression. The threat of annihilation is clearly in that category.

When the stressor on the family is social or political, therapeutic change must include moves into the social or political arena. It has been well established, for example, that there is no sense in analyzing a man's abusive impulses toward his wife unless the reality of the abuse is first eliminated. The same holds true if nuclear fears enter family discussions. Once the taboo is broken, what are the adults actually ready to do? The oft-repeated question "What shall we tell the children?" is a disguised wish for a magic formula to make the issue go away, because the parents cannot imagine what to do about their helplessness once the problem has been broached. In a sense, empty talk is worse than no talk. It taps the emotions without moving toward a less-threatening reality and, thus, no matter how well intentioned, it becomes a betrayal. It is particularly acute if the children in the family are adolescents, because they are naturally skeptical of adults, and are also vulnerable to disillusionment with parental failures. Far more than young children, they will react with bitterness and alienation if they sense that the adults offer nothing more than high-sounding talk.

Political or social action may occur on a spectrum of intensity appropriate to the individual and to his or her age and life circumstances. It might be just joining a local association of concerned citizens or receiving a newsletter from an appropriate organization. Or it might involve full-scale political activity, such as joining in demonstrations and letter writing (Lifton, 1985). Whatever the scale of involvement, the therapist may be needed as a catalyst, because any move into a new personal arena can use support and encouragement. In addition, an important change in the real-life activities of a family member is likely to unbalance the relationship system. For example, an adolescent girl responding to a perceived need for political action might become more assertive and thus stimulate her mother to greater assertiveness, as well—which could cause problems in the marital dyad. This is the kind of change that any systemically oriented therapist would be alert to, but the most important thing here is not the consequences of change but the necessity for action. Once the subject is uncovered by the family, discussion by itself is not sufficient. Empowerment for the parents to act, provided by the therapist, becomes empowerment from the parents to their children.

WHY IT DOES NOT HAPPEN

The foregoing discussion applies when the family, in some way, legitimizes nuclear anxiety as a discussion topic. But in actuality, without the push of a media event or other outside influence, this does not happen. Even Halflife's committed and resourceful members failed to develop a way of introducing the issue in the clinical setting. At present, they all rely solely on cues from the family—cues that never arise. Halflife alumni have remained active in antiwar organizations, so their failure to find a clinical application cannot simply be a manifestation of psychic numbing. They are also inventive and experienced therapists, so lack of innovative talent is also unlikely as an explanation. One is left with the conclusion that there must be something about family therapy itself—at least in its present form—that argues against the emergence of nuclear fears.

It seems clear that the problem is epistemological, not technical. From this point of view, the issue could be addressed not only directly but also by analogy. For example, parents could be counseled to direct their runaway daughter to a political action group "because your daughter needs to know that you can offer her some hope in this frightening world." But few, if any, therapists today would make such a move, because there is no accepted linkage between delinquent behavior and nuclear fear. The daughter's running away might be linked to hidden problems between the parents, or to rebalancing a conflict between her brother and her father, *but it cannot be legitimized in the mind of today's therapist as a response to world events or to the uncertainty of the human future.*

Then, too, we must consider how the act of family therapy is structured. ("Act" is used here to denote the therapeutic encounter as an entity in itself, distinguished from content issues such as the therapist's school of thought, the family's dynamics, or its relationship with the therapist.) From this perspective, family therapy has a formal context:

1. It is specifically purchased from the therapist. This is true whether the family pays a fee for service or the purchase is made by an agency paying a salary to the therapist. (Low-cost clinics generally aspire to deliver the equivalent of private care, although at a reduced rate.)

2. Family members bring to the therapy not only their problems, but also their underlying loyalty to each other. With respect to nuclear fears, parents will not subject their children to frightening speculations about the end of the world, and children—likewise loyal—will not confront their parents on a topic they think them to be helpless about.

3. The sessions are time limited, thus imposing the necessity to set priorities among the topics for discussion.

4. The therapist's input, it is tacitly agreed, will be applied "to the head" only. It is considered improper to meddle in clients' politics, religion, financial decisions, and so on, except under extraordinary circumstances. Therapists, of course, are not really expected to be value-free; on the contrary, value judgments are expected to be present and to be inwardly recognized, like countertransference feelings. But recognizing them is in the service of *neutralization*, not promoting them with the clients.

5. The basis for the contract is the expectation that a certain problem is to be solved, for instance, getting a son in his 20s to find a job. Problem definition may be open to negotiation at both the beginning and during the course of therapy, but whatever is finally agreed to be the problem is expected to improve in order for the consumers to feel that their time and money have not been wasted. This is a binding mandate for the therapist. Violations of problem definition on his or her part are considered at least circumspect, and perhaps intrusive. A familiar example of this principle would be a student therapist, assigned the case of that nonfunctioning young man, immediately confronting the parents' marital conflicts. As a result, the case is lost, because the parents

do not see their marital stresses (if they are aware of any) as being the problem.

The same fate awaits the nuclear-aware therapist who would unilaterally bring the issue into the therapy session without some invitation from family members or from a current event such as *The Day After*. What ethical therapist (i.e., one adhering to accepted standards of practice) would work from a hypothesis based on the index patient's despair for the global future, and resentment of the parents' failure to act in a responsible way politically? We see volumes of published cases in which the parents of such a man are instructed to be firm with him; to research their families of origin; to go out for the evening without letting him know their whereabouts, and so on. We have yet to see a case in which they were urged to attend an antiwar rally. The point is not that this would necessarily be the correct intervention, but that the thought of it is so foreign to conventional practice. How would a family therapist even ask about the issue? Parents might be prepared, however warily, to answer questions about their sex life, but would they answer questions about political commitments? True to its roots in psychoanalysis, family therapy is primarily a program for interior redesign. It legitimizes discussion of such items as loyalty, system balance, the struggle for independence, and other aspects of selfhood, but it has no recognized place for political activism. And since the family (or the agency on behalf of the family) has purchased the therapist's time in order to work on "the problem," it is a serious breach of therapeutic ritual to put the discussion on a plane that no one was expecting and no one wants to think about.

"*Eppure, il muove.*" Thus muttered Galileo after the Inquisition forced him to recant the idea that the earth moves around the sun. "Nevertheless, it moves." We have, of course, reached an absurd conclusion in theory and practice: that the most overwhelming reality of our age, and probably of all the human future, is inadmissable in psychotherapy unless brought into focus by the media or by current events.

The situation is made all the more absurd by the well-documented fact that the same family members will reveal their nuclear concerns quite readily when interviewed in the context of the peer group (Eisenbud et al., 1986; Escalona, 1982; Mack, 1981; Physicians for Social Responsibility, 1982; Schwebel, 1982). And the same would apply to the therapist in private life, since he or she could also be queried in a peer group setting. Therefore, the issue cannot be absent when the family assembles for therapy. As we have seen, discussion is blocked on the family's side by the family members' covert loyalty to each other, and on the therapist's side by a lack of rationale for introducing the topic unilaterally.

It seems that family therapy's theoretical—and, therefore, clinical—base is just not large enough to encompass the issue of nuclear war. This is not a new discovery; the preceding chapters document a number of big issues that, until recently, have had no clear place in the field despite their importance in the personal lives of therapists and clients. Until the nuclear issue engenders such theory building, it will continue to need outside stimuli in order to enter the consulting room. This theory building is going on all the time, indirectly, as economic, sexual, and political realities become incorporated into treatment planning. Certain issues that we recognized in contemporary family therapy have overtones of the nuclear age, for example:

●Just how important are territory, possession, and power? Some forms of family therapy are recognizably linked to these metaphors. A detailed critique is beyond the scope of this chapter, but the field must consider whether some approaches to therapy are undesirably isomorphic with concepts that have set the political system on its present risky course.

●Is force necessary in family life? Family therapists do not advocate beating children or spouses into submission, but there are many kinds of force and many kinds of beatings. To take one popular concept as an example, where does hierarchy end and bullying begin? This is a particularly sensitive issue in raising adolescents. What lessons do forceful parents teach children about conflict resolution, and will they eventually be expressed in the voting booth as well as in the next generation?

●What is the proper role of the family in the political system? The particular dilemmas posed by the question were explored above.

●Do women know something that might be unique when told in the corridors of power?

The last question raises the issue of feminism—specifically, the current feminist revision of psychological theory—as a potential for developing family therapy in a direction that can more fully address the issue of nuclear war.† This connection goes deeper than simply equating the female sex with such clichés as "gentleness" or "caring," which would imply—quite wrongly—that women are just too nice to drop the bomb. The hard-nosed political views of Golda Meir, Indira Gandhi, and Margaret Thatcher also contradict such sentimentality. As Sara Ruddick (1984) has expressed it:

> Out of maternal practice *a distinctive kind of thinking* arises that is incompatible with military strategy but consonant with pacifist commitment to non-violence. The peacefulness of mothers, however, is not now a reliable source for peace. In order for motherly peacefulness to be publicly significant . . . maternal thinking would have to be transformed by a feminist politics. (p. 223)

That public significance still has to be achieved is documented by Peggy Penn's "The Women at Greenham Common" (1984). This paper illustrates the considerable problems involved in finding a political voice for the antiwar feeling inherent in what Ruddick calls "maternal practice." Penn describes, in a personal, free-flowing narrative, how these passive protesters and their children lived from day to day, and how they organized their membership and planned their formal demonstrations. Their doubts, anxieties, and missteps are interwoven with the author's parallel feelings. Her narrative format—so different from the accepted norms of scientific journals—repeats, on a smaller scale, the Greenham women's determination not to be caught up in Establishment clichés of how thinking is to be organized. This isomorphism is important, because it suggests a link between a way of being in the family context, a way of being in the world, and an approach to political realities that does not separate them from personal or family experience.

† See the appropriate chapters in this volume.

> The real danger facing the women and the life of this protest would be if they abandoned their own proliferative myth and adopted a power myth, an apocalyptic myth. . . . What the women have understood for the last two years is that a premise based on power is false, and they have shown us, through nonviolent actions in behalf of peace, the real power attainable in the giving up of power. (p. 78)

Penn recognizes that this attitude toward thought and action is not a feminine monopoly, and it certainly should not become a solely feminine responsibility.† Characterizing it as feminist underscores its roots in the differing cognitive and moral development of men and women. As Ruddick (1984) puts it:

> Separating moral and human significance from other aspects of a plan or action is an aspect of abstraction. It is often said that men are more apt to engage in this sort of moral dissociation than women. . . . Women are . . . less concerned with claiming rights, more with sharing responsibilities. They do not value independence and autonomy over connection and the restraints of caring, but rather assume that the conflict between rightful self-assertion and responsible interdependence is at the heart of moral life. (p. 250)

Perhaps the new "feminist" epistemology, based on the inherent moral power of motherhood, may give us the link between a way of being in the family context and a way of being in the world. We will know if it does because the connections of clinical work and the prevention of war will no longer seem so elusive. Attacking a clinical problem through pacifism and political activism will have achieved an accepted and comfortable rationale. We will be able to question the tacit assumption of all therapy that there is sure to be a future, and we will be able to face latent doubts about that future. Part of that direction is the expansion of clinical thought suggested by this book, that is, including the externals of life in our understanding of a personal and family psychology.

Eppure, il muove.

REFERENCES

Bloch, D. (1984). What do we tell the children? *Family Networker, 8*, 30.

Eisenbud, M., Van Hoorn, J., & Gould, B. (1986). Children, adolescents, and the threat of nuclear war. *Advances in International Maternal and Child Health, 6.*

Escalona, S. (1982). Growing up with the threat of nuclear war: Some indirect effects on personality development. *American Journal of Orthopsychiatry, 52,* 600–607.

Greenwald, S., & Zeitlin, S. (1987). *No reason to talk about it: Families confront the nuclear taboo.* New York: Norton.

Lifton, R. (1983). *The broken connection: On death and the continuity of life.* New York: Basic Books.

Lifton, R. (1985, Aug.). Toward a nuclear-age ethos. *Bulletin of the Atomic Scientists.*

---

†Robert J. Lifton's (1985) similar statements further argue against identifying this position only with women: "To renounce nuclearism is to renounce the nuclear illusions of limit and control, preparation, protection, stoic behavior under attack, and recovery, and to recognize nuclear weapons as instruments of genocide and that the continuity of human life—hope itself—lies only in prevention."

Mack, J. (1981, Apr.). *Psychosocial effects of the nuclear arms race. Bulletin of the Atomic Scientists*, 2–7.

Penn, P. (1984). The women at Greenham Common: An observation. *Family Systems Medicine*, 2, 66–79.

Physicians for Social Responsibility (1982). *Preparing for nuclear war: The psychological effects.* New York: Physicians for Social Responsibility.

Ruddick, S. (1984). Preservative love and military destruction: Some reflections on mothering and peace. In J. Treblicot (Ed.), *Mothering: Essays in feminist theory*. Totowa, N.J.: Rowman & Allanheld.

Schell, J. (1982) *The fate of the earth*. New York: Alfred A. Knopf.

Schwebel, M. (1982). Effects of the nuclear war threat on children and teenagers: Implications for professionals. *American Journal of Orthopsychiatry*, 52, 608–618.

Simon, R. (1984). The nuclear family. *Family Networker*, 8, 22.

Wetzel, N., & Winawer, H. (1986). The psychosocial consequences of the nuclear threat from a family systems perspective. *International Journal of Mental Health*, 15, 298–313.

20

FAMILY THERAPY IN THE NUCLEAR AGE: FROM CLINICAL TO GLOBAL*

Jonathan W. Reusser, A.C.S.W.
and Bianca Cody Murphy, Ed.D.

> A professional social science that loses concern for the larger society cannot do even its professional job, for there is too much of reality with which it cannot deal. (Bellah, Madsen, Sullivan, Swindler, & Tipton, 1985, p. 3)

One of the most pressing social issues confronting us today is the threat of nuclear holocaust. With the advent of nuclear arsenals, we have acquired the ability to destroy the world as we know it. Never before have humans been capable of such destruction. As Jonathan Schell (1982) has eloquently expressed it, today "the fate of the earth" lies in the balance. "Nuclear weapons radically alter our existence. Nothing we do or feel in working, playing and living, and in our private, family and public lives is free of this influence. The threat they pose has become the context of our lives, a shadow that persistently intrudes upon our mental ecology" (Lifton & Falk, 1982, p. 3).

Family therapists have recently become involved in applying their theoretical and clinical skills to the challenges of the nuclear threat. Over the past five years, there is a growing body of literature in which family therapists discuss the impact of the nuclear threat on families and children. More recently, a handful of family therapists have attempted to address the effect family therapists might have on the social and political context in which the threat is embedded, on both the national and the international level. In this chapter, we undertake to describe some of the work currently being done by family therapists to address the nuclear threat, ranging from interventions made in the clinical setting to those made in the international global arena.

*The authors wish to thank Richard Chasin, Margaret Herzig, Terry Real, and Steven Zeitlin for their helpful comments on earlier drafts of this chapter.

PSYCHOLOGISTS' INVOLVEMENT IN NUCLEAR ISSUES

The broader field of psychology has long been committed to looking at the application of psychological concepts to issues in the nuclear age (Morawski & Goldstein, 1985). In the late 1950s and early 1960s, such eminent psychologists as Urie Bronfenbrenner (1961), Morton Deutsch (1961, 1963), Jerome Frank (1960, 1967), Herbert Kelman (1965), and Charles Osgood (1959, 1962) were writing about international relations in the nuclear age. Psychological concepts such as aggression, attribution, cognition, conflict resolution, game theory, group psychology, mirror image, negotiation, perception, personality theory, and psychoanalysis were applied to understanding nuclear strategy and international relations.

There was a decline in interest in nuclear issues on the part of psychologists in the 1970s, perhaps reflecting the decreased interest on the part of the public as a whole after the trauma of the Cuban missile crisis, the ensuing test-ban treaty of 1963, and the upsurge in other social issues, such as poverty, racism, and the war in Vietnam (Morawski & Goldstein, 1985).

However, the 1980s have seen a resurgence on the part of the psychological community in both research and publications relating to nuclear issues. Psychologists have continued their writings about international relations (Blight, 1987, 1988; Deustch, 1983; Frank, 1987; Jervis, Lebow, & Stein, 1985: Kelman, 1986; Lifton & Falk, 1982; Mack, 1985; White, 1984,1986). Psychologists have also focused attention on the psychological effects of living in the nuclear age. Many researchers (Beardslee & Mack, 1982; Escalona, 1982; Goodman, Mack, Beardlsee, & Snow, 1983; Schwebel, 1982) have studied the impact of the nuclear threat on children in particular. Others have begun to research the effects on family functioning (Greenwald & Zeitlin, 1987). There has been so much writing in this area that it has even been proposed that there is a newly emergent field that might be called "nuclear psychology."

FAMILY THERAPISTS' INVOLVEMENT IN NUCLEAR ISSUES

What comparable work is being done by family therapists? Relative to their colleagues in individual psychology, who have been active on the nuclear question since the 1940s, family therapists have only recently begun to address these issues.

In 1982, the American Family Therapy Association (AFTA) established the Nuclear Issues Task Force. It is preparing a monograph that will explore how to use family systems thinking to better understand international relations. A second goal of the AFTA task force is to lend support to those addressing nuclear issues in their professional roles.

It was also in 1982 that Don Bloch and Peggy Penn organized a session at the annual meeting of the other major family therapy organization, the American Association of Marriage and Family Therapists (AAMFT), to explore the role family therapists could play in preventing nuclear holocaust. During discussions that took place at that meeting, it was pointed out that "family therapy concepts like reframing, paradox, symmetrical escalation, and systems and cybernetics theory . . . [might be] valuable tools for understanding the nuclear threat, and thus somehow could be our contribution toward finding a solution" (Fine, 1984, p. 69).

Family therapists have also been active in the Nuclear Issues Study Group of the American Orthopsychiatric Association (Ortho). The annual meetings of Ortho have had nuclear issues as a focus in plenary sessions since the beginning of the 1980s. The annual Ortho program contains numerous workshops, papers, and panels addessing nuclear concerns from a family therapy perspective.

As family therapists, we are faced with the dilemma of the nuclear threat in our role both as clinicians and as citizens. How are we to help families discover affirmative ways of facing a situation that seems overwhelming, life threatening, and often unthinkable? How can we use our skills as creators of context in which dialogue can occur to foster meaningful and novel exchange between nations, while as nations we are engaged in recursive threat and counterthreat?

The work in which family therapists are engaged to meet the challenge of the nuclear threat can be divided into three types: those that focus on the clinical arena; those that attempt to make an educational intervention; and those that explore how family concepts can be applied to international conflict and global relations.

Clinical Approaches

Many family systems therapists who have addressed nuclear issues have been working in the context of the clinical setting. In their clinical work, they have helped clients focus on the effects of living in the nuclear age—anxiety, fear, depression, numbness, a sense of powerlessness and isolation. Their work has been both responsive and evocative. Some family therapists have responded to clients' nuclear worries as they appear in the clinical setting. For example, it is not uncommon for the adolescent girl engaged in a struggle with her parents over her school performance to announce that there is no point to studying, as the world could blow up any day. Although it is tempting to treat this as an evasive maneuver on her part, the alert family therapist can also see it as an opportunity for dialogue about very real fears shared by the entire family. A sensitive inquiry about the impact of such a statement on the rest of the family can assist all the family members to draw upon their collective strength in facing serious obstacles to productive living. Nuclear concerns often surface in the form of sardonic humor about the end of the world, or in allusions to unnerving dreams of global disaster. The family therapist concerned with responding to these worries will ask how much the client worries about nuclear war, to whom the client talks about it, and how it affects his or her vision of their future.

Other family therapists have begun initiating discussions with clients about these concerns. Wetzel and Winower (1986) state:

The threat of global nuclear extinction constitutes a danger to the survival of every family, couple, or individual who come into our practice. The consequences of this danger for the physical and mental health, for the general well-being, of our clients, particularly the children and young adults, are becoming increasingly evident. This threat is therefore of immediate therapeutic concern and should be part of our professional responsibilities. (p. 305)

Many family therapists agree with their view that it is, therefore, appropriate for the family therapist to initiate discussion of the nuclear threat with clients, just as the therapist inquires about such issues as money, sex, or religion, which are of pressing concern to the family while they may at first be reluctant to discuss them. The therapist's willingness to speak openly about the nuclear threat can offer the family the opportunity for enhanced dialogue in a previously taboo area. Chapter 18 presents examples of such clinical intervention in more detail.

As family therapists have struggled with the ethical and personal dilemmas of addressing the nuclear threat in the clinical setting, the necessity for support of one's peers has become evident. Many informal support groups have become active in recent years, such as the Halflife program described in Chapter 19. Indeed, the Nuclear Issues Study Group of Ortho devoted an entire two-day preconference workshop at the 1988 annual meeting to the task of helping clinicians work with issues of nuclear threat in therapy.

Educational Approaches

In addition to focusing on the nuclear threat with individuals and families in the clinical setting, many family therapists believe we have a responsibility that extends beyond therapy into the larger community. An increasing number of projects are being undertaken by family therapists that address the effect of the nuclear threat on our daily lives in a nonclinical, educational context (Berger-Gould, 1987; Eisenbud, Van Hoorn, & Berger-Gould, 1986; Greenwald & Forman, 1987; Reusser, 1987; Simon, 1984; Zeitlin, 1984). Although educational workshops, seminars, and family interviews have been designed in a wide variety of formats, several are described in more detail below for the purpose of illustration.

In gathering data for their research, Greenwald and Zeitlin (1987) asked families to have a conversation about their feelings and thoughts about the possibility of nuclear war. These conversations were powerful educational interventions, frequently resulting in parents and children talking with each other in a new way. In follow-up interviews, some of the families studied had the opportunity to view the videotapes of their interview. These interviews were even more exciting in some ways than the initial ones. Family members now had the opportunity to see themselves as they appeared to others, and, more important, to share their reactions to their own statements and behavior. These interviews usually led to both an enhanced acknowledgment of shared feelings of vulnerability and an affirmation of the family's caring for each other.

Another approach taken by many family therapists involves direct work with parents on the difficulties they feel in dealing with their children about the nuclear threat. A wide variety of educational seminars and parenting workshops have been developed for use with school, community, and religious groups. A typical example of this type of workshop has been described by Reusser (1987). In these workshops, groups of parents met without their children, comparing their own experiences as they became aware of the nuclear threat and the beliefs they developed in response. The parents role-played conversations with their children about the nuclear threat, providing them with the opportunity both to play out the question they dreaded being asked by their own child and to compare their fears with those of other parents. The dialogue generated in such workshops usually had the effect of alleviating the sense of isolation felt by many parents around this issue, clarifying the areas in which some parents felt blocked, and affirming many parents' resolve to face squarely their own feelings and those of their families about the nuclear threat.

Berger-Gould and her colleagues (1986) have developed a series of multi-generational family workshops in which they bring together four or five families with children of various ages "to facilitate communications between family members of different generations about the nuclear threat and to redefine nuclear anxiety as a normal shared feeling" (p. 115). Berger-Gould found that it was easier for children to talk to parents other than their own. As a result of their experiences, Berger-Gould and her colleagues (1986) developed a series of guidelines entitled "How to Talk to Your Children About Nuclear War."

The efforts of these and other family therapists to educate and assist families focus on the painful sense of vulnerability experienced by family members in relation to the nuclear threat. Greenwald and Zeitlin (1987) delineate three processes with which families typically respond when this vulnerability emerges during family discussions of the nuclear threat. The first such process is one in which families minimize both the danger of the nuclear threat and the extent of their feelings about it, or attempt to keep their thoughts and feelings hidden from each other. In a second process, families acknowledge the vulnerability they feel and concentrate on locating its "cause" and blaming the guilty person or institution. The third process involves family members acknowledging the vulnerable and troubling feelings they are experiencing about the nuclear threat, and doing so in a manner that affirms their caring for and connectedness with each other. In families in which the latter process is operating, family members often have a sense of being strengthened by their connections to their family, and, in some cases, feel greater clarity about how to proceed in their own lives.

These projects share an underlying belief that increased opportunity for open dialogue about thoughts and feelings about the nuclear threat will have an enhancing effect on the depth and quality of participants' relationships, and that the process of such exchanges can open the door to an increased sense of social connectedness and responsibility.

International Approaches

Family systems thinking has been useful on the clinical and educational level, helping to cope with the effects of the nuclear threat. What are family systems therapists doing in the international sphere, not only to deal with the effects of living with the nuclear deadlock, but also to explore the underlying international conflicts and the belief systems that perpetuate them? In reviewing the literature and conducting interviews with five family therapists involved in nuclear issues, we have found two broad categories in which family therapists are attempting to have an impact in the international/global arena: efforts in Track II diplomacy, and attempts to apply family therapy concepts to international relations.

Track II diplomacy

Many family therapists have become involved in international exchanges which have come to be known as Track II diplomacy. Track II diplomacy involves the creation of opportunities for personal contact and dialogue between citizens of different countries beyond the bounds of traditional diplomatic channels. Family therapist Benina Berger-Gould (1985) explains Track II diplomacy in terms of Bateson's (1971) ideas on difference. "If new information and energy proceed from the study of differences, it is logical to conclude that information taken in from visiting another culture will change our way of thinking about that culture" (p. 68).

Within the family therapy community, family therapists have been working with their colleagues in international professional organizations to address the roles that family therapists can take in response to the nuclear threat. At the International Family Therapy Conference: The Pattern Which Connects, held in Prague in May 1987, an entire half-day was devoted to nuclear issues. One panel of representives from both East and West discussed nuclear issues and their psychological effect on the family. A number of papers were presented and participants were able to meet in small international groups (Winawer, personal communication, 1987). An expanded program is planned for another international family therapy conference planned for Budapest in 1989 (Bloch, personal communication, 1987)

In addition, a group of American family therapists is preparing to travel to the Soviet Union under the auspices of the Association for Humanistic Psychology in 1988. Their expressed purpose is to provide training in family therapy to Soviet colleagues, but it is also hoped that this type of exchange will lead to discussions of nuclear issues (Berger-Gould, personal communication, 1987).

The Philadelphia-Leningrad Space Bridge Project, organized by a group of family therapists, involves the joint production by Soviet and American video journalists of a television program, or perhaps a series of programs, that would chronicle a lengthy exchange process between a Soviet and an American family, each including parents, children, and grandparents (Fishman, Fishman, Foreman, & Greenwald, 1987). After initial correspondence, videotapes about daily life in each family will be exchanged. Included in the videotapes will be a comparison of concerns shared by members of corresponding generations in each family. For example, the American and Soviet grandparents will be asked to compare their memories of World War II and their thoughts about aging, and the American and Soviet parents would share dilemmas in leisure activities, the presures of day-to-day life, and parenting. The process will culminate with a live satellite television link between the two families, in which they will talk face to face. All aspects of the exchange process will be recorded and produced as a television program for widespread distribution in both countries. The planning stages of the Space Bridge Project have already afforded considerable opportunity for Track II contact between American and Soviet citizens. These contacts have involved not only working out the technical cooperation necessary, but also addressing the question of how images of the enemy are formed and perpetuated, and how these affect national policy and decision making.

Since family therapists believe that changes at any point in the system reverberate throughout the system, those working in the area of Track II diplomacy expect that meaningful contact between Soviet and American citizens, and the changes in their beliefs about each other that can be stimulated by such exchanges, will begin to effect changes in the beliefs held in the wider cultures of each country about the other. Ultimately, they would argue that these changes may also be felt at the level of international policy and decision making.

Applications of systems concepts to international relations

Many family therapists have noted the parallel between behavior we see in families and observations we can make about the behavior of nations. Berger-Gould (1986) suggests that the United States and the Soviet Union resemble an estranged couple in a trial separation, while conflict between third world nations resembles attempts of the offspring to fight out the family battle among themselves, thereby avoiding the ultimate dissolution of the family. (While her idea is useful in terms of looking at international relations in family systems terms, we feel she inadvertently relates a mistaken notion of third world countries as subordinate to the superpowers that have legitimate rights as parents to control them.) In a more humorous piece, Fine (1984) imagines himself as a "family therapist to the world" who receives consultations from various family therapy luminaries.

Chasin and Herzig (1987) offer a thoughtful application of systems theory to the patterns of geopolitical conflict and the belief systems that underlie this conflict. The notion of circular causality is a pivotal family systems concept with clear application to the nuclear threat. Circular causality refers to the belief that events that occur in complex systems, such as the global community, reciprocally influence each other, with each event existing as both cause and effect of the others. An example of this principle familiar to most family therapists is that of the couple in which one member showers his or her partner with affection, wishing to become more intimate. The partner, feeling smothered and invaded, becomes unresponsive and withdrawn. The first partner, alarmed at this distancing, redoubles his or her attentions. And so on, indefinitely. In the international arena, a parallel relationship sometimes can be seen between a superpower nation and client state.

Chasin highlights two related notions. One is the idea that "action patterns and belief systems have a circular relationship to each other: actions are justified by beliefs and beliefs rationalize actions" (Chasin & Herzig, 1987, p. 2). For example, the American belief that the Soviets seek nuclear superiority justifies American initiatives in building a new generation of space weapons. These actions reinforce Soviet beliefs that Americans seek nuclear superiority. These beliefs, in turn, justify Soviet initiatives in space weaponry. These Soviet actions, in turn, reinforce the American beliefs with which we began. In this way, we can see that the belief systems and action patterns of both parties have a reciprocal and reinforcing influence on each other.

A second related concept is that of punctuation, the way in which we construct complex circular realities into simple linear causes and effects. In trying to make sense out of a set of complex related behaviors, such as the arms race, we tend to see the behavior as having starting points (causes) and stopping points (effects). However, the choice of specific events as starting or stopping points is an arbitrary one. Chasin points out that the way in which we designate certain events as causes and others as effects—that is, the way in which we punctuate events—flows from our belief systems, and also tends to support them. The process of punctuation has profound significance in our understanding of conflict, and in our attempts to move beyond it. On the global level, powerful beliefs about the malevolence of the adversary are maintained by both Soviet and American punctuations of the arms race. Each nation sees its own hostile actions as responses to provocations by the other, both supported by and justifying beliefs that the other country embodies dangerous and untrustworthy attributes.

Another family therapy concept applied by Chasin to the international arena is that of symmetrical escalation. In our work with families, we often see communications, and hence relationships, as either complementary or symmetrical. In complementary relationships, the participants occupy significantly different positions, typically with one more powerful and the other less so. Typical examples of this type of relationship are the boss-underling system, the pursuer-distancer system, and the persecutor-victim system. In the symmetrical relationship however, the participants hold roughly equivalent power, and behave toward each other in a similar manner. In families, we see this manifested, for example, in the blamer-blamer system. When one partner finds fault with the other, the second is likely to respond in kind, to which the first will react with a counterresponse, and so on. This can lead to a process of symmetrical escalation, which Chasin points out "has the potential for great destructiveness" (Chasin & Herzig, 1987, p. 4). On the international level, this process is all too familiar. This type of interaction is the exact nature of the arms race: we build more arms, because they built more arms, because we built more arms, and so on. Chasin and Herzig suggest that not only the actions of nations, but also the belief systems they hold about each other, can develop in a process of symmetrical escalation.

Chasin makes a final point: just as the family therapist "explores the negative consequences of apparently positive change, . . . we must make that inquiry, also, in our study of obstacles to true international security" (Chasin & Herzig, 1987, p. 5). For example, there is the possibility that if there were no nuclear standoff between the United States and the U.S.S.R., the currently stable NATO and Warsaw Pact alliances might destabilize.

A different application of family therapy concepts to the nuclear dilemma on the international level was made by Wetzel and Winawer (1986). They point out that families can collectively exhibit self-destructive behavior that does not reside in a single family member. In a similar manner, the global community appears to have self-destructive elements that are not inherent in particular nations or in particular decision-making bodies of either superpower. They note that change can originate and flow from anywhere in the system, not just at the level of the governing group. Wetzel and Winawer are hopeful that changes that family therapists are able to effect in smaller systems will ultimately bear fruit in the international arena.

Other family therapists are interested in the usefulness of family therapy concepts to defense strategists. Block (1987) is attempting to devise a context within which systems thinkers could join with nuclear policy makers and strategists, creating, it is hoped, the opportunity for unexpected solutions to emerge. He imagines that the knowledge held by systems thinkers that would be appealing to strategists would be precisely in the area of the unanticipated or counterintuitive behavior of complex human systems—that is, how to understand why and predict when elaborate strategies produce unpredictable kinds of change (Bloch, personal comminication, 1987).

Systems interventions on the international level

While much of what has been written about the applications of family therapy concepts to the global arena is theoretical in nature, Chasin and others have designed two interventions on the international level that apply systemic concepts to nuclear issues.

Together with Roger Fisher and Frank Sander at the Negotiation Project at Harvard Law School, Chasin has developed the notion of "opposite-positives" (Chasin & Herzig, 1987):

> One way to challenge current belief systems is to use language that casts societal differences in terms of oppositite-positives rather than "good and evil." This mode of positive description might be likened to benign conotation. Such language would acknowledge the strengths of both societies and would have an impact similar to embracing circular causality. Opposite-positives remove the punctuation of blame and leave us with a diverse set of valuable characteristics. (p. 7)

Chasin illustrates this concept with examples of the kind of paired statements this would entail. He lists the following examples of opposite positive statements that could be made by Americans about the United States and the U.S.S.R. (Chasin & Herzig, 1987, p. 7):

> Ours is a land of opportunity; theirs is a land of security.
> We offer maximum flexibility; they offer maximum predictability.
> We value the individual; they value the collective.
> We reward the successful; they protect the weak.
> We value freedom to get ahead; they value equality.
> We promote experimentation; they promote stability.

Finally, Chasin has developed a workshop, which he conducted with Marat Vartanyan, a Soviet colleague, at the 1987 International Physicians for the Preventions of Nuclear War (IPPNW) Congress in Moscow. The workshop was designed to discover the assumptions that members of national groups make about one another, which may constitute some of the psychological factors that contribute to the arms race. Chasin's IPPNW excerise is a form of cicular questioning called "mind reading," often used in couples work. It is a method used to stimulate a variety of beliefs in areas where there has been a fair amount of rigid thinking.

The attendees were divided into five groups U.S.S.R., United States, U.S.S.R. allies, U.S. allies, and unaligned. The United States and U.S. allies were given the following instructions (Chasin, 1987):

> List six assumptions that the Soviets have about Americans. Two of these should be Soviet assumptions about American personal, social or cultural qualities, characteristics or values. Two of these should be Soviet assumptions about American (national) internal goals or intentions. Two of these should be Soviet assumptions about American international goals or intentions. All of these Soviet assumptions about Americans should be factors that could be fueling the arms race. For each assumption specify which subgroup of Soviets make the assumption and specify what they might believe to be evidence and specify what they might believe to be evidence supporting the assumption. (pp. 3–4)

The Soviets and their allies were given a similar task—to list assumptions that Americans hold about Soviets, and participants from the unaligned countries were given both tasks. Ultimately, two lists were produced, one of 16 American attributes and one of 16 Soviet attributes.

In the second phase of the workshop, the United States and its allies were given the following instructions (Chasin, 1987):

> Study the list of sixteen characteristics attributed to Americans. Working alone, without discussion, select the four attributes which you think are least widely held by Americans or are least true of Americans and write down the code numbers. For one of these "least true" attributes, the one you feel most strongly about, write a sentence of no more than 20 words. This sentence should express one reason or one bit of evidence which shows that attribute to be false or inadequate. (p. 7)

The Soviets were given similar directions for the characteristics attributed to Soviets, while the unaligned were told to do both tasks; that is, to disavow the two Soviet attributes and the two American attributes they thought were least true and to write a sentence about the Soviet attribute and the American attribute that they felt most strongly about.

When dealing with people who are stuck because their belief systems restrain them from thinking broadly and restrain their repertoire of actvities, one approach used by family therapists is to flood them with information that is not directly contrary to their belief systems. This is done in a nonconfronting manner that evokes a thoughtful or curious response rather than a defensive one. The effect is to induce a sort of "benign confusion" (Chasin, personal communication, 1987). In this atmosphere, new information can be considered in a way that opens the belief systems to question and modification. Described here is one of the principles applied in the workshop. The participants in this excerise were exposed to an array of new information, presented in a format that avoided any contradiction of their own belief systems, as the information consisted only of reports of beliefs about the thoughts of others. For example, American participants learned directly how their Soviet counterparts imagined that the Americans saw the Soviets, and conversely. Participants also had the opportunity to learn what their counterparts thought about these imagined attributes. All of this was accomplished without a direct challenge to the belief system of any participant, in an atmosphere of curiosity rather than accusation, of conversation rather than escalation.

CONCLUSION

Family therapists are working in widely varied arenas to address the challenge posed by the nuclear dilemma, but their work shares some common themes.

Whether their focus is in the clinical, the educational, or the international sphere, family therapists working on nuclear issues share a belief that in seeking new responses to the nuclear threat, it is crucial that we direct attention into arenas that have previously been unexplored or unnoticed. This is clearly seen in the efforts of those family therapists who are attempting to enable families to move beyond the taboo against acknowledging their reactions to the nuclear threat. It can also be observed in the efforts of family therapists who, in the international sphere, are exploring the ways in which our belief systems evolve and are maintained, and how they might be transformed.

A second shared belief is in the creative potential of dialogue. It is through true dialogue, the juxtaposition of multiple perspectives and descriptions, that we can move above the limitations of linear beliefs in which the nuclear dilemma is embedded. Family therapists are often specialists in the creation of contexts in which dialogue can take place in novel ways between people with different, and sometimes conflicting, experiences and beliefs. Whether the dialogue is between parents and children, Russian and American citizens, or the policy makers who shape our nuclear policy, the interventions we have discussed all suggest the importance of true conversations and dialogue.

Finally, as most family therapists recognize that intervention in any part of a system will have reverberations for the entire system, the work of family therapists in nuclear issues shares the idea that whether one is working with individual clients, with parents, or with national leaders, all are working to affect the global arena; that is, to prevent nuclear destruction. The work in all these areas is important and mutually reinforcing. Working in the clinical sphere can be seen as having an international impact; applications of family therapy concepts in the global context inform our educational efforts, and so on around the circle.

The challenge presented by the nuclear threat is overwhelming; it raises extremely high levels of anxiety and often results in apathy and despair. Linear approaches to problem solving tend to reinforce despair, as so many steps seem necessary to be taken in a sequential fashion before one reaches a solution. We have attempted to present an overview of the variety of ways in which family therapists are using their skills to address the nuclear threat in various arenas: the clinical, educational, and international/global. Family therapy concepts, which are often circular and ecological, highlight the interconnections among elements in complex systems. Family therapists, therefore, recognize that transformations can take place in a large system by an effective intervention in any of its subsystems. This recognition can help empower those of us who might otherwise be overwhelmed and incapacitated by the magnitude of the nuclear challenge.

REFERENCES

Bateson, G. (1971). The cybernetics of "self"; A theory of alcoholism. *Psychiatry, 34*, 1–8.

Beardslee, W., & Mack J. (1982). The impact on children and adolescents of nuclear developments. In American Psychiatric Association Task Force Report no. 20, *Psychosocial Aspects of Nuclear Development* (pp. 64–93). Washington D.C.: American Psychiatric Association.

Bellah, L., Madsen, R., Sullivan, W., Swindler, A., & Tipton, S. (1985). *Habits of the heart: Individualism and commitment in American life.* New York: Harper and Row.

Berger-Gould, B. (1985). Large systems and peace. *Journal of Strategic and Systemic Therapies, 4*(2), 64–64.

Berger-Gould, B. (1986). Siblings in the same race: Family therapists and the nuclear issue. In M. Ault-Riche (Ed.), *Women and family therapy* (pp. 112–116). Rockville, Md.: Aspen.

Blight, J. (1987). Toward a policy-relevant psychology of avoiding nuclear war: Lessons for psychologists from the Cuban missile crisis. *American Psychologist, 4*(1), 12–29.

Blight, J. (1988). Can psychology help reduce the risk of nuclear war? Reflections of a "little drummer boy" of nuclear psychology. *Journal of Humanistic Psychology, 28*(2), 7–58.

Bronfenbrenner, V. (1961). The mirror-image in Soviet-american relations: A social psychologist's report. *Journal of Social Issues, 16*(3), 45–56.

Chasin, D. (1987). Notes on a workshop called "Assumptions and perceptions which fuel the arms race." Held at the 1987 Congress of the International Physicians for the Prevention of Nuclear War, Moscow. Unpublished paper.

Chasin, D., & Herzig, M. (1987). A systems theory approach to U.S./Soviet relations. A working paper of the Project on Assumptions and Perceptions that Fuel the Nuclear Arms Race. Cambridge: Center for Psychological Studies in the Nuclear Age.

Chasin, R. and Herzig, M. (1988). Correcting misperceptions in Soviet-American relations. *Journal of Humanistic Psychology. 28*(3), 88–97.

Deutsch, M. (1961). Some considerations relevant to national policy. *Journal of Social Issues, 17*(3), 57–68.

Deutsch, M. (1963). On changing an adversary. *American Journal of Orthopsychiatry, 33*, 244–246.

Deutsch, M. (1983). The prevention of World War II: A psychological perspective. *Political Psychology, 4*(1), 3—31.

Eisenbud, M. M., Van Hoorn, J. L., & Berger-Gould, B. (1986). Children, adolescents and the threat of nuclear war: An international perspective. In D. Jellifee (Ed.), *Advances in International Material and Child Health* (Vol. b). Fairlawn, N.J.: Oxford University Press.

Escalona, S. K. (1982). Growing up with the threat of nuclear war: Some indirect effects on pesonality development. *American Journal of Orthopsychiatry, 52*, 600–607.

Fine, M. (1984). Family therapists and symmetrical nuclear escalation. *Journal of Strategic and Systemic Therapies, 3*(1), 66–71.

Fishman, H. C., Fishman, T., Foreman, W., & Greenwald, D. (1987). Countering the images of the enemy: Family to family space bridge. Paper presented at the Annual

Meeting of American Orthopsychiatric Association, Washington, D.C.

Frank, J. (1967). *Sanity and survival: Psychological aspects of war and peace*. New York: Vintage Books.

Frank, J. (1987). The drive for power and the nuclear arms race. *American Psychologist, 42*(4), 337–344.

Frank, J. D. (1960. Breaking the thought barrier: Psychological challenge in the nuclear age. *Psychiatry, 23*, 245–266.

Goodman, L. A., Mack, J. E., Beardslee, W. R., & Snow, R. M. (1983). The threat of nuclear war and the nuclear arms race: Adolescent experience and perceptions. *Political Psychology, 4*, 501–530.

Greenwald, D., & Forman, W. (1987). Families communicating about nuclear threat. Paper presented at Annual Meeting of American Orthopsychiatric Association, Washington, D.C.

Greenwald, D., & Zeitlin, S. (1987). *No reason to talk about it: Families confront the nuclear taboo*. New York: Norton.

Jervis, R., Lebow, R. N., & Stein, J. G. (1985). *Psychology and deterrence*. Baltimore, Md.: John Hopkins University Press.

Kelman, H. (Ed.), (1965). *International behavior: A social-psychological analysis*. New York: Holt.

Kelman, H. (1986). An interactional approach to conflict resolution. In R. White (Ed.), *Psychology and the prevention of nuclear war* (pp. 171–193). New York: New York University Press.

Lifton, R. J., & Falk, R. (1982). *Indefensible weapons: The political and psychological case against nuclearism*. New York: Basic Books.

Mack, J. (1985). Toward a collective psychopathology of the nuclear arms competition. *Political Psychology, 6*(2), 291–321.

Morawski, J. G., & Goldstein, S. C. (1985). Psychology and nuclear war: A chapter in our legacy of social reponsibility. *American Psychologist, 40*, 276–284.

Osgood, C. (1959). Suggestions for winning the real war with communism. *Journal of Conflict Resolution, 3*, 295–325.

Osgood, C. (1962). *An Alternative to war or surrender*. Urbana, Ill.: University of Illinois Press.

Reusser, J. (1987). Working with parents around nuclear threat. Paper presented at the Annual Meeting of American Orthopsychiatric Association, Washington, D.C.

Schell, J. (1982). *The fate of the earth*. New York: Avon.

Schwebel, M. (1982). Effects on nuclear war threat on children and teenagers: Implications for professionals. *American Journal of Orthopsychiatry, 52*, 608–618.

Simon, R. (1984). The nuclear family. *The Family Therapy Networker, 8*(2), 22.

Simon, R. (1988). Does nuclear war have a place in family therapy? In M. Merkin (Ed.), *The social and political context of family therapy*. New York: Gardner Press.

Wetzel, N., & Winawer, H. (1986). The psychological consequences of the nuclear threat from a family systems perspective. *International Journal of Mental Health, 15*(1-3), 298–313.

White, R. K. (1984). *Fearful warriors: A psychological profile of U.S.-Soviet relations*. New York: Free Press.

White, R. K. (Ed.), (1986). *Psychology and the prevention of nuclear war*. New York: New York University Press.

Zeitlin, S. (1984). What do we tell mom and dad? *the Family Therapy Networker, 31*, 38–39, 62.

Name Index

Subject Index